Postoperative Nausea and Vomiting

A Practical Guide

Postoperative Nausea and Vomiting

A Practical Guide

Edited by

Tong Joo Gan
Stony Brook University, Stony Brook, New York, USA

and

Ashraf S. Habib
Duke University Medical Center, Durham, North Carolina, USA

CAMBRIDGE
UNIVERSITY PRESS

CAMBRIDGE
UNIVERSITY PRESS

University Printing House, Cambridge CB2 8BS, United Kingdom

Cambridge University Press is part of the University of Cambridge.

It furthers the University's mission by disseminating knowledge in the pursuit of education, learning and research at the highest international levels of excellence.

www.cambridge.org
Information on this title: www.cambridge.org/9781107465190

First published 2016

A catalogue record for this publication is available from the British Library

Library of Congress Cataloguing in Publication data
Names: Gan, Tong Joo, editor. | Habib, Ashraf S., editor.
Title: Postoperative nausea and vomiting : a practical guide / edited by Tong Joo Gan and Ashraf S. Habib.
Description: Cambridge; New York: Cambridge University Press, 2016. | Includes bibliographical references and index.
Identifiers: LCCN 2015046516 | ISBN 9781107465190 (paperback)
Subjects: | MESH: Postoperative Nausea and Vomiting – prevention & control | Postoperative Nausea and Vomiting–therapy | Antiemetics – therapeutic use | Anesthesia – adverse effects
Classification: LCC RD98.4 | NLM WO 184 | DDC 617.9/195–dc23
LC record available at http://lccn.loc.gov/2015046516

ISBN 978-1-107-46519-0 Paperback

To

My wife
Audrey

My kids
Zoe, Sophie and Julia

My parents
Kim Hoe and Siew Yiah

For their support and inspiration

Tong Joo Gan

To my wife Faten and my children Lina and Sami
Thank you for your love, encouragement and support

Ashraf Habib

Contents

Contributors

Keith A. Candiotti
Department of Anesthesiology, Perioperative Medicine and Pain Management at the University of Miami, FL, USA

John Carlisle
Consultant in Anaesthesia, Intensive Care and Perioperative Medicine, Torbay Hospital, Devon, UK

Jessica Carter
Anesthesia Resident, Duke University Medical Center, Durham, NC, USA

Enisa M.F. Carvalho
Department of Anesthesiology, Perioperative Medicine and Pain Management at the University of Miami, FL, USA

Matthew T.V. Chan
Professor at the Department of Anaesthesia and Intensive Care, The Chinese University of Hong Kong, Shatin, New Territories, Hong Kong Special Administrative Region

Michelle Dalton
Department of Anesthesiology, Baylor College of Medicine, Texas Children's Hospital, Houston, TX, USA

Gildasio De Oliveira
Associate Chair for Research, Department of Anesthesiology, Northwestern University, Evanston, IL, USA

Brian Donnenfeld
Division Chief, Ambulatory/Gynecologic/Robotic Surgery at the Department of Anesthesiology, Brigham and Women's Hospital, and Instructor in Anesthesia at Harvard Medical School, Boston, MA, USA

Tong Joo Gan
Professor and Chairman at the Department of Anesthesiology, Stony Brook University, Stony Brook, NY, USA

Tony Gin
Professor at the Department of Anaesthesia and Intensive Care, The Chinese University of Hong Kong, Prince of Wales Hospital, Shatin, New Territories, Hong Kong

Ashraf S. Habib
Professor of Anesthesiology, Chief, Division of Women's Anesthesia, Department of Anesthesiology, Duke University Medical Center, Durham, NC, USA

Vallire D. Hooper
Manager, Nursing Research at Mission Health System, Asheville, NC, USA

Anthony L. Kovac
Kasumi Arakawa Professor of Anesthesiology at the University of Kansas Medical Center, Kansas City, KS, USA

Peter Kranke
Professor at the Department of Anaesthesia and Critical Care, University Hospitals of Wuerzburg, Wuerzburg, Germany

Linda M.L. Lai
Associate Consultant at the Yan Chai Hospital, Tsuen Wan, Hong Kong Special Administrative Region

Anna Lee
Department of Anaesthesia and Intensive Care, The Chinese University of Hong Kong, Shatin, New Territories, Hong Kong

Amy Mauritz
Anesthesia Fellow, Duke University Medical Center, Durham, NC, USA

Ana C. Mavarez
Department of Anesthesiology, Perioperative Medicine and Pain Management at the University of Miami, FL, USA

Russell K. McAllister
Program Director, Anesthesiology Residency Program and Assistant Dean of Quality and Patient Safety, Scott & White Health, Temple, TX, USA

Tricia A. Meyer
Regional Director of Pharmacy at Baylor Scott & White Health and Associate Professor of Anesthesiology at Texas A&M College of Medicine, Temple, TX, USA

Paul S. Myles
Director, Department of Anaesthesia and Perioperative Medicine, Alfred Hospital, and Professor and Chair at the Department of Anaesthesia and Perioperative Medicine at Monash University, VIC, Australia

Jacob Nouriel
Research Volunteer, Department of Anesthesiology, Northwestern University, Evanston, IL, USA

Beverly K. Philip
Vice President for Scientific Affairs at the American Society of Anesthesiology, Professor of Anesthesia at Harvard Medical School, and Founding Director, Day Surgery Unit, Brigham and Women's Hospital, Boston, MA, USA

Johan Raeder
Department of Anaesthesiology, Oslo University Hospital, Ullevaal, Oslo, Norway

Aaron Skolnik
Medical Student at the Department of Anesthesiology, Duke University Medical Center, Durham, NC, USA

Imelda Tjia
Department of Anesthesiology, Baylor College of Medicine, Texas Children's Hospital, Houston, TX, USA

Mehernoor F. Watcha
Department of Pediatric Anesthesiology at the Texas Children's Hospital, Houston, TX, USA

William K.K. Wu
Assistant Professor at the Department of Anaesthesia and Intensive Care, The Chinese University of Hong Kong, Shatin, New Territories, Hong Kong Special Administrative Region

Foreword

During the last decade, there has been increased interest worldwide in perioperative medicine and techniques to improve postoperative recovery as condensed into the "enhanced recovery (ER) programs" or "fast-track surgery." In this context, the common problem of postoperative nausea and vomiting (PONV) plays a prominent role, since it does not only delay recovery but also has inherent side effects with subjective discomfort and dissatisfaction, both of which subsequently lead to a longer hospital stay or less successful outpatient procedures.

It is therefore both laudable and timely that Dr. Tong Joo Gan and Dr. Ashraf Habib have compiled this multiauthor textbook for the perioperative management of PONV. The many chapters cover all relevant aspects to be used for perioperative physicians and nurses involved in daily practiced PONV management. Undoubtedly, this comprehensive text will not only be helpful for PONV prevention and management, but also emphasize its role in a successful ER program.

Henrik Kehlet, Prof., MD, PhD
Section for Surgical Pathophysiology, Rigshospitalet,
Copenhagen University, Denmark

Preface

About 240 million surgeries are performed each year worldwide. Postoperative nausea and vomiting (PONV) is one of the most common and distressing problems facing patients after surgery. Many patients fear PONV more than pain after surgery and are willing to pay a substantial amount out-of-pocket to avoid this problem. PONV causes extreme patient discomfort, prolonged recovery, a decrease in satisfaction with surgery, an increase in the length of stay in the recovery room, and unexpected hospital admission following day surgery and healthcare costs. PONV can extend beyond discharge from the day surgery center and can delay patient return to normal activity. Successful management of PONV is also an essential component of enhanced recovery after surgery and perioperative surgical home protocols, which are gaining widespread popularity and are being increasingly used to optimize recovery following a wide range of surgical procedures. Many clinicians underappreciate the extent of the problem and may not be familiar with effective treatment strategies.

Written by world experts in the field, this book provides up-to-date information on various aspects of this common problem, including the incidence and mechanism of PONV, risk factors, pharmacologic and nonpharmacologic treatment options, implementation of successful treatment strategies, genomics, research methodology and cost effectiveness.

This book is one of the most comprehensive in its field and provides the readers with indepth understanding of this common problem in the perioperative period. It is a valuable resource to many healthcare providers managing this ubiquitous problem, such as nurses, pharmacists, nurse anesthetists, anesthesiologists and surgeons, as well as researchers in this field. Patients undergoing surgery would also benefit by gaining a better understanding of this common problem and education on successful management strategies.

Chapter 1

History of postoperative nausea and vomiting

Johan Raeder

Nausea and vomiting for species survival

Throughout the evolution of species, some vital ways of protecting the organism against dangerous material and impact from the surroundings have developed. The pain response is well known; if an animal gets in contact with noxious stimuli, the pain response will initiate an immediate withdrawal and subsequent learning of protective behavior for the future. Similarly, if the skin gets in contact with harmful agents, a rash may develop and in case of contaminated food or water, a strong smell may sometimes act as an important warning sign. If by accident or ignorance we ingest dangerous items, there are systems to help us, such as the strong cough reflex when solids or fluids get into the airway. If we eat or drink substances that may be poisonous, diarrhea may help to clean the gastrointestinal cavities from substances otherwise absorbed. Nausea and vomiting also fit into this context. If we eat something potentially toxic, the rapid and very forceful expulsion of gastric and duodenal contents will remove the potentially dangerous substance before absorption into the blood. For this reason we need receptors, such as the serotonin 5-hydroxytryptamine type 3 (5-HT_3) receptors on the intraluminal surface of the gastric canal, to register potentially toxic contents inside the gut. Further, it may be of help to have receptors in close contact with the systemic circulation if a toxic substance starts to be absorbed from the gut into the blood. In such cases, vomiting may limit the amount of substance that presents for absorption and also stop the oral intake of a larger amount. Whereas vomiting is a somewhat automatic, forceful, brainstem response not requiring intellectual or deliberate decision-making, nausea as a subjective experience is different. For obvious reasons we do not know if animals have developed the feeling of being nauseated, but in humans nausea may be a strong source for learning. The prolonged, unpleasant feeling of being nauseated will tell us about food and situations we should avoid in the future. The general feeling of nausea during hypoxia, hypotension and many cases of systemic disease, may also be an important warning about the inappropriateness of eating or drinking in situations where the body is not ready for what was ingested. From a learning point of view, it is interesting to see that younger individuals have a stronger nausea and vomiting response than the elderly, who may supposedly have learnt lessons throughout previous experiences. It is also a little intriguing that nausea is so common in the first trimester of pregnancy, a phase where the fetus is particularly vulnerable to substances in the mothers' blood, which may cause damage to the genetic transmission and subsequent organ formation.

Postoperative Nausea and Vomiting: A Practical Guide, eds. Tong Joo Gan and Ashraf S. Habib. Published by Cambridge University Press.

The body has developed very useful physiologic responses to external poisons, somewhat like the well-designed physiologic nociceptive responses to trauma. These responses have obviously not been modified by the slow process of species evolution to fit into the development of surgery and anesthesia throughout the last two centuries. In this context, the trauma response, and particularly the postoperative nausea and vomiting (PONV) response, are mostly inappropriate as they may cause extra hazards for the patients and obviously great discomfort if they are not prevented or relieved.

Three facets of PONV: danger, discomfort and economic cost

The three important aspects of most problems or measures in modern medicine are the danger, the discomfort and the economic cost, and it may be helpful to view PONV in this context. The priority and ranking of these three aspects have varied throughout history, but also as a result of standpoint and philosophy of the player in question.

In the early days of surgery and anesthesia, mortality was high and obviously the potential for improving safety was large. Even during the very first cases of general anesthesia with ether in the 1840s, some patients vomited gastric contents into the lungs and subsequently died from suffocation or aspiration pneumonia. From this experience the concept of having an empty stomach before surgery evolved and probably saved many lives. For this reason, a review by Smith in 1934 designated vomiting as the most feared complication with general anesthesia[1], a conclusion repeated by Morton and Wylie in 1951[2]. In a survey of 1,000 anesthetic deaths as late as in 1956, Edwards et al. reported 110 cases (11%!) with vomiting and aspiration as the main causative factor[3].

From a safety point of view, vomiting is definitely the key issue; nausea is unpleasant but not so dangerous. Thus, most of the early reports were only concerned with the incidence of vomiting. Also in the past, a subjective symptom, such as nausea, was more or less not registered as the patients were very drowsy and had amnesia for a prolonged period after surgery. In the 1930s and 1940s, there were vivid discussions on whether ether and cyclopropane should be abandoned in favor of new intravenous (IV) agents such as the barbiturates, which were introduced by 1927. Vomiting was a strong argument against the old inhalational agents, whereas the dangers of hypotension and strong respiratory depression were arguments against the IV drugs.

The development of the first successful local anesthetic block by Carl Koller in eye surgery may be regarded as a result of quality improvement as early as in 1884. The eye surgeons noted the very high frequency of vomiting associated with eye surgery under ether anesthesia, with subsequent straining of the delicate structures of the newly operated eye as well as great discomfort for the patients. Thus, the development of cocaine for local anesthetic eye blocks and the subsequent development of locoregional anesthetic drugs and techniques in general, may also be viewed as a result of concern regarding vomiting as a quality problem. Hence, as general anesthesia became much safer after the Second World War and also through developments of new drugs and equipment in the 1980s and 1990s, the importance of quality became stronger. As safety problems arose much less frequently, focus turned into other issues such as quality; as patients were more customer-orientated, they started to ask not only for safety but also for improvement in quality. As numerous different techniques and means to address the PONV problem became available, the interest in this issue clearly increased.

Until the last 20–30 years, most limitations in healthcare in the Western World were caused by lack of evidence-based knowledge and drugs. This has dramatically changed in the last few decades. The vast development of effective, but often expensive, methods for diagnosis and treatment in many areas combined with an increasing elderly population have widened the scope of potential medical services extensively, putting economy or more precisely value for money, into the forefront. As PONV is not currently regarded as a safety issue but merely a short-lasting quality problem, the cost–benefit discussions in this area have been quite extensive. Some of the new specific antiemetic drugs, such as 5-hydroxytryptamine type 3 and neurokinin type 1 (NK_1) antagonists, have been regarded as expensive, and the potential gain in terms of better quality and less need of nursing care is weighted against drug acquisition costs. Of note, many of the 5-HT_3 antagonists are now available in generic formulation, and hence less costly.

PONV in science: epidemiology, basic science and clinical research

Nausea and vomiting are very common symptoms, experienced by virtually all individuals throughout a lifespan, although with very different duration and intensity. In spite of this fact, the research into this area has been limited and not highly ranked in priority. The reasons may be numerous: the symptoms rarely cause death or permanent disability; the economic interests in terms of profit from drugs have, until recently, been quite limited; and experimental or animal models of vomiting have been difficult to develop. Rats and mice do not vomit, and behavior and sensitivity in terms of vomiting show species differences in ferret, shrew and dog.

However, by the turn of the nineteenth century, theories were present for both gastric emetic receptors and a vomiting center in the brain. In 1891, Thomas abolished the emetic response to apomorphine in dogs by destroying a portion in the medulla oblongata[4]. Authoritative reviews on the physiology of vomiting were written in 1924 by Hatcher[5] and in 1953 by Borison and Wang [6], summing up the knowledge present at the time. In the first half of the century, there were vivid discussions as to the location and nature of the vomiting center from somewhat conflicting animal data. Some clarification of these issues were provided by the description in 1939 by Wang and Borison of the chemoreceptor trigger zone in the area postrema as a receptor site for emetic agents in the blood[7]. Attempts were made to put the emetic actions of anesthetics into the map laid out by basic scientists. In 1912, Ferguson had discussions on whether ether caused vomiting by diffusing into the intestinal lumen, thus acting on localized receptors in the wall, or whether a systemic emetic effect of ether in the blood reaching the brain was more important[8]. Based on these theories, there were some controversial reports on the use of olive oil to protect the intestinal receptors, potentially reducing vomiting if ingested before general anesthesia. Telford and Falconer launched another theory in 1906, pointing to acidosis as a cause of emesis, being relieved by an infusion of glucose with insulin. It was not until the 1950s and 60s when causative pathways of PONV were laid out. However, the current detailed knowledge of receptor involvement in PONV is still quite new and the elucidation of intracellular mechanisms even younger and still not completely understood. Although the antiemetic action of anticholinergics was already noted by Brown Seguard in 1883 and later by Fraser, the histamine and dopamine receptors role was not described until the 1950s. The important clinical observation of high-dose metoclopramide being significantly more effective against nausea during chemotherapy treatment[9] led to the search for a new receptor with a low metoclopramide affinity being stimulated only by high doses. This resulted in the discovery of the 5-HT_3 receptor as an important player in the etiology of PONV. During the 1980s, the technology of radioligand techniques for identification and study of protein receptors and ligands was developed. Such techniques became important tools in identification, localization and classification of antiemetic drugs and mechanisms.

Further studies of basic emetic physiology also identified the NK_1 receptor as an interesting target for antiemetic treatment[10,11]. NK_1 antagonists have gained widespread use in cancer chemotherapy and are presently being explored successfully for PONV. They seem to have fairly similar efficacy and duration on nausea compared with the 5-HT_3 blockers, but a somewhat better effect against vomiting. Aprepitant is best documented at present[12], but other substances of this drug class seem to be equally promising.

Another area of interesting research is the elucidation of the cannabinoid receptors, which, in contrast to others receptors involved with PONV, seem to provide antiemesis by agonist action rather than antagonism[13]. This has led to the search for an endogenous antiemetic substance, as well as interest in developing drugs from the cannabis family[14], which are known to be effective antiemetics when smoked for recreation or as a part of terminal care in cancer patients.

Basic research into nausea and vomiting has evolved substantially during recent years[15]. A potential role of a calcium block in the attenuation of vomiting[15] has been shown, surprisingly also shared by a dual effect of opioids: high opioid dose that penetrates into deeper central nervous system structures may actually have an antiemetic effect[16]. The role of serotonin is also very complex; some of the seven subclasses of receptors may be emetic, whereas others are potentially antiemetic[15,17]. Excellent reviews with many papers on the basic physiology of nausea and vomiting are found in a recent dedicated issue of the *European Journal of Physiology*[18].

Much of the knowledge about PONV has emerged through epidemiologic observations. These have been relatively simple to perform because so many surgical patients experienced PONV, and therefore it has been easier to account for some possible causative factors of PONV. In 1883 Fraser and Brown Seguard reported that morphine, ether and cyclopropane caused emesis per se, and in 1899, Blumfeld and Cantab[19] made the observation that the type of surgical procedure had an influence on the incidence. In this report there was an incidence of 75% of vomiting after ether anesthesia, with a higher frequency after intraperitoneal surgery. In a review from 1934, Smith provided a list of risk factors: travel sickness, intra-abdominal surgery, preoperative hunger, preoperative anxiety and elective (!) surgery[1]. He also discussed the impact of anesthetic drugs, noting that chloroform and ether were the worst agents in this aspect, but best in an overall evaluation of anesthetic quality in terms of relaxed muscles and adequate ventilation, respectively. In 1928, Scrager reported more frequent vomiting in patients with gallbladder distention, and in 1941, Davis made the observation of more vomiting in women than males[20]. In a review from 1954, Dent et al. add hypoxia, dehydration, toxins in blood and stimulation of the brain nerves to previous lists of causative factors[21].

It is interesting in this context to note that the publications throughout the first 100 years of general anesthesia in humans almost exclusively deal with vomiting, mostly because of the association with aspiration into the lungs as the only life-threatening aspect, but probably also because vomiting is very easy and objective to record, whereas nausea may have been considered a minor symptom and not worth much attention. However, in one area nausea was recognized quite early on as a major problem, namely the area of chemotherapy treatment for cancer. As effective IV chemotherapeutics became in use as prolonged infusions for several days in many patients, the problems of nausea causing insufficient oral intake as well as diminished patient motivation and compliance with the treatment came into focus. Also, during the 1950s and 1960s, the increased use of more rapidly cleared anesthetic drugs, such as barbiturates, new opioids and halothane, made nausea a specific problem in awake postoperative patients more evident in the recovery areas. The development of neuroleptic anesthesia was important in this aspect, as the addition of fairly high doses of neuroleptic drugs to opioids led to progress in terms of reducing the incidence of PONV. It was then realized that high doses of neuroleptics frequently caused dysphoria and low doses of droperidol were equally effective in an antiemetic context. Subsequently, in recent years a black box warning was put on droperidol by the US Food and Drug Administration due to very rare reports of potential association with QT prolongation leading to arrhythmias. This problem was hardly considered in Europe and other places, and also in the USA there is an ongoing debate on the validity of this issue[22].

A further major step in the direction of more rapid and clear-headed recovery was the marketing of modern drugs by the end of the twentieth century with even more rapid decline of effect after use, such as midazolam, sevoflurane, desflurane, propofol, alfentanil and remifentanil.

A dramatic shift towards ambulatory surgery during the 1980s and 1990s was another important trend, made possible by the development of new surgical methods, new anesthetic drugs, and a general change in attitude and reimbursement model in the USA. This put forward the aspects of PONV: apart from pain and surgical complications, PONV became the most frequent obstacle in early ambulation and discharge. As safety is almost 100% maintained in modern ambulatory anesthetic care, the aspects of patient quality and comfort have been put at the forefront, with absence of PONV as a very important goal. The frequently cited statement of Kapur in an editorial in 1991 makes a good sum-up of this development: PONV – the big "little problem"[23].

PONV in children has also been increasingly addressed as there are some pediatric surgical procedures with a very high frequency of PONV, and aspects of heredity have been highlighted as a useful tool in individual PONV prediction[24].

Specific antiemetic drugs

Although anticholinergics, especially atropine, have been known to be effective antiemetics for more than 100 years, it was during the 1950s that interest in drugs for treatment and prophylaxis of PONV became more evident[25]. In a nonrandomized study from 1955, Dent noted a reduction in overall PONV from 27% to 21% in 3000 patients when the antihistamine cyclizine was used for prophylaxis[21]. One reason for this low incidence of PONV may have been that a high fraction of patients received regional or spinal anesthesia, and it was noted that these techniques resulted in less PONV than barbiturates, which again was better than cyclopropane or ether. In a randomized double-blind study of 554 patients from 1956, Knapp and Beecher reported a significant beneficial effect of using barbiturate for general anesthesia, particularly when combined with chlorpromazine prophylaxis[26]. However, it was also noted that the gain in terms of less

PONV was at the cost of a higher incidence of hypotension and postoperative fatigue. In a study of 2500 cases in 1957, Burtles and Peckett reported less PONV after prophylaxis with either promethazine or chlorpromazine[27]. He also noted that the younger patients had a higher tendency for PONV than the elderly. Further, throughout the 1950s and 60s, there was an increasing number of publications refining the use of neuroleptics, anticholinergics and antihistamines for PONV[28]. In 1970, Lind and Breivik published a double-blind study on the effect of metoclopramide, which soon became a drug of choice for first-line treatment of PONV[29].

During the 1980s and 90s, much effort and money was put into the development and documentation of ondansetron, and later other 5-HT$_3$ antagonists, as effective antiemetics[30]. In 2004, Apfel et al. published a very important, large and impressive paper on risk factors and antiemetic drug effects, stating an equal and additive effect of neuroleptic, glucocorticoid and 5-HT$_3$ prophylaxis[31].

Although anesthetic drugs such as ether, desflurane[32] and opioids are usually associated with causing PONV, propofol was soon recognized to result in less PONV than other agents, and evidence in the late 1980s actually suggested that it had a specific antiemetic action[33,34].

The 5-HT$_3$ receptor antagonists story

The development of specific serotonin 5-HT$_3$ antagonists became a milestone in the treatment and prophylaxis of PONV in many ways[35] – not because these drugs provide a solution to the problems of PONV (when carefully reviewing the data, these drugs are not substantially better than neuroleptics that were already being used for the management of PONV), but because the 5-HT$_3$ antagonists represent a class of drugs specially designed by the industry to deal with PONV as well as emesis during chemotherapy. Further, they represent very clean drugs with a specific action and very few serious side effects[36], as well as presenting a major step forward in the understanding of the receptor physiology and mechanisms of PONV. Although some small groups made the first satellite publications on these drugs[37], the introduction of ondansetron as the first representative for this drug class made way for large, well-designed and well-controlled multicenter trials of PONV[38]. Some criticism was raised, however, as to the handling of drug and therapy development by a single pharmaceutical company: the studies were mostly versus placebo and not versus viable alternatives; the studies were mostly in high-risk patients with sometimes suboptimal (in terms of reducing PONV) anesthetic care; and some negative studies were not published. However, as ondansetron became released for general use and a lot of new "-setrones" have made their way to clinical use (e.g., tropisetron, granisetron, dolasetron, palonosetron, etc.), the research and marketing of these drugs became more balanced. Although ondansetron was developed and investigated mostly in the western countries, the Fujii group from Japan was very active in testing granisetron[39]. However, the validity of their research was severely questioned and their publications on this issue have later been withdrawn by most major journals[40].

A further development with 5-HT$_3$ receptor antagonists was the introduction of long-acting drugs, such as palonosetron, with an elimination half-life of almost 2 days. This may be very useful in the setting of postdischarge nausea and vomiting, but the studies have so far probably been underpowered to show a significant prolonged antiemetic effect beyond 24 h[15,41].

Adjunctive drugs and other therapy

Apart from using specific antiemetic drugs, a lot of observations and research has been done with many drugs and nonpharmacologic measures to reduce the incidence of PONV. In the 1860s, Snow used morphine premedication in order to relieve anxiety and risk of vomiting in his patients[42]. Although opioids are basically emetogenic, the observations of Snow fits with the study of Andersen and Krohg from 1976 showing the antiemetic effect of treating concomitant pain and nausea with opioids[43]. Another conflicting observation is that while stress, anxiety and catecholamines may induce PONV, ephedrine is a very effective antiemetic, not only as a means to prevent hypotension but possibly through a specific antiemetic effect[44]. Adrenergic stimulation and activation is a complex area in physiology with a somewhat dual action in the PONV context[15]. The antiemetic effect of corticosteroids was first noticed by oncologists treating brain edema from metastases. Subsequently, the antiemetic effect of these drugs for PONV has been widely reported, although the mechanism is still debated[45,46]. The groups of Liu and Wang have published extensively on dexamethasone, elucidating the effective dose in different clinical settings[45,47].

Another exciting area is the nonpharmacologic measures. It has been known that classical Chinese acupuncture at the P6 point (the sixth point along the pericardial meridian) is effective against seasickness. This has later been confirmed to be an effective measure in the treatment and prophylaxis of PONV[48]. More modern applications of the same concept have been sought for and demonstrated to be effective, such as transcutaneous electrical stimulation by a dedicated device[49].

Further, it is also an ongoing discussion as to whether sedative drugs, such as the benzodiazepines, are true antiemetics or merely result in less reports of the subjective feeling of nausea due to their general effects on well-being[50].

PONV in anesthetic training and practice

PONV is a well-defined clinical entity and has a lot of "classical" aspects such as: mechanisms, etiology, epidemiology, pharmacology, economy, clinical effects and side effects. For this reason, the topic lends itself easily to reviewing, and throughout the last 70 years a lot of authoritative and frequently cited reviews have been published in the major journals. One of the first was by Smith in the *British Journal of Anaesthesia* in 1934, dealing only with vomiting[1]. Dent et al. (1955)[21], Riding (1960)[51], Belleville et al. (1960)[52], Purkis (1964) [53], Dundee et al.[54] and Janhunen et al.[55] also address vomiting, whereas Palazzo and Strunin in 1984 made one of the first extensive and authoritative reviews on the whole concept of postoperative emesis, including nausea[56,57].

The term PONV first appeared in the literature in 1992 in a review paper by Bunce on 5-HT_3 mechanisms. The term rapidly became very popular, probably because it is short, easy to spell and precise.

In 1992, an extensive review was published by Watcha and White[58], which is still cited and used in teaching, and as a source of knowledge for clinical use. In 2002, an extensive update was published by Gan[59] putting together all knowledge with the ambiguous goal of actually eliminating the problem. A very important concept in this context is the multimodal use of different methods with different targets in order to attack the problem from many angles[33,60]. This concept has been very successful as most antiemetics have a ceiling effect, and at best a 50% efficacy when used alone. During the last 10 years, the Society for Ambulatory Anesthesia has put a lot of effort into creating guidelines for prophylaxis and treatment of PONV[61], being revised recently[62]. A recent review of Skolnik and Gan also sum up these guidelines[63].

A new trend in reviewing, the meta-analyses, evolved throughout the 1990s as a result of the development of statistical methods, and particularly the potential of modern high-powered data technology. The group of McQuay and Tramer has been especially active in using this method in order to provide evidence-based knowledge from all the small or intermediately sized studies that have been performed with quite standardized measures of outcome[38, 64–68]. As in other areas of anesthesia, the use of meta-analyses has been criticized as the selection of trials and influence from one dominating center may also put bias into this method[69].

The new development: focus on cost-effectiveness

As modern medicine has so many potential options, increasing focus has been put on limiting the use of methods that carry high cost with minor or intermediate improvements in health effects. The area of PONV lends itself readily to those kinds of discussions as some drugs are expensive, some are very cheap and the condition is not life-threatening. There are, however, a lot of indirect costs involved, such as increased need of nursing care and rescue medication, as well as delayed discharge or re-admission if a patient experiences PONV. Many of the recent papers on this issue point out the importance of reducing PONV, as the indirect costs may be quite high. Further, there seems to be little rationale for using the most expensive drugs instead of the less costly, classical drugs from a cost-effectiveness point of view[70–74].

An important aspect of this discussion is the issue of whether to use drugs prophylactically or to wait and treat patients when they have established symptoms[75]. Prophylactic use carries the risk of introducing side effects to patients not needing the drug as well as extra costs by giving a drug to all patients. On the other hand, as PONV is very unpleasant, patients may prefer prophylaxis instead of waiting for puking and subsequently continuing to experience symptoms while waiting for the onset of action of rescue agents.

Identification of patients at risk

As a spin-off from the cost-effectiveness discussion, the ideal concept would be to reliably predict which patient will develop PONV and who will not, and administer prophylaxis in a dedicated, individualized way. A large amount of data about etiology, epidemiology and clinical research may be used for this purpose, and throughout the 1990s many formulas and guidelines were published for this purpose[75]. Both complicated mathematical algorithms and simple yes/no statements on 3–5 risk factors have been suggested by the groups of Toner[76], Koivuranta[77], Apfel[78–80], Raeder[81] and many others. The most used and best documented is the simple 0–4 score developed in parallel by Apfel and Koivuranta; the risk factors being the female gender, nonsmoking, use of opioids and a history of either PONV or motion sickness[82]. There is an ongoing debate as to whether risk assessment should be done individually in all patients and prophylactic antiemetics administered accordingly, or whether the simpler approach is to administer a standardized prophylaxis to all patients.

Recently, there has been a growing interest in genetics, both in mapping genes for potential individual susceptibility to have PONV, and also genetic variations in drug effects and metabolism[15].

Summary

The history of PONV is a fascinating journey through many aspects of anesthetic development since the first successful demonstration of ether by William T.G. Morton in 1846. It involves aspects of fundamental evolution, physiology, epidemiology and pharmacology together with very important daily applications in clinical practice. Although a good armamentarium for understanding PONV and application of knowledge and drugs into prophylaxis and treatment has been developed, there is still a lot to learn from the history in this field. And the story goes on …

References

1. Smith GFR. Post-operative vomiting. *Br J Anaesth* 1934; 11:132–9.
2. Morton HJV, Wylie WD. Anaesthetic deaths due to regurgitation or vomiting. *Anaesthesia* 1951; 6:190–205.
3. Edwards G, Morton HJV, Pask EA, et al. Deaths associated with anaesthesia. A report on 1000 cases. *Anaesthesia* 1956; 11:194–220.
4. Thomas LJ. Uber da Brechcentrum und uber die Wirkung einiger pharmakologischer Mittel auf dasselbe. *Virchows Arch pat Anat* 1891; 123:44–69.
5. Hatcher RA. Mechanism of vomiting. *Physiol Rev* 1924; 4:479–504.
6. Borison HL, Wang SC. Physiology and pharmacology of vomiting. *Pharmacol Rev* 1953; 5:193–230.
7. Wang SC, Borison HL. A new concept of organization of the central emetic mechanism. *Gastroenterology* 1952; 22:1–12.
8. Ferguson RH. The use of olive oil to prevent or relieve postanesthetic vomiting. *NY Med J* 1912; 95:1359–61.
9. Gralla RJ, Itri LM, Pisko SE, et al. Antiemetic efficacy of high-dose metoclopramide: randomized trials with placebo and prochlorperazine in patients with chemotherapy-induced nausea and vomiting. *N Engl J Med* 1981; 305:905–9.
10. Gesztesi Z, Scuderi PE, White PF, et al. Substance P (Neurokinin-1) antagonist prevents postoperative vomiting after abdominal hysterectomy procedures. *Anesthesiology* 2000; 93:931–7.
11. Rojas C, Raje M, Tsukamoto T, et al. Molecular mechanisms of 5-HT(3) and NK(1) receptor antagonists in prevention of emesis. *Eur J Pharmacol* 2014; 722:26–37.
12. George E, Hornuss C, Apfel CC. Neurokinin-1 and novel serotonin antagonists for postoperative and postdischarge nausea and vomiting. *Curr Opin Anaesthesiol* 2010; 23:714–21.
13. Lewis IH, Campbell DN, Barrowcliffe MP. Effect of nabilone on nausea and vomiting after total abdominal hysterectomy. *Br J Anaesth* 1994; 73:244–6.
14. Sharkey KA, Darmani NA, Parker LA. Regulation of nausea and vomiting by cannabinoids and the endocannabinoid system. *Eur J Pharmacol* 2014; 722:134–46.
15. Horn CC, Wallisch WJ, Homanics GE, et al. Pathophysiological and neurochemical mechanisms of postoperative nausea and vomiting. *Eur J Pharmacol* 2014; 722:55–66.
16. Smith HS, Laufer A. Opioid induced nausea and vomiting. *Eur J Pharmacol* 2014; 722:67–78.
17. Johnston KD, Lu Z, Rudd JA. Looking beyond 5-HT(3) receptors: a review of the wider role of serotonin in the pharmacology of nausea and vomiting. *Eur J Pharmacol* 2014; 722:13–25.
18. Darmani NA. Preface. New vistas in the pharmacology and neurochemistry of diverse causes of nausea and vomiting. *Eur J Pharmacol* 2014; 722:1.

19. Blumfeld J, Cantab MD. The prevention of sickness after anaesthetics. *Lancet* 1899; 77:833–5.

20. Davies RM. Some factors affecting the incidence of post-anaesthetic vomiting. *Br Med J* 1941; 578–80.

21. Dent SJ, Ramachandra V, Stephen CR. Postoperative vomiting: incidence, analysis, and therapeutic measures in 3000 patients. *Anesthesiology* 1955; 16:564–72.

22. White PF, Abrao J. Drug-induced prolongation of the QT interval: what's the point? *Anesthesiology* 2006; 104:386–7.

23. Kapur PA. The big "little problem". *Anesth Analg* 1991; 73:243–5.

24. Eberhart L, Morin A, Kranke P. [Nausea and vomiting after anaesthesia for children – big problems for little patients]. *Anasthesiol Intensivmed Notfallmed Schmerzther* 2014; 49:24–9.

25. Didier EP, Barila TG, Slogum HC, et al. An evaluation of antiemetic drugs in the control of postoperative nausea and vomiting. *Surg Forum* 1954; 5:707–12.

26. Knapp MR, Beecher HK. Postanesthetic nausea, vomiting, and retching. *JAMA* 1956; 160:376–85.

27. Burtles R, Peckett BW. Postoperative vomiting. Some factors affecting incidence. *Br J Anaesth* 1957; 29:114–23.

28. Dyrberg V, Johansen SH. Pre-anaesthetic medication with chlorpromazine. *Acta Anaesthesiol Scand* 1958; 2:133–47.

29. Lind B, Breivik H. Metoclopramide and perphenazine in the prevention of postoperative nausea and vomiting. *Br J Anaesth* 1970; 42:614–7.

30. Gan TJ. Selective serotonin 5-HT3 receptor antagonists for postoperative nausea and vomiting: are they all the same? *CNS Drugs* 2005; 19:225–38.

31. Apfel CC, Korttila K, Abdalla M, et al. A factorial trial of six interventions for the prevention of postoperative nausea and vomiting. *N Engl J Med* 2004; 350:2441–51.

32. Raeder JC, Mjaland O, Aasbo V, et al. Desflurane versus propofol maintenance for outpatient laparoscopic cholecystectomy. *Acta Anaesthesiol Scand* 1998; 42:106–10.

33. Hammas B, Thorn SE, Wattwil M. Superior prolonged antiemetic prophylaxis with a four-drug multimodal regimen – comparison with propofol or placebo. *Acta Anaesthesiol Scand* 2002; 46:232–7.

34. Borgeat A, Stirnemann HR. [Antiemetic effect of propofol]. *Anaesthesist* 1998; 47:918–24.

35. Bunce KT, Tyers MB. The role of 5-HT in postoperative nausea and vomiting. *Br J Anaesth* 1992; 69:60S–2S.

36. Hindle AT. Recent developments in the physiology and pharmacology of 5-hydroxytryptamine. *Br J Anaesth* 1994; 73:395–407.

37. Larijani GE, Gratz I, Afshar M, et al. Treatment of postoperative nausea and vomiting with ondansetron: a randomized, double-blind comparison with placebo. *Anesth Analg* 1991; 73:246–9.

38. Tramer MR, Reynolds DJ, Moore RA, et al. Efficacy, dose–response, and safety of ondansetron in prevention of postoperative nausea and vomiting: a quantitative systematic review of randomized placebo-controlled trials. *Anesthesiology* 1997; 87:1277–89.

39. Fujii Y, Tanaka H, Toyooka H. Prophylactic antiemetic efficacy of granisetron in patients with and without previous postoperative emesis. *Can J Anaesth* 1997; 44:273–7.

40. Hanaoka K. Notice of formal retraction of articles by Dr. Yoshitaka Fujii. *Masui* 2013; 62:1029–30.

41. Yang LP, Scott LJ. Palonosetron: in the prevention of nausea and vomiting. *Drugs* 2009; 69:2257–78.

42. Ellis RH. The case books of Dr John Snow. *Med Hist Suppl* 1994; 14: i–1vii, 1–633.

43. Andersen R, Krohg K. Pain as a major cause of postoperative nausea. *Can Anaesth Soc J* 1976; 23:366–9.

44. Hagemann E, Halvorsen A, Holgersen O, et al. Intramuscular ephedrine reduces emesis during the first three hours after

abdominal hysterectomy. *Acta Anaesthesiol Scand* 2000; 44:107–11.

45. Wang JJ, Ho ST, Lee SC, et al. The prophylactic effect of dexamethasone on postoperative nausea and vomiting in women undergoing thyroidectomy: a comparison of droperidol with saline. *Anesth Analg* 1999; 89:200–3.
46. Aasboe V, Raeder JC, Groegaard B. Betamethasone reduces postoperative pain and nausea after ambulatory surgery. *Anesth Analg* 1998; 87:319–23.
47. Liu K, Hsu CC, Chia YY. The effect of dose of dexamethasone for antiemesis after major gynecological surgery. *Anesth Analg* 1999; 89:1316–8.
48. Dundee JW, McMillan CM. P6 acupressure and postoperative vomiting. *Br J Anaesth* 1992; 68:225–6.
49. Zarate E, Mingus M, White PF, et al. The use of transcutaneous acupoint electrical stimulation for preventing nausea and vomiting after laparoscopic surgery. *Anesth Analg* 2001; 92:629–35.
50. Rodola F. Midazolam as an anti-emetic. *Eur Rev Med Pharmacol Sci* 2006; 10:121–6.
51. Riding JE. Post-operative vomiting. *Proc R Soc Med* 1960; 53:671–7.
52. Belleville WJ, Irwin DJ, Howland WS. Postoperative nausea and vomiting IV: factors related to postoperative nausea and vomiting. *Anesthesiology* 1960; 21:186–93.
53. Purkis IE. Factors that influence postoperative vomiting. *Anaes Soc J* 1964; 11:335–53.
54. Dundee JW, Kirwan MJ, Clarke RS. Anaesthesia and premedication as factors in postoperative vomiting. *Acta Anaesthesiol Scand* 1965; 9:223–31.
55. Janhunen L, Tammisto T. Postoperative vomiting after different modes of general anaesthesia. *Ann Chir Gynaecol Fenn* 1972; 61:152–9.
56. Palazzo MG, Strunin L. Anaesthesia and emesis. II: Prevention and management. *Can Anaesth Soc J* 1984; 31:407–15.
57. Palazzo MG, Strunin L. Anaesthesia and emesis. I: Etiology. *Can Anaesth Soc J* 1984; 31:178–87.
58. Watcha MF, White PF. Postoperative nausea and vomiting. Its etiology, treatment, and prevention. *Anesthesiology* 1992; 77:162–84.
59. Gan TJ. Postoperative nausea and vomiting – can it be eliminated? *JAMA* 2002; 287:1233–6.
60. Scuderi PE, James RL, Harris L, et al. Multimodal antiemetic management prevents early postoperative vomiting after outpatient laparoscopy. *Anesth Analg* 2000; 91:1408–14.
61. Gan TJ, Meyer T, Apfel CC, et al. Consensus guidelines for managing postoperative nausea and vomiting. *Anesth Analg* 2003; 97:62–71.
62. Gan TJ, Diemunsch P, Habib AS, et al. SAMBA Consensus guidelines for the management of postoperative nausea and vomiting. *Anesth Analg* 2014; 118:85–113.
63. Skolnik A, Gan TJ. Update on the management of postoperative nausea and vomiting. *Curr Opin Anaesthesiol* 2014; 27:605–9.
64. Tramer MR, Phillips C, Reynolds DJ, et al. Cost-effectiveness of ondansetron for postoperative nausea and vomiting. *Anaesthesia* 1999; 54:226–34.
65. Tramer MR, Fuchs-Buder T. Omitting antagonism of neuromuscular block: effect on postoperative nausea and vomiting and risk of residual paralysis. A systematic review. *Br J Anaesth* 1999; 82:379–86.
66. Tramer M, Moore A, McQuay H. Omitting nitrous oxide in general anaesthesia: meta-analysis of intraoperative awareness and postoperative emesis in randomized controlled trials. *Br J Anaesth* 1996; 76:186–93.
67. Henzi I, Walder B, Tramer MR. Metoclopramide in the prevention of postoperative nausea and vomiting: a quantitative systematic review of randomized, placebo-controlled studies. *Br J Anaesth* 1999; 83:761–71.

68. Tramer MR. A rational approach to the control of postoperative nausea and vomiting: evidence from systematic reviews. Part I. Efficacy and harm of antiemetic interventions, and methodological issues. *Acta Anaesthesiol Scand* 2001; 45:4–13.

69. Kranke P, Apfel CC, Eberhart LH, et al. The influence of a dominating centre on a quantitative systematic review of granisetron for preventing postoperative nausea and vomiting. *Acta Anaesthesiol Scand* 2001; 45:659–70.

70. Adriani J, Summers FW, Antony SO. Is the prophylactic use of antiemetics in surgical patients justified? *JAMA* 1961; 175:666–71.

71. Subramaniam B, Madan R, Sadhasivam S, et al. Dexamethasone is a cost-effective alternative to ondansetron in preventing PONV after paediatric strabismus repair. *Br J Anaesth* 2001; 86:84–9.

72. Hill RP, Lubarsky DA, Phillips-Bute B, et al. Cost-effectiveness of prophylactic antiemetic therapy with ondansetron, droperidol, or placebo. *Anesthesiology* 2000; 92:958–67.

73. Tang J, Watcha MF, White PF. A comparison of costs and efficacy of ondansetron and droperidol as prophylactic antiemetic therapy for elective outpatient gynecologic procedures. *Anesth Analg* 1996; 83:304–13.

74. Watcha MF, Smith I. Cost-effectiveness analysis of antiemetic therapy for ambulatory surgery. *J Clin Anesth* 1994; 6:370–7.

75. Sinclair DR, Chung F, Mezei G. Can postoperative nausea and vomiting be predicted? *Anesthesiology* 1999; 91:109–18.

76. Toner CC, Broomhead CJ, Littlejohn IH, et al. Prediction of postoperative nausea and vomiting using a logistic regression model. *Br J Anaesth* 1996; 76:347–51.

77. Koivuranta M, Laara E, Ranta P, et al. Comparison of ondansetron and droperidol in the prevention of postoperative nausea and vomiting after laparoscopic surgery in women. A randomised, double-blind, placebo-controlled trial. *Acta Anaesthesiol Scand* 1997; 41:1273–9.

78. Apfel CC, Greim CA, Haubitz I, et al. A risk score to predict the probability of postoperative vomiting in adults. *Acta Anaesthesiol Scand* 1998; 42:495–501.

79. Apfel CC, Kranke P, Greim CA, et al. What can be expected from risk scores for predicting postoperative nausea and vomiting? *Br J Anaesth* 2001; 86:822–7.

80. Apfel CC, Kranke P, Eberhart LH, et al. Comparison of predictive models for postoperative nausea and vomiting. *Br J Anaesth* 2002; 88:234–40.

81. Trope A, Raeder JC. [Can postoperative nausea or vomiting be predicted?]. *Tidsskr Nor Laegeforen* 2000; 120:2423–6.

82. Apfel CC, Laara E, Koivuranta M, et al. A simplified risk score for predicting postoperative nausea and vomiting: conclusions from cross-validations between two centers. *Anesthesiology* 1999; 91:693–700.

Chapter 2

Mechanisms of nausea and vomiting

Anthony L. Kovac

A patient's postoperative nausea and vomiting (PONV) are caused by a variety of mechanisms, which are specific stimuli due to the patient, surgery and anesthesia, resulting in an anatomic and physiologic response. Multiple causes of nausea and vomiting are listed in Table 2.1[1–4]. Gastrointestinal (GI) physiology is an important peripheral mechanism. Nausea is a subjective feeling of the need to vomit. Vomiting is an objective response to a noxious stimulus and is the actual oral passage of GI contents. Retching is the objective muscular event of vomiting without passage of vomit[1]. GI retroperistalsis is initiated at the pyloric sphincter and in the small intestine. To protect teeth enamel from stomach acids, an increase in salivary gland fluid occurs. In order to prevent aspiration, an individual takes a deep breath and the epiglottis closes over the glottis. As inspiration occurs, there is a decrease in intrathoracic pressure. One or multiple retching acts may occur, followed by vomiting and an increased physiologic sympathetic response of sweating and increased heart rate (Figure 2.1)[1,5].

Anatomical areas of nausea and vomiting

Emetic afferent and efferent impulses stimulate nausea and vomiting peripherally via the GI tract and centrally via the central nervous system (CNS). These stimuli control the initiation and degree of nausea and/or vomiting that a patient may experience. Stimulation of afferent pathways to the vomiting center occurs from the GI tract via the vagus nerve. Central CNS pathways act via neural networks through different areas of the brain. Neural pathways of nausea and vomiting with CNS inputs, CNS integration and physiologic outputs are listed in Table 2.2[1,5].

Mechanical and chemical receptors reside in the GI tract. Mechanical expansion or contraction of the stomach, intestine and esophagus, as well as the abdomen and heart, can cause nausea and vomiting by directly stimulating the vagus nerve. Medications such as chemotherapeutic agents (i.e., cisplatin, methotrexate, etc.) cause the release of serotonin (5-hydroxytryptamine) from enterochromaffin cells of the duodenum to directly cause nausea and vomiting[6,7].

Central CNS pathways causing nausea and vomiting appear to be more interrelated and complex than GI pathways. The main CNS areas involved with nausea and vomiting are located in the cerebral cortex, thalamus, hypothalamus, meninges, cerebellum, pons and medulla oblongata. Specific vomiting areas that are located below the pons and next to the fourth ventricle include the medulla oblongata, vomiting center and chemoreceptor zone

Postoperative Nausea and Vomiting: A Practical Guide, eds. Tong Joo Gan and Ashraf S. Habib. Published by Cambridge University Press.

Table 2.1 Multiple causes of nausea and vomiting

Disease or condition	Cause
Gastrointestinal diseases	Obstruction Inflammation, hepatitis, pancreatitis, enteritis Gastritis Gastric irritants
Intracranial disease	Malignant hypertension Increased intracranial pressure (cancer, hemorrhage)
Infections	Bacterial Viral
Pregnancy	Hyperemesis gravidarum Morning sickness
Migraines	
Metabolic diseases	Diabetic ketoacidosis Addison's disease
Vestibular and labyrinthine disorders	Motion sickness Vestibular neuritis Labyrinthitis
Pain	
Exogenous emetic substances	Drugs, opioids, anesthesia Poisons Radiation Chemotherapy – cisplatin/methotrexate (acute versus delayed)

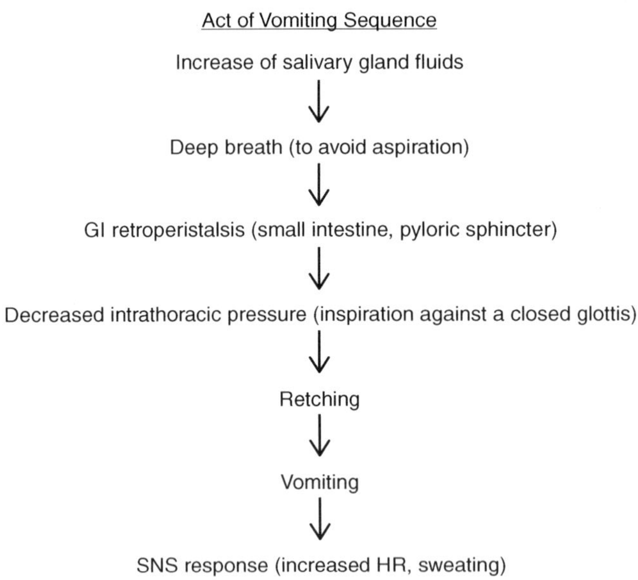

Figure 2.1 Act of vomiting sequence. GI, gastrointestinal; HR, heart rate; SNS, sympathetic nervous system.

Table 2.2 Neural pathways

Stimulus	Neural pathway
CNS inputs	Cerebral Vestibular system Area postrema, chemoreceptor trigger zone Abdominal vagal afferents Serotonin release from duodenum
CNS integration	Nucleus tractus solitaries Salivary nuclei Ventral lateral medulla Dorsal motor nucleus Retrofacial nucleus Respiratory
Physiologic outputs	Prodromal signs Muscles – retching/vomiting (sequence of muscles used in retching is different from vomiting)

Table 2.3 CNS neuroanatomical areas and receptors associated with nausea and vomiting

CNS neuroanatomical areas	Receptors
Vestibular system	Muscarinic: M_3, M_5 Cholinergic: ACh_1 H_1
Area postrema, chemoreceptor trigger zone	Opioid: mu (μ) 5-HT_3 D_2: substance P NK_1; cholinergic – ACh_1
Nucleus of the solitary tract	Opioid: mu (μ) 5-HT_3 NK_1

5-HT_3, serotonin 5-hydroxytryptamine type 3; ACh_1, acetylcholine muscarinic type 1; D_2, dopamine type 2; H_1, histamine type 1; NK_1, neurokinin type 1.

(CTZ). The CTZ and area postrema are considered to be synonymous areas. The CTZ is located in the area postrema on the floor of the fourth ventricle in the medulla oblongata. In addition, the vestibular system and cerebellum lie in close proximity to the vomiting centers at the base of the pons. Nerve connections extend from the cerebellum to the pons. The actual act of vomiting is initiated by neurochemical and receptor actions originating from the CTZ. The CTZ can be stimulated concurrently by the CNS, peripheral nervous system and peripheral GI motor pathways[1,6,8].

Neuropharmacologic targets and receptor areas associated with nausea and vomiting are listed in Table 2.3. The area postrema is connected to the nucleus of the solitary tract as well as to other autonomic control centers in the brain stem. The blood–brain barrier is located between the area postrema and the nucleus tractus solitarius. Opioids affect the area postrema, nucleus tractus solitarius, brain stem, spinal receptors and alter GI motility[9]. Inhaled anesthetics affect the area postrema, nucleus tractus solitarius and vagal afferents [5,6,10]. The vestibular system is involved with a patient's sense of balance and the

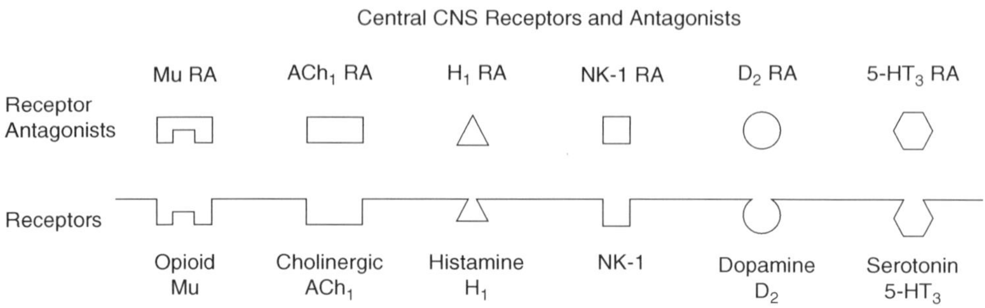

Figure 2.2 Central nervous system receptors and antagonists. 5-HT_3, serotonin 5-hydroxytryptamine type 3; ACh_1, acetylcholine; CNS, central nervous system; D_2, dopamine; H_1, histamine; NK, neurokinin; RA, receptor antagonists.

sensation of motion sickness. Abnormalities or diseases of the vestibular system can directly cause motion sickness. Histamine type 1 (H_1) and acetylcholine muscarinic type 1 (ACh_1) receptors are located in the vestibular system. Activation and deactivation of these receptors are the result of stimulation and blockade, respectively, with histamine or cholinergic medications[10,11].

Chemoreceptors located in the CTZ include dopamine type 2 (D_2), substance P neurokinin type 1 (NK_1), serotonin 5-hydroxytryptamine type 3 (5-HT_3), acetylcholine type 1 (ACh_1) and opioid (mu) receptors. The vomiting center includes the nucleus of tractus solitarius. Receptors in the vomiting center include H_1, ACh_1, NK_1 and serotonin 5-HT_3 receptors. Each specific receptor in the area postrema and CTZ has a corresponding agonist and antagonist (Figure 2.2)[6,11].

Mechanical effects, such as GI tract distention from air, fluids or nitrous oxide, cause nausea and vomiting via stimulation by the vagus nerve to the vomiting center and the vestibular part of the vestibulocochlear eighth cranial nerve, which is also affected by opioids[6,11].

Vomiting can be caused by a variety of single or multiple stimuli working at or via many parallel and corresponding neural pathways, which eventually reach the vomiting center. Because of this complex interaction, a "silver bullet, one drug fits all" universal antiemetic medication has not been found for PONV or postdischarge nausea and vomiting (PDNV)[12]. Stimuli from the vagal abdominal afferent pathway appear to be one of the better understood peripheral pathways. NK_1 and 5-HT_3-receptor antagonists are present in peripheral and central locations (Figure 2.3). Combination blockade of peripheral and central emetogenic receptors is needed to successfully find the universal antiemetic medication or technique[3,12].

Inputs to the vomiting center

The CTZ is located at the base of the fourth ventricle with input from the vomiting center. The vestibular system of the inner ear has input by H_1 receptors to the vomiting center via the vestibulocochlear eighth cranial nerve resulting in nausea and motion sickness. When the pharynx is stimulated, the glossopharyngeal tenth cranial nerve is correspondingly stimulated, resulting in the gag reflex. In addition, when activated, the enteric nervous system and vagal nerve fibers around the gut transfer stimuli to the vomiting center. Stress and anxiety input stimuli to the vomiting center directly from the CNS via dopaminergic receptors[6,12].

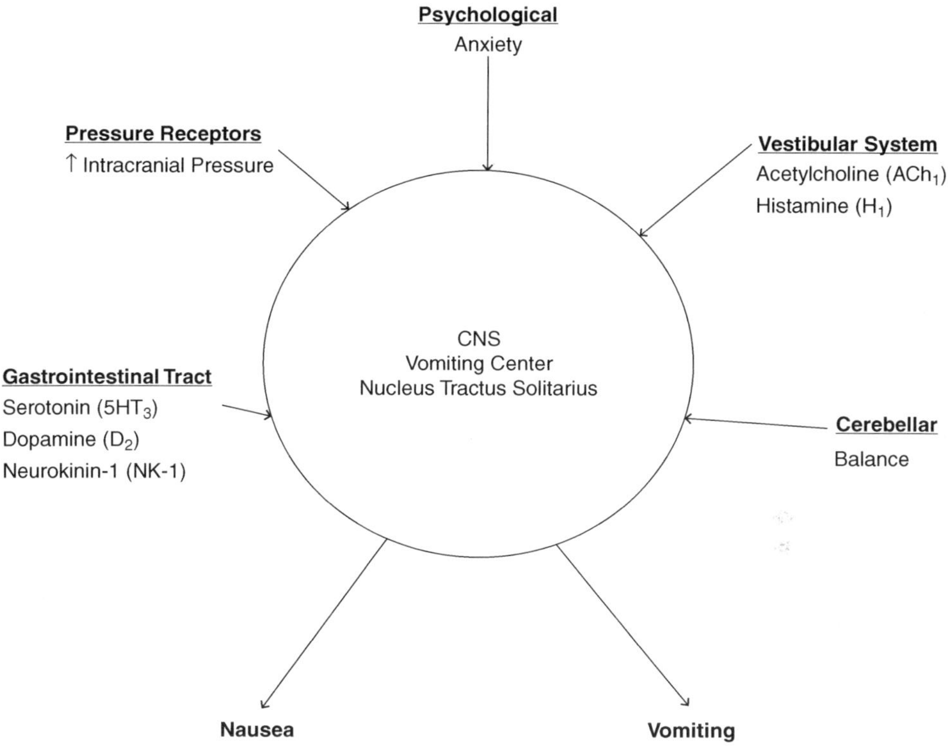

Figure 2.3 Receptor antagonists in peripheral and central locations. CNS, central nervous system.

Animal models of nausea and vomiting

Animal studies of the mechanism of nausea and vomiting have involved various species with the ferret, musk shrew and dog as the most frequently studied[13,14]. The ferret has been a standard model for chemotherapy-induced nausea and vomiting (CINV). However, while ferrets are insensitive to the nausea and vomiting effects of a volatile agent such as isoflurane, they are sensitive to opioids, specifically morphine[14]. This opioid effect can be reversed by administration of naloxone. The musk shrew is sensitive to the effects of halothane, isoflurane and nitrous oxide. Dogs are sensitive and exhibit vomiting and regurgitation following administration of halothane, isoflurane or sevoflurane. Interestingly, rats do not exhibit a vomiting reflex[13].

Emetogenic CNS areas reside on both sides of the blood–brain barrier. Intrinsic primary afferent neurons transmit stimuli to the vomiting center. Vagal efferent motor neurons reside in the esophagus, stomach and intestine. Spinal somatomotor neurons are located in the anterior abdominal muscles and the diaphragm. Stimulation of the airway, heart, skin, salivary gland and GI tract causes prodromal effects leading to symptoms of pallor, sweating, salivation and alterations of gastric and GI function[1,13].

The primary practical physiologic function of vomiting is to empty noxious stimuli such as drugs, chemicals and foreign objects from the upper GI tract. Vomiting itself serves as a defense mechanism to rid the body of dangerous noxious substances. Diarrhea empties noxious stimuli from the lower GI tract[1,5].

The severity of drug-induced emesis can be controlled with antiemetics, such as the NK_1 and 5-HT_3 receptor antagonists. Nausea is more difficult to control and is a more persistent problem. The D_2 receptor antagonists appear to have a greater effect on nausea than on vomiting[3].

Fluid volume/hypotension

The status of a patient's circulatory volume and blood pressure effects, such as hypotension, can cause nausea and vomiting after administration of a spinal or epidural block due to vasodilatation with a decrease in blood pressure and blood flow to the brain's CNS vomiting centers. This decrease in blood flow as well as orthostatic changes that may occur in the operating room and/or postanesthesia care unit initiates the release of CNS emetogenic neurochemicals causing nausea and/or vomiting in the awake patient. Intravenous fluid replacement and administration of a vasopressor, such as ephedrine, are useful measures to treat this cause of nausea and vomiting. Gut ischemia also causes the release of emetogenic substances such as serotonin[3,10,11,15].

Antiemetics according to receptor areas and mechanisms of action

Corticosteroids

Dexamethasone is one of the more common steroid medications given for its antiemetic effect. Methylprednisolone also has been shown to have similar antiemetic properties[16–18]. Glucocorticoids have a central effect on corticosteroid receptors in the nucleus tractus solitarius. Not much is known about the mechanism of action of steroids to decrease PONV. The central antiemetic mechanism of corticosteroids is not fully understood as there is no known central steroid receptor. It is hypothesized that the antiemetic effect of steroids is due to their ability to decrease inflammation and edema. Dexamethasone decreases the release of arachidonic acid, which in turn decreases the synthesis of mediators of inflammation that sensitizes nerves. However, this effect takes time to work and can be as long as 3–4 h for an effect to occur[12,19].

Metoclopramide

Metoclopramide is a competitive antagonist at dopaminergic (D_2) receptors and a weak competitive antagonist at 5-HT_3 receptors. Metoclopramide exerts its effect at multiple receptors in the CNS and periphery, depending on the dose administered. At doses greater than 20 mg, it acts on multiple D_2, H_2 and 5-HT_3 receptors in the area postrema as well as having a prokinetic effect in the GI tract, specifically the stomach and intestines, by antagonism of D_2 and 5-HT_4 receptors. However, extrapyramidal side effects, such as tardive dyskinesia, increase with an increase in number of treatments and dose. Metoclopramide increases gastric motility as an acetylcholine mediator[7,20].

Dopamine antagonists

Phenothiazines, such as prochlorperazine and chlorpromazine, act on dopamine D_2 receptors in the CTZ and the periphery. However, the extrapyramidal effects of prochlorperazine and the anticholinergic side effects of chlorpromazine limit the usefulness of these medications. Butyrophenones, such as droperidol and haloperidol, act on D_2 receptors in the area postrema and CTZ. The US Food and Drug Administration (FDA) black box warning related to concerns about the electrocardiogram (ECG) effects of the butyrophenones on QTc interval prolongation has limited their use[6,7].

Antihistamines

Histamine H_1 receptors are located in the CTZ, vestibular nuclei and vomiting center of the medulla. Blockade of H_1 receptors is a nonspecific antihistaminergic mechanism of antihistamine medications. Antihistamines have been found useful as a treatment method to attenuate PONV effects following ear, mastoid or operations on the vestibular system. However, H_2-receptor antagonists have not been found to be effective for PONV prophylaxis[6,7].

Anticholinergics

Anticholinergics, such as transdermal scopolamine, are useful antiemetic agents to prevent or treat vestibular causes of PONV. Similar to antihistamines, they are useful for operations on the ear, mastoid and vestibular system. Transdermal scopolamine exerts its effect at postganglionic muscarinic receptors in the peripheral nervous system; its CNS action antagonizes cholinergic M_3 and M_5 receptors, blocking transmission to vestibular nuclei. Possible side effects include a dry mouth on the first operative day and vision disturbances such as diplopia on the second day[7,21].

NK_1-receptor antagonists

Aprepitant, the only FDA-approved NK_1-receptor antagonist for PONV, exhibits its antiemetic effect by antagonism of NK_1 receptors. Blockade of NK_1 receptors occurs in the nucleus tractus solitarius and the reticular formation of the CNS as well as having an effect on the GI tract. Aprepitant has more of an effect on emesis than nausea.

Serotonin 5-HT_3-receptor antagonists

The 5-HT_3 receptor is a subtype of the 5-HT serotonin receptor that is present centrally in the CNS and vagus nerve and peripherally in the small intestine. The nausea and vomiting related to chemotherapy is peripherally activated by the release of serotonin from enterochromaffin cells of the duodenum. The 5-HT_3 antagonists can effectively block this release of serotonin and decrease or prevent CINV[6,7]. PONV due to serotonin release is more complex and involves blockade of both the peripheral and central CNS 5-HT_3 receptors. The first-generation 5-HT_3-receptor antagonists include ondansetron, dolasetron, granisetron, tropisetron and ramosetron[3]. Palonosetron has a long-acting, 40-h half-life and is a second-generation 5-HT_3 receptor antagonist, which exerts its effect to block the 5-HT_3 receptor by non cooperatively binding to allosteric rather than orthosteric sites[22–24]. "Allo" refers to "other." Ortho refers to the normal competitive binding sites. Allosteric binding occurs at a site other than the active site[25]. Palonosetron also exhibits positive cooperativity among serotonin receptors and binding sites. Binding of the initial first palonosetron molecule allows for subsequent binding of palonosetron molecules to occur more easily[24].

Pharmacogenetics

A patient's individual genetic makeup helps control and predict multiple disease and drug processes. Racial differences may exist in vestibular hypersusceptibility and sensitivity to motion sickness between Asian (Chinese) compared to non-Asian populations[26]. Differences in genetic makeup and sequencing can alter a patient's drug response with possible change in absorption, transport and/or metabolism[27,28], resulting in a medication's success or failure. Genes help regulate individual drug therapy regarding whether or not a patient may or may not respond to a specific medication. A patient's individual drug response may be due to differences in their DNA gene sequencing or in the control of proteins that regulate specific metabolic receptors and processes. A change or duplication of a specific gene allele can increase or decrease metabolism, altering an antiemetic's serum blood level and thus the therapeutic response. Ultra-rapid metabolism can result in a lower than desired blood level and reduced drug effectiveness. Alternately, decreased metabolism can lead to a higher than desired blood level with a corresponding increased potential for drug interactions and adverse events[29]. Genetic variability of protein transporters has been determined to alter ondansetron's ability to cross the blood–brain barrier. The 3435TT and 2677TT genotypes have been determined to increase ondansetron's transport across the blood–brain barrier, resulting in higher ondansetron concentrations to interact with more CNS 5-HT_3 receptors[15]. An increased antiemetic response occurs resulting in a lower degree of PONV. Genetic interindividual variability has been shown to occur in the multidrug resistance 1 (MDR1) glycoprotein, which is important in drug metabolism and disposition. Genetic polymorphisms and ethnic differences have been determined in the CYP3A, CYP249, CYP2D6 and MDR1/ABC1 enzymes, which are important in the metabolism of the 5-HT_3-receptor antagonists[30]. These effects are discussed in more detail in Chapter 5.

Summary

The mechanisms causing PONV and PDNV are multiple and interrelated. Anesthetics, medications, blood pressure changes (hypotension), motion and balance (position changes, ambulation), mechanical effects and genetics all play a part. Stimuli can occur from the periphery or be centrally activated. In the difficult patient, multiple antiemetic agents and methods/techniques may be needed using a multimodal technique to prevent and/or treat PONV and PDNV. While research in this area is evolving, further research is needed to help solve the problems of PONV and PDNV.

References

1. Becker DE. Nausea, vomiting, and hiccups: a review of mechanisms and treatment. *Anesth Prog* 2010; 57(4):150–6.
2. Keeley PW. Nausea and vomiting in people with cancer and other chronic diseases. *BMJ Clin Evid* 2009; 2406.
3. Gan TJ, Diemunsch P, Habib AS, et al. Consensus guidelines for the management of postoperative nausea and vomiting. *Anesth Analg* 2014; 118(1):85–113.
4. Chow CM, Leung AKC, Hon KL. *Acute gastroenteritis: From guidelines to real life.* Macclesfield, UK: Dove Medical Press; 2010; 97–112.
5. Horn CC. Why is the neurobiology of nausea and vomiting so important? *Appetite* 2008; 50(2–3):430–4.
6. Bashashati M, McCallum RW. Neurochemical mechanisms and pharmacologic strategies in managing nausea and vomiting related to

cyclic vomiting syndrome and other gastrointestinal disorders. *Eur J Pharmacol* 2014; 722:79–94.

7. Gordon P, LeGrand SB, Walsh D. Nausea and vomiting in advanced cancer. *Eur J Pharmacol* 2014; 722:187–91.
8. Miller AD, Nonaka S, Jakus J. Brain areas essential or non-essential for emesis. *Brain Res* 1994; 647(2):255–64.
9. Smith HS, Laufer A. Opioid induced nausea and vomiting. *Eur J Pharmacol* 2014; 722:67–78.
10. Horn CC, Wallisch WJ, Homanics GE, et al. Pathophysiological and neurochemical mechanisms of postoperative nausea and vomiting. *Eur J Pharmacol* 2014; 722:55–66.
11. Watcha MF, White PF. Postoperative nausea and vomiting. Its etiology, treatment, and prevention. *Anesthesiology* 1992; 77(1):162–84.
12. Sanger GJ, Andrews PL. Treatment of nausea and vomiting: gaps in our knowledge. *Auton Neurosci* 2006; 129(1–2):3–16.
13. Andrews PL, Horn CC. Signals for nausea and emesis: implications for models of upper gastrointestinal diseases. *Auton Neurosci* 2006; 125(1–2):100–15.
14. Horn CC, Meyers K, Pak D, et al. Post-anesthesia vomiting: impact of isoflurane and morphine on ferrets and musk shrews. *Physiol Behav* 2012; 106(4):562–8.
15. Ho KY, Gan TJ. Pharmacology, pharmacogenetics, and clinical efficacy of 5-hydroxytryptamine type 3 receptor antagonists for postoperative nausea and vomiting. *Curr Opin Anaesthesiol* 2006; 19(6):606–11.
16. Miyagawa Y, Ejiri M, Kuzuya T, et al. Methylprednisolone reduces postoperative nausea in total knee and hip arthroplasty. *J Clin Pharm Ther* 2010; 35(6):679–84.
17. Romundstad L, Breivik H, Roald H, et al. Methylprednisolone reduces pain, emesis, and fatigue after breast augmentation surgery: a single-dose, randomized, parallel-group study with methylprednisolone 125 mg, parecoxib 40 mg, and placebo. *Anesth Analg* 2006; 102(2):418–25.
18. Weren M, Demeere JL. Methylprednisolone vs. dexamethasone in the prevention of postoperative nausea and vomiting: a prospective, randomised, double-blind, placebo-controlled trial. *Acta Anaesthesiol Belg* 2008; 59(1):1–5.
19. De Oliveira GS Jr, Almeida MD, Benzon HT, et al. Perioperative single dose systemic dexamethasone for postoperative pain: a meta-analysis of randomized controlled trials. *Anesthesiol* 2011; 115(3):575–88.
20. Henzi I, Walder B, Tramer MR. Metoclopramide in the prevention of postoperative nausea and vomiting: a quantitative systematic review of randomized, placebo-controlled studies. *Br J Anaesth* 1999; 83(5):761–71.
21. Apfel CC, Zhang K, George E, et al. Transdermal scopolamine for the prevention of postoperative nausea and vomiting: a systematic review and meta-analysis. *Clin Ther* 2010; 32(12):1987–2002.
22. Yang LP, Scott LJ. Palonosetron: in the prevention of nausea and vomiting. *Drugs* 2009; 69(16):2257–78.
23. Wallenborn J, Kranke P. Palonosetron hydrochloride in the prevention and treatment of postoperative nausea and vomiting. *Clin Med Insights Ther* 2010; 2:387–99.
24. Rojas C, Stathis M, Thomas AG, et al. Palonosetron exhibits unique molecular interactions with the 5-HT3 receptor. *Anesth Analg* 2008; 107(2):469–78.
25. Davies PA. Allosteric modulation of the 5-HT(3) receptor. *Curr Opin Pharmacol* 2011; 11(1):75–80.
26. Stern RM, Hu S, Uijtdehaage SH, et al. Asian hypersusceptibility to motion sickness. *Hum Hered* 1996; 46(1):7–14.
27. Coulbault L, Beaussier M, Verstuyft C, et al. Environmental and genetic factors associated with morphine response in the postoperative period. *Clin Pharmacol Ther* 2006; 79(4):316–24.

28. Wallden J, Lindberg G, Sandin M, et al. Effects of fentanyl on gastric myoelectrical activity: a possible association with polymorphisms of the mu-opioid receptor gene? *Acta Anaesthesiol Scand* 2008; 52(5):708–15.

29. Hahm TS, Ko JS, Choi SJ, et al. Comparison of the prophylactic anti-emetic efficacy of ramosetron and ondansetron in patients at high-risk for postoperative nausea and vomiting after total knee replacement. *Anaesthesia* 2010; 65(5):500–4.

30. Candiotti KA, Birnbach DJ, Lubarsky DA, et al. The impact of pharmacogenomics on postoperative nausea and vomiting: do CYP2D6 allele copy number and polymorphisms affect the success or failure of ondansetron prophylaxis? *Anesthesiology* 2005; 102(3):543–9.

Chapter 3

Risk factors and their impact on postoperative nausea and vomiting

Anthony L. Kovac

The impact of postoperative nausea and vomiting (PONV) and the effectiveness of antiemetic therapy play an important part in the recovery of patients from anesthesia. All antiemetic medications have various possibilities of introducing benefits (efficacy) and/or harm (side effects). From the degree of efficacy and side effects, respectively, are derived concepts of number needed-to-treat and number needed-to-harm[1]. A decision to add or omit a specific antiemetic medication or therapy should be made after determining the possible benefits and/or harm of the therapy. In order to make a decision regarding the proper use of single or combination prophylactic or treatment therapy for PONV, it is important to estimate each patient's risk to develop either PONV, postoperative vomiting (POV) and/or postdischarge nausea and vomiting (PDNV)[2]. Specific factors directly affect the risk of an adult or pediatric patient developing PONV (Table 3.1), POV (Table 3.2) or PDNV (Table 3.3). These factors are characteristics related to the type of (a) surgery, (b) patients, (c) anesthetic medications and agents/techniques and (d) postoperative effects[2–6].

Risk factors for PONV include:

- Female gender
- History of PONV and/or motion sickness
- Nonsmoking history
- Postoperative opioids

Risk factors for POV include:

- Strabismus surgery
- Age ≥3 years
- Surgery >30 min
- History of POV or PONV in relatives (mother, father, siblings).

Factors contributing to PDNV include:

- Female gender
- Age <50 years
- History of nausea and/or vomiting after previous anesthesia
- Opioid administration in the postanesthesia care unit (PACU)
- Nausea in the PACU.

Postoperative Nausea and Vomiting: A Practical Guide, eds. Tong Joo Gan and Ashraf S. Habib. Published by Cambridge University Press.

Table 3.1 Simplified risk score for predicting PONV in adults[a]

Number of risk factors present	PONV % incidence	PONV risk
0	10	Low
1	21	Mild
2	39	Moderate
3	61	High
4	79	Extremely high

[a] PONV % incidence increases as the total number of risk factors increases. Each additional risk factor increases the incidence of PONV by approximately 20%.

Table 3.2 Simplified risk score for predicting POV in children[a]

Number of risk factors	POV risk (%)
0	10
1	10
2	30
3	50
4	70

[a] POV % incidence increases as the total number of risk factors increases. Each additional risk factor increases the incidence of POV by approximately 20%.

Table 3.3 Simplified risk score for predicting PDNV in adults

Number of risk factors	PDNV % incidence
0	7
1	20
2	28
3	53
4	60
5	89

Surgery-related PONV risk factors

Risk factors are associated with numerous aspects of a particular surgery and include the duration of surgery. Surgical time has a direct correlation with anesthesia exposure. Operations with a surgical time of more than 30 min have an increased incidence of PONV[5]. Sinclair et al.[4] determined that the frequency of PONV increased from 2.8% for adult patients having surgery less than 30 min to 27.7% for operations of more than 3 h. Eberhart et al.[6] indicated that children undergoing surgery lasting more than 30 min also had a greater risk of POV.

Specific surgeries associated with a higher risk for PONV may include operations on the eye, ear, nose, throat, teeth, oral cavity, brain, urologic, gynecologic and gastrointestinal

(GI) tract[7–16]. Operations on the head and neck, including the upper airway, nose, throat, oral, pharyngeal and dental areas as well as esophagus and/or stomach, can cause upper airway or GI bleeding resulting in swallowed blood and an increase in nausea and vomiting[17]. Operations on the brain, airway and neck may stimulate central nervous system (CNS) vomiting center receptors as well as the vagus and/or glossopharyngeal nerves to cause nausea and vomiting[8,18,19]. A decrease in CNS blood flow due to hypotension secondary to blood loss, inadequate fluid replacement or a sympathetic nerve block following spinal or epidural anesthesia may stimulate vomiting center receptors resulting in nausea and/or vomiting in the PACU. Hypovolemia causing hypotension can also lead to gut ischemia and nausea and/or vomiting due to the release of serotonin from the GI tract[2,20–22]

Surgeries, such as laparoscopic procedures (hysterectomy or cholecystectomy) in adults as well as strabismus repair and tonsillectomy in children can be especially emetogenic[2,23–27]. PONV is of special concern following distension of the abdomen in patients having laparoscopic procedures with insufflation of carbon dioxide gas into the abdominal cavity. Similarly, middle ear surgery and surgery on or manipulation of the esophagus, stomach, small or large intestine can lead to nausea and vomiting[23–27]. Even if a particular surgery has a low PONV risk, prophylactic antiemetics should still be considered because, should PONV occur, the physical and/or physiologic effects could be devastating to the patient[2,28].

Patient-related PONV risk factors

Patient-related factors include age <50 years, female gender, nonsmoking status, prior history of motion sickness or PONV and the administration of postoperative opioids[2,29–32] (Tables 3.1 and 3.3). There appears to be weak evidence for the use of intraoperative opioids as a cause for PONV[2]. Apfel et al.[29,30] described an increased PONV risk for females compared to males, which occurs following puberty with an increase in the hormones estrogen and progesterone[33]. History of motion sickness is an important patient-related risk factor, as motion can affect the degree and amount of histamine type 1 (H_1) and muscarinic receptors stimulated in the vestibular system[2,34].

Nonsmoking status is an important risk factor to recognize, as patients who do not smoke have an increased PONV incidence[2,34]. The fact that nonsmokers have more PONV than patients who smoke could possibly be explained by the induction of P450 enzymes; the increased metabolism of anesthetics and opioids in patients who smoke allows these patients to become more tolerant to emetogenic substances in tobacco smoke[35–38]. Receptors in the CNS causing PONV include the dopamine (D_2), cholinergic, H_1, serotonin 5-hydroxytryptamine type 3 (5-HT_3) and neurokinin type 1 (NK_1) receptors[2]. The antiemetogenic effect of tobacco smoke may act at one of these receptors to decrease the receptor's response. Smoking status appears to be related to a reduced PONV response with the patient becoming "acclimated" to the toxic chemicals in smoke, a result of CNS receptor adaption to repeated emetogenic smoke stimulation[5,29,39]. In addition, many of the strongly toxic chemical substances in cigarette smoke are metabolized via enzyme detoxification in the cytochrome P450 (CYP450) pathway. Smoking results in elevated CYP1A2 and CYP2E1 enzyme activity causing increased metabolism of opioid and volatile agents. Consequently, this leads to lower levels of opioid and volatile agents resulting in a more rapid emergence from anesthesia[40–42]. Nicotine patches do not increase hepatic CYP1A2 enzyme activity or result in the same drug interactions caused by smoking cigarettes[43].

Risk factors that have been disproven or have limited clinical relevance include: obesity, anxiety and preoperative fasting. Conflicting evidence of risk factors that cause PONV are American Society of Anesthesiologists physical status and menstrual cycle[2,30,34,39,44–47].

Pediatric patients

The incidence of POV in children has been reported to be 42.3% when prophylaxis was not used[2]. There is an approximately equal occurrence in boys and girls older than 3 years of age until they reach puberty[2]. At puberty, girls overtake boys with an increased incidence that is approximately three times more frequent in adult females compared to males. The most common operations causing PONV or POV in the pediatric population are strabismus surgery and tonsillectomy. Strabismus surgery is thought to cause nausea and vomiting following traction of the extraocular muscles and tonsillectomy due to the swallowing of blood. Other surgeries causing POV in children include GI procedures and craniotomy[2,48].

Anesthetic medications and agents/techniques

Anesthesia-related factors that contribute to PONV include the use of gases, such as nitrous oxide, volatile anesthetics, such as isoflurane, sevoflurane and desflurane, and the use of postoperative opioids[30,49,50]. Sinclair et al.[4] found a five-times increase in PONV incidence in patients having a general anesthetic compared with other types of anesthesia. Orthostatic hypotension in the PACU with a drop in cerebral perfusion pressure and blood flow to the CNS emetic centers can initiate nausea and vomiting. More than 45 min of anesthesia exposure (correlating to more than 30 min of surgery) contributes to PONV, as more time is available for the absorption of volatile (sevoflurane, desflurane, isoflurane) and gas (nitrous oxide) agents[51]. Use of regional instead of general anesthesia results in decreased PONV due to a decreased requirement for volatile/gas agents and opioids[52]. Eliminating the need for volatile and gas agents along with the use of propofol during total intravenous anesthesia results in a decrease of PONV[50, 53]. It appears that the perioperative use of proton pump inhibitor medications, intraoperative use of a nasogastric tube or application of intraoperative oxygen have a limited or no effect on PONV[44,45,47]. There is also conflicting evidence regarding menstrual cycle, perioperative fasting and muscle relaxant reversal[30,34,54]. Decreasing the dose of muscle relaxant reversal with an anticholinesterase medication, such as neostigmine, has not proved to decrease PONV[2,55,56].

Postoperative factors

Animal studies[57] and the clinical use of postoperative analgesics[29] have shown that opioids are a definite triggering mechanism for nausea and vomiting[58]. It is believed that exogenous opioids stimulate mu-receptors in the vestibular system and CNS chemoreceptor trigger zone[2,59]. In addition, opioids can cause alterations of GI dysfunction with inhibition of intestinal mobility, delayed gastric emptying and an increase of GI transit time, respectively, resulting in stomach bloating and constipation[58]. Opioid use can cause further GI dysfunction with a decrease in GI peristalsis and motility. A decrease in GI motility can cause postoperative ileus, bowel distention and cramping, leading to nausea and/or vomiting. Opioids also cause a decrease of GI secretions and relaxation of the colon's longitudinal muscles with decreased propulsion and drying of stool[58,60,61].

PONV, POV and PDNV risk-scoring methods

Various risk-scoring methods have been described and proposed for PONV and PDNV in adults and POV in children (Tables 3.1–3.3)[5,29,62–64]. Scoring methods for PONV, PDNV and POV have been described by Apfel et al.[29,30], Van den Bosch et al.[63], Koivuranta et al.[65] and Eberhart et al.[6]. Risk in adults and children can be estimated with various scoring methods using independent predictors that have been statistically corrected for confounding variables[5,64,66]. While a number of factors are associated with a high PONV incidence, their specific association is not necessarily one of cause and effect. For example, the high PONV incidence after gynecological surgery is thought to be most likely related to the increased susceptibility of women (gender-specific) rather than the specific type of surgery (gynecologic)[5].

Van den Bosch et al.[63] described a risk score evaluating the variables of gender, history of PONV or motion sickness, smoking status, surgery type, anesthetic technique and age. Koivuranta et al.[65] described a simpler PONV scoring method evaluating gender, PONV history, motion sickness history, smoking status and duration of surgery (≥60 min). Eliminating the surgery duration variable, Apfel et al.[3] proposed a further, simpler score evaluating four factors: gender, smoking status, PONV/motion sickness history and anticipated postoperative administration of opioids. The simplified Apfel score (Table 3.1) appears to be the most widely evaluated and used PONV risk-scoring method for both clinical and research use[29].

PONV/POV risk score in children

Eberhart et al.[6] have described the only currently available PONV/POV risk score for children undergoing surgery. In their scoring method, the risk factors evaluated are: (a) strabismus surgery; (b) surgery longer than 30 min; (c) age ≥3 years; and (d) history of POVN or POV in parents or siblings (Table 3.2)[67]. Numerous other clinicians and researchers have included tonsillectomy as a surgical procedure that may increase the risk of POV in children[17, 68–71]. This has been validated in surgeries other than strabismus repair[6,72,73].

Risk score for PDNV

Apfel et al. have extended their predictive work on PONV to further evaluate the risk for PDNV (Table 3.3)[74]. Five independent risk factors were determined to be important for PDNV: (a) female gender; (b) age <50 years; (c) history of PONV; (d) nausea in the PACU; and (e) administration of opioids in the PACU. While most PDNV has resolved after 3 days, PDNV may also be related to the patient becoming more ambulatory, advancing their diet (clear liquids to solid food) with the use of oral opioids, antibiotics and/or other oral medications or herbals.

Use of risk-scoring methods for PONV and PDNV

With the relatively low side-effect profile of the 5-HT_3 receptor antagonists and the introduction of "generic" ondansetron at a cost far less than the "trade name" Zofran

(GlaxoSmithKline, Philadelphia, PA, USA) formulation, a change in antiemetic use for PONV developed, particularly with regard to ambulatory surgery. There has been increased discussion regarding how and when risk scores and antiemetic medications actually should be applied for everyday clinical use[5,75,76]. Should one or two routine antiemetics be given to all patients in spite of a low patient PONV risk (10–20%) and the low possibility of antiemetic side effects? In some patients this would be no problem. However, in other patients, this approach could cause problems as low- and high-risk patients would be exposed to unnecessary risk for rare but possible side effects.

The use of simplified PONV algorithms should lead to an increased benefit for a larger proportion of patients as the patients at risk could be easily identified[77–79]. Eberhart et al. noted that "risk scores" are useful and should be used in clinical practice to predict PONV or POV[76]. In general, using a risk-dependent approach based on a simple risk score should help avoid giving antiemetics to patients with a low PONV risk. However, implementation of PONV guidelines and algorithms in clinical practice appears to be more variable and difficult to accomplish[77,80].

Pierre et al.[81] noted that rather than focusing on the criticism of a specific PONV risk score in order to change an anesthesia provider's clinical behavior, one should concentrate one's attention on promoting and explaining the usefulness of clinical algorithms and encourage the implementation of these PONV "reminders." Kranke and Eberhart[66,77] mention that the weakest link in the chain from research to patient benefit is the implementation of proven strategies (see Chapter 16). A risk-score dependent approach can effectively reduce PONV[75,82]. However, PONV risk algorithms need to be customized to local patient populations in order to have the best value for the patient and be most efficient for the provider[66]. Use of risk scores can help predict which patients are at moderate-to-high risk (80%) for PONV. Treatment of PONV appears to be more cost-effective in patients with a PONV risk of 40% or greater (two or more of the Apfel risk factors)[50].

Using PONV risk assessment has been shown to reduce an institution's PONV rate. A properly implemented plan is important as poorly implemented protocols fail, and it is difficult to maintain protocol compliance in a busy clinical practice. In one study, providers failed to follow a simple algorithm that suggested that one antiemetic be used for each identified risk factor[83]. Instead, almost all patients received a single antiemetic despite their risk for PONV. PONV symptoms, particularly nausea, are often missed in a busy clinical practice with only 42% of PONV episodes detected in the PACU[83]. It appears that a simpler and more practical PONV risk assessment with a liberal prevention strategy are better than a complex PONV prevention protocol with a detailed risk and treatment plan[5,29].

Studies have suggested that electronic medical record reminders improve clinical compliance[84,85]. Automated reminders in the electronic medical record help increase adherence to guidelines for prophylactic PONV administration. There is also a need to accurately collect PONV data to provide feedback to clinical providers, such as nurses and physicians, in addition to monitoring the impact of antiemetic interventions on the overall incidence of PONV. Ongoing personal performance feedback helps improve guideline performance[80]. An improvement of provider PONV "behavior" can occur through: (a) education, such as conferences, lectures and meetings; (b) PONV risk-assessment documentation in the preoperative note; (c) preoperative and postoperative order sets; and (d) PONV quick-reference guides posted in the operating room and connected to the anesthesia machine. To improve and solidify anesthesia provider human behavior regarding PONV, it may be necessary to require mandatory completion of a preoperative PONV risk assessment and postoperative orders in the electronic medical record. Postoperative order sets should reflect the best evidence-based clinical practice available. This hopefully will eliminate inappropriate antiemetic redosing by allowing for the appropriate use of antiemetics.

Summary

Patients undergoing a variety of outpatient or inpatient procedures may experience nausea and/or vomiting depending on individual patient-, surgery- and anesthesia-related factors. Children and adults present with different PONV/POV incidences and etiologies. While patient- and surgery-related factors are often unchangeable, anesthesia and pharmacologic-related risk factors can be altered or eliminated. Volatile and gas anesthetic agents and opioids are among the most emetogenic factors that a patient may receive in the perioperative period. However, other factors can also cause PONV and PDNV. Risk assessment can help decrease an institution's PONV incidence rate. Improved acceptance and adherence to PONV protocols and algorithms can occur through proper and regular education as well as electronic medical record reminders via preoperative and postoperative order sets.

References

1. Tramer M. A rational approach to the control of postoperative nausea and vomiting: evidence from systemic reviews. Part 1. Efficacy and harm of antiemetic interventions, and methodological issues. *Acta Anaesthesiol Scand* 2001; 45:4–13.
2. Gan TJ, Diemunsch P, Habib AS, et al. Consensus guidelines for the management of postoperative nausea and vomiting. *Anesth Analg* 2014; 118:85–113.
3. Apfel CC Läärä E, Koivuranta M, et al. A simplified risk score for predicting postoperative nausea and vomiting. *Anesthesiology* 1999; 91:693–700.
4. Sinclair DR CF, Mezei G. Can postoperative nausea and vomiting be predicted? *Anesthesiology* 1999; 91:109–18.
5. Apfel CC, Kranke P, Eberhart LH, et al. Comparison of predictive models for postoperative nausea and vomiting. *Br J Anaesth* 2002; 88:234–40.
6. Eberhart LH, Morin AM, Guber D, et al. Applicability of risk scores for postoperative nausea and vomiting in adults to paediatric patients. *Br J Anaesth* 2004; 93:386–92.
7. Ebrahim Soltani A, Mohammadinasab H, Arbabi S, et al. Prophylactic P6 acupressure, ondansetron, metoclopramide and placebo for prevention of vomiting and nausea after strabismus surgery. *Eur J Anaesthesiol* 2009; 26:129.
8. Ghosh JS, Das. Comparision of granisetron and ondansetron for prevention of PONV in patients undergoing elective craniotomy – a randomized, double-blind study. *J Neurosurg Anesthesiol* 2009; 21 (4):388.
9. Kolodzie K, Apfel CC. Nausea and vomiting after office-based anesthesia. *Curr Opin Anaesthesiol* 2009; 22:532–8.
10. Abreu MPd, Vieira JL, Silva IFd, et al. [Efficacy of ondansetron, metoclopramide, droperidol and dexametasone in preventing post-gynecological videolaparoscopy nausea and vomiting in outpatient setting. Comparative study.]. *Revista Brasileira de Anestesiologia* 2006; 56:8–15.
11. Akin A, Esmaoglu A, Gunes I, et al. The effects of the prophylactic tropisetron-propofol combination on postoperative nausea and vomiting in patients undergoing thyroidectomy under desflurane anesthesia. *Mt Sinai J Med* 2006; 73:560–3.

12. Bilgin TE, Birbicer H, Ozer Z, et al. A comparative study of the antiemetic efficacy of dexamethasone, ondansetron, and metoclopramide in patients undergoing gynecological surgery. *Med Sci Monit* 2010; 16:CR336–41.
13. Manahan MA, Basdag B, Kalmar CL, et al. Risk of severe and refractory postoperative nausea and vomiting in patients undergoing diep flap breast reconstruction. *Microsurgery* 2014; 34:112–21.
14. Peixoto AJ, Celich MF, Zardo L, et al. Ondansetron or droperidol for prophylaxis of nausea and vomiting after intrathecal morphine. *Eur J Anaesthesiol* 2006; 23:670–5.
15. Jung JSa, et al. Effect of midazolam upon the prevention of nausea and vomiting after middle ear surgery. *Korean J Anesthesiol* 2007; 52:550–5.
16. Apfel CC, Kranke P, Eberhart LH, et al. Comparison of surgical site and patient's history with a simplified risk score for the prediction of postoperative nausea and vomiting. *Anaesth Intensive Care* 2004; 59:1078–82.
17. Moiniche S, Rømsing J, Dahl JB, et al. Non-steroidal anti-inflammatory drugs and the risk of operative site bleeding after tonsillectomy – a quantitative systematic review. *Anesth Analg* 2003; 96:68–77.
18. Frost F, Dailler F, Duflo F. [Ondansetron: a meta-analysis on its efficacy to prevent postoperative nausea and vomiting after craniotomy in adults and children]. *Annales Francaises d Anesthesie et de Reanimation* 2010; 29:19–24.
19. Latz B, Mordhorst C, Kerz T, et al. Postoperative nausea and vomiting in patients after craniotomy: incidence and risk factors. *J Neurosurg* 2011; 114:491–6.
20. Tarhan O, Canbay O, Celebi N, et al. Subhypnotic doses of midazolam prevent nausea and vomiting during spinal anesthesia for cesarean section. *Minerva Anestesiol* 2007; 73:629–33.
21. Shifman EM, Pogodin AM. Prevention of intraoperative nausea and vomiting during spinal anaesthesia for caesarean section: dexamethasone vs. metoclopramide. *Int J Obstet Anesth* 2010; 19:S23.
22. Le TP, Gan TJ. Update on the management of postoperative nausea and vomiting and postdischarge nausea and vomiting in ambulatory surgery. *Anesthesiol Clin* 2010; 28:225–49.
23. Bhatia N, Katyal S, Grewal A, et al. Antiemetic prophylaxis with granisetron, ondansetron and metoclopramide in ambulatory gynaecological laparoscopic surgery: a comparison. *J Anaesthesiol Clin Pharmacol* 2008; 24:303–6.
24. Mitsunari H, Ashikari E, Tanaka K. The use of droperidol decreases postoperative nausea and vomiting after gynecological laparoscopy. *J Anesth* 2007; 21:507–9.
25. Saerens L, Teunkens A, Van de Velde M, et al. Alizapride versus ondansetron in preventing postoperative nausea and vomiting in laparoscopic gynaecological surgery: intermittent analysis of a randomized, double-blind trial. *Reg Anesth Pain Med* 2010; 35(5):E167.
26. Liu ZQ. Multimodal antiemetic therapy for postoperative nausea and vomiting in patients receiving gynecological laparoscopic surgery. [Chinese]. *Acad J Second Military Med Uni* 2011; 32:447–9.
27. Boehler M MG, Schlager A. Korean hand acupressure reduces postoperative nausea and vomiting after gynecological laparoscopic surgery. *Anesth Analg* 2002; 94:872–5.
28. Gold BS, Kitz DS, Lecky JH, et al. Unanticipated admission to the hospital following ambulatory surgery *JAMA* 1989; 262:3008–10.
29. Apfel CC, Laara E, Koivuranta M, et al. A simplified risk score for predicting postoperative nausea and vomiting: conclusions from cross-validations between two centers. *Anesthesiology* 1999; 91:693–700.
30. Apfel CC, Heidrich FM, Jukar-Rao S, et al. Evidence-based analysis of risk factors for postoperative nausea and vomiting. *Br J Anaesth* 2012; 109:742–53.

31. Roberts GW, Bekker TB, Carlsen HH, et al. Postoperative nausea and vomiting are strongly influenced by postoperative opioid use in a dose-related manner. *Anesthes Analg* 2005; 101:1343–8.

32. Chimbira W, Sweeney BP. The effect of smoking on postoperative nausea and vomiting. *Anaesthesia* 2000; 55:540–4.

33. Kloth DD. New pharmacologic findings for the treatment of PONV and PDNV. *Am J Health Syst Pharm* 2009; 66:S11–8.

34. Gan TJ. Risk factors for postoperative nausea and vomiting. *Anesth Analg* 2006; 102:1884–98.

35. Brattwall M, Warren Stomberg M, Rawal N, et al. Postoperative impact of regular tobacco use, smoking or snuffing, a prospective multi-center study. *Acta Anaesthesiol Scand* 2010; 54:321–7.

36. Hough M, Sweeney B. The influence of smoking on postoperative nausea and vomiting. *Anaesthesia* 1998; 53:932–3.

37. Heffernan AM, Rowbotham DJ. Postoperative nausea and vomiting – time for balanced antiemesis? *Br J Anaesth* 2000; 85:675–7.

38. Sweeney BP. Why does smoking protect against PONV? *Br J Anaesth* 2002; 89:810–3.

39. Apfel CC, Roewer N. [Risk factors for nausea and vomiting after general anesthesia: fictions and facts]. *Der Anaesthesist* 2000; 49:629–42.

40. Miller LG. Cigarettes and drug therapy: pharmacokinetic and pharmacodynamic considerations. *Clin Pharm* 1990; 9:125–35.

41. Schein JR. Cigarette smoking and clinically significant drug interactions. *Ann Pharmacother* 1995; 29:1139–48.

42. Zevin S, Benowitz NL. Drug interactions with tobacco smoking. An update. *Clinical Pharmacokinet* 1999; 36:425–38.

43. Czarnetzki C, Schiffer E, Lysakowski C, et al. Transcutaneous nicotine does not prevent postoperative nausea and vomiting: a randomized controlled trial. *Br J Clin Pharmacol* 2011; 71:383–90.

44. Kranke P, Apfel CC, Papenfuss T, et al. An increased body mass index is no risk factor for postoperative nausea and vomiting. A systematic review and results of original data. *Acta Anaesthesiol Scand* 2001; 45:160–6.

45. Orhan-Sungur M, Sessler D, Kranke P, et al. Supplemental oxygen does not reduce postoperative nausea and vomiting: a systematic review of randomized controlled trials. *Anesthesiology* 2005; 103:A626.

46. Grabowska-Gawel A, Porzych K, Piskunowicz G. [Risk factors and frequency of postoperative nausea and vomiting in patients operated under general anesthesia]. *Przeglad lekarski* 2006; 63:72–6.

47. Raeder J, Dahl V, Bjoernestad E, et al. Does esomeprazole prevent post-operative nausea and vomiting? *Acta Anaesthesiol Scand* 2007; 51:217–25.

48. Wagner DS, Gauger V, Chiravuri D, et al. Ondansetron oral disintegrating tablets for the prevention of postoperative vomiting in children undergoing strabismus surgery. *Ther Clin Risk Manag* 2007; 3:691–4.

49. Apfel CC, Kranke P, Katz MH, et al. Volatile anaesthetics may be the main cause of early but not delayed postoperative vomiting: a randomized controlled trial of factorial design. *Br J Anaesth* 2002; 88:659–68.

50. Apfel CC, Korttila K, Abdalla M, et al. A factorial trial of six interventions for the prevention of postoperative nausea and vomiting. *N Engl J Med* 2004, 350:2441–51.

51. Apfel CC KM, Kranke P, et al. Volatile anaesthetics may be the main cause of early but not delayed postoperative vomiting: a randomized controlled trial of factorial design. *Br J Anaesth* 2002; 88:1–10.

52. Akcaboy EY, Akcaboy ZN, Gogus N. Comparison of paravertebral block versus fast-track general anesthesia via laryngeal mask airway in outpatient inguinal herniorrhaphy. *J Anesth* 2010; 24:687–93.

53. Visser K, Hassink EA, Bonsel GJ, et al. Randomized controlled trial of total intravenous anesthesia with propofol versus inhalation anesthesia with isoflurane-nitrous oxide: postoperative nausea with vomiting and economic analysis. *Anesthesiology* 2001; 95:616–26.

54. Eberhart LH, Morin AM, Georgieff M. [The menstruation cycle in the postoperative phase. Its effect of the incidence of nausea and vomiting]. *Der Anaesthesist* 2000; 49:532–5.

55. Watcha MF, White PF. Postoperative nausea and vomiting. Its etiology, treatment, and prevention. *Anesthesiology* 1992; 77:162–84.

56. Cheng CR SD, Apfel CC. Does neostigmine administration produce a cliically important increase in postoperative nausea and vomiting? *Anesthes Analg* 2005; 101:1349–55.

57. Rudd JA, Cheng CH, Naylor RJ, et al. Modulation of emesis by fentanyl and opioid receptor antagonists in *Suncus murinus* (house musk shrew). *Eur J Pharmacol* 1999; 374:77–84.

58. Smith HS, Laufer A. Opioid induced nausea and vomiting. *Eur J Pharmacol* 2014; 722:67–78.

59. Golembiewski J, Tokumaru S. Pharmacological prophylaxis and management of adult postoperative/postdischarge nausea and vomiting. *J Perianesth Nurs* 2006; 21:385–97.

60. Sanger GJ, Andrews PL. Treatment of nausea and vomiting: gaps in our knowledge. *Auton Neurosci* 2006; 129:3–16.

61. Andrews PL, Horn CC. Signals for nausea and emesis: implications for models of upper gastrointestinal diseases. *Auton Neurosci* 2006; 125:100–15.

62. Biedler A, Wermelt J, Kunitz O, et al. A risk adapted approach reduces the overall institutional incidence of postoperative nausea and vomiting. *Can J Anaesth* 2004; 51:13–9.

63. van den Bosch JE, Kalkman CJ, Vergouwe Y, et al. Assessing the applicability of scoring systems for predicting postoperative nausea and vomiting. *Anaesthesia* 2005; 60:323–31.

64. Eberhart LH, Hogel J, Seeling W, et al. Evaluation of three risk scores to predict postoperative nausea and vomiting. *Acta Anaesthesiol Scand* 2000; 44:480–8.

65. Koivuranta M, Läärä E, Snare L, et al. A survey of postoperative nausea and vomiting. *Anaesthesia* 1997; 52:443–9.

66. Kranke P, Schuster F, Eberhart LH. Recent advances, trends and economic considerations in the risk assessment, prevention and treatment of postoperative nausea and vomiting. *Exp Opin Pharmacother* 2007; 8:3217–35.

67. Eberhart LH, Geldner G, Kranke P, et al. The development and validation of a risk score to predict the probability of postoperative vomiting in pediatric patients. *Anesth Analg* 2004; 99:1630–7.

68. Montazeri K, Okhovat A, Honarmand A, et al. Pre-incisional infiltration of tonsils with dexamethasone dose not reduce posttonsillectomy vomiting and pain in children. *Saudi J Anaesth* 2009; 3:53–6.

69. Splinter W, Roberts DJ. Prophylaxis for vomiting by children after tonsillectomy: dexamethasone versus perphenazine. *Anesth Analg* 1997; 85:534–7.

70. Splinter WM, Rhine EJ. Prophylaxis for vomiting by children after tonsillectomy: ondansetron compared with perphenazine. *Br J Anaesth* 1998; 80:155–8.

71. Sukhani R, Pappas A, Lurie J, et al. Ondansetron and dolasetron provide equivalent postoperative vomiting control after ambulatory tonsillectomy in dexamethasone-pretreated children. *Anesth Analg* 2002; 95:1230–5.

72. Kranke P, Eberhart LH, Toker H, et al. A prospective evaluation of the POVOC score for the prediction of postoperative vomiting in children. *Anesth Analg* 2007; 105:1592–7.

73. Eberhart LH, Geldner G, Kranke P, et al. The development and validation of a risk score to predict the probability of postoperative vomiting in pediatric patients. *Anesth Analg* 2004; 99:1630–7.

74. Apfel CC, Philip BK, Cakmakkaya OS, et al. Who is at risk for postdischarge nausea and vomiting after ambulatory surgery? *Anesthesiology* 2012; 117:475–86.

75. Kranke P, Eberhart LH. [Postoperative nausea and vomiting: rational algorithms for prevention and treatment based on current evidence]. *Anasthesiologie, Intensivmedizin, Notfallmedizin, Schmerztherapie: AINS*. 2009; 44:286–94; quiz 95.

76. Eberhart LHJ, Morin AM. Risk scores for predicting postoperative nausea and vomiting are clinically useful tools and should be used in every patient: Con – Life is really simple, but we insist on making it complicated. *Eur J Anaesthesiol* 2011; 28:155–9.

77. Kranke P, Eberhart LH. Possibilities and limitations in the pharmacological management of postoperative nausea and vomiting. *Eur J Anaesthesiol* 2011; 28:758–65.

78. Kooij FO, Klok T, Hollmann MW, et al. Automated reminders increase adherence to guidelines for administration of prophylaxis for postoperative nausea and vomiting. *Eur J Anaesthesiol* 2010; 27:187–91.

79. Kooij FO, Klok T, Hollmann MW, et al. Decision support increases guideline adherence for prescribing postoperative nausea and vomiting prophylaxis. *Anesth Analg* 2008; 106:893–8.

80. Frenzel JC, Kee SS, Ensor JE, et al. Ongoing provision of individual clinician performance data improves practice behavior. *Anesth Analg* 2010; 111:515–9.

81. Pierre S, Corno G, Benais H, et al. A risk score-dependent antiemetic approach effectively reduces postoperative nausea and vomiting – a continuous quality improvement initiative. *Can J Anaesth* 2004; 51:320–5.

82. Pierre S, Corno G, Benais H, et al. A risk score-dependent antiemetic approach effectively reduces postoperative nausea and vomiting – a continuous quality improvement initiative. *Can J Anaesth* 2004; 51:320–5.

83. White PF, O'Hara JF, Roberson CR, et al. The impact of current antiemetic practices on patient outcomes: a prospective study on high-risk patients. *Anesth Analg* 2008; 107:452–8.

84. Kooij FO, Klok T, Hollmann MW, et al. Decision support increases guideline adherence for prescribing postoperative nausea and vomiting prophylaxis. *Anesth Analg* 2008; 106:893–8.

85. Kooij FO, Klok T, Hollmann MW, et al. Automated reminders increase adherence to guidelines for administration of prophylaxis for postoperative nausea and vomiting. *Eur J Anaesthesiol* 2010; 27:187–91.

Chapter 4

Patients' experience and nursing perspective

Vallire D. Hooper

Introduction

Many in the healthcare environment perceive postoperative and postdischarge nausea and vomiting (PONV/PDNV) as the big "little problem"[1,2]. A minor inconvenience that, though stressful at the time of encounter, is relatively harmless in the long term ... and certainly not life-threatening. As such, the phenomenon gains little attention outside of the anesthesia and surgical specialties. Whilst funding for medication development and drug trials may be readily obtainable, funding to support the exploration of the patient experience of PONV/PDNV draws little financial support. The patient experience of PONV/PDNV and the nursing perspective of the prevention and/or management of these phenomena, however, are of significant importance to the patient and their family's overall psychologic and physical experience of an anesthesia/surgical encounter.

Incidence and outcomes associated with PONV/PDNV

An estimated 234 million patients annually undergo major surgical procedures on a worldwide basis, approximately 75 million of which include general anesthesia[3]. Depending on country, 10–80% of these procedures will be conducted in an ambulatory surgical setting, with approximately 60% of all US surgeries being conducted on an ambulatory basis[4]. The general incidence of postoperative vomiting (POV) across all populations is approximately 30%; with the incidence of nausea around 50%. High-risk patients, however, may experience an incidence as high as 80%[5,6]. Incidence of PDNV, defined as nausea and vomiting occurring after discharge from the ambulatory surgery facility[7], is highest on the day of surgery, with a reported incidence as high as 57%. PDNV may persist as long as 7 days postoperatively, with incidence ranging from 56.9% on the day of surgery to 12% on postoperative day 2 and 6% on postoperative day 7. PDNV can be particularly incapacitating as the patient does not have ready access to medical resources and is often resigned to home treatment remedies, many of which are ineffective and not evidence-based[4,8,9].

Although risk of PONV and PDNV is high, the incidence of adverse outcomes, such as aspiration, airway compromise, wound dehiscence, esophageal rupture, subcutaneous emphysema and pneumothorax are relatively low[1,3,7,10]. PONV and PDNV, however, are associated with numerous other costly outcomes. PONV is associated with increased length of postanesthesia care unit (PACU) stay, with every emesis episode extending PACU stay by as much as 20 min. Protracted PONV is one of the most common reasons for unplanned

Postoperative Nausea and Vomiting: A Practical Guide, eds. Tong Joo Gan and Ashraf S. Habib. Published by Cambridge University Press.

hospital admission after ambulatory surgery. PDNV increases the risk of postoperative emergency department visits and subsequent hospitalization. Return to normal activities, to include return to work, can also be delayed. The annual costs for PONV and PDNV have been estimated to be several million in US dollars, a number that should justify this complication as an important public health concern[3,4,6,8].

Patient perspective

The patient-family centered care (PFCC) movement has transformed healthcare by bringing the needs, concerns and priorities of patients and families to the forefront of patient care. The PFCC movement has revealed that the priorities of healthcare providers often differ drastically from those of the patient. A "good" outcome for the surgical/anesthesia team may be an "uncomplicated" procedure with a safe transition across the surgical services continuum, coupled with an uneventful recovery period. Patient/family expectations, however, are often more specific and focused.

The anesthesia/surgical team often consider PONV and PDNV as "minor" complications that are frequently unavoidable[3]. Patients, on the other hand, fear PONV more than shivering and postoperative pain[4,9,11,12]. PDNV has been shown to adversely impact quality of life and patient functioning, as well as decreasing patient satisfaction with the overall anesthesia and surgery experience[4].

Research supports that patients who have experienced nausea are willing to pay up to $73 US dollars out-of-pocket for an antiemetic prior to surgery; those who have experienced emesis are willing to pay $100 out-of-pocket[4,9,13,14]. A study examining the parental response to PONV in children found that parents were willing to pay up to $80 out-of-pocket to prevent POV for their children[4,15].

The experience of PDNV can be particularly problematic and impactful on the anesthesia/surgical experience, as the patient no longer has immediate access to fast-acting antiemetic medications and may be unable to tolerate oral medications. These patients are more likely to manage their symptoms with self-care strategies that are often ineffective and not evidence-based[4,8,9]. Odom-Forren[4] examined patient management strategies and outcomes associated with PDNV over a 7-day period. Whilst the total incidence of PDNV was 56.9% (141 patients), only 14.9% (21 patients) recorded antiemetic use at home. A wide variety of nonpharmacologic methods, such as gradual diet progression (liquid to solid), taking medication with food, drinking carbonated beverages, laying down/resting, cool washcloths/air, etc., was reported. Only one patient reported use of evidence-based, nonpharmacologic methods such as acupressure. Some patients reported stopping their pain medications. Whilst opioid medications are associated with PONV/PDNV, uncontrolled pain can also contribute to the development of PONV/PDNV.

As the impact of the patient experience and patient satisfaction on hospital/ambulatory setting reimbursement continues to grow and evolve, it will be critical to capture the multifaceted patient experience of PONV/PDNV. Traditional outcome measures have focused on incidence or cost measures, such as length of PACU stay, unplanned hospital admissions and/or visits to the emergency department. PONV/PDNV incidence is typically measured by number of incidents of nausea or retching, the level of nausea is rated using a subjective visual analog scale, numerical rating scale or verbal rating scale[5]. Whilst these instruments capture important trends regarding PONV/PDNV, they fail to capture the patient experience and perspective of this symptomology.

Table 4.1 Ambulatory Surgery Index of Nausea, Vomiting and Retching (AS-INVR)[17]

Since discharge	How many times did you vomit?
	How much distress have you felt from retching or dry heaves?
	How much distress did you have from vomiting?
	How long have you felt nauseated or sick to your stomach?
	How much distress have you felt from nausea or being sick to your stomach?
	How much did you vomit?
	How many times have you felt nausea or sick to your stomach?
	How many times have you had periods of retching or dry heaves?

Hocking et al.[16] developed and validated an instrument designed to capture the *patient's* perspective of a high-quality anesthesia experience. Patients and members of the general public were asked to identify attributes that they considered to be associated with a "high quality" anesthesia experience. Eleven items were consolidated to five factors, accounting for 72% of the variance in perceived anesthesia experience quality. These factors included:

- attention/gentleness
- pain management
- information/confidence
- PONV
- concerns addressed.

Questions with the highest quality index and accounting for the greatest single item variance in patient perception of anesthesia quality were pain management (11% of the variance) and PONV (9% of the variance).

Other instruments and techniques can be useful in evaluating the patient experience of PONV/PDNV[5]. Diaries and surveys can be useful in capturing the full patient experience of PONV/PDNV across the extended recovery continuum. The patient perception of nausea duration, nausea and vomiting frequency, distress from nausea, and amount of vomiting can be captured using the Ambulatory Surgery Index of Nausea, Vomiting and Retching (AS-INVR) questionnaire, modified from the Rhodes Index for use in ambulatory surgery[17]. The patient is asked to self-report on their experience with eight items since discharge from the surgical center; the items are scored using a Likert scale (Table 4.1). The Functional Living Index-Emesis (FLIE) questionnaire[18], originally developed to capture the impact of chemotherapy-induced nausea and vomiting on daily living, can also be useful in capturing the impact of PDNV on patient functioning and return to normal activities postambulatory surgery. Also scored on a Likert scale (Table 4.2), the instrument asks the patient to retrospectively rank the impact of nausea and vomiting on their daily living experience over a timeframe designated by the researcher, usually 3, 5 or 7 days.

Nursing perspective

The prevention and management of PONV and PDNV require a multidisciplinary team approach incorporating both pharmacologic and nonpharmacologic interventions. The healthcare team lead who has the most contact with the patient and family, and as such

Table 4.2 Functional Living Index-Emesis (FLIE) items[18]

How much nausea have you had?
Has nausea affected your ability to maintain usual recreation or leisure activities?
Has nausea affected your ability to make a meal or do minor household repairs?
How much has nausea affected your ability to enjoy a meal?
How much has nausea affected your ability to enjoy liquid refreshment?
How much has nausea affected your willingness to see and spend time with family and friends?
Has nausea affected your daily functioning?
Rate the degree to which your nausea has imposed a hardship on you (personally)
Rate the degree to which your nausea has imposed a hardship on those closest to you
How much vomiting have you had?
Has the vomiting affected your ability to maintain usual recreation or leisure activities?
Has vomiting affected your ability to complete your usual household tasks?
How much has vomiting affected your ability to enjoy a meal?
How much has vomiting affected your ability to enjoy liquid refreshment?
How much has vomiting affected your willingness to see and spend time with friends?
Has vomiting affected your daily functioning?
Rate the degree to which your vomiting has imposed a hardship on you (personally)
Rate the degree to which your vomiting has imposed a hardship on those closest to you

serves as the patient advocate and the care coordinator is the nurse. One of the few studies[1] examining the nurse's perspective of the care of the patient with PONV reported that nurses derive their care from four sets of tools at their disposal: listen and understand, information, the clinical eye and availability.

"Listen and understand" implies that nurses are observant and *listen* to the patient by using all of their senses, by being fully present in their care. Nurses support their patients to talk about their feelings, thoughts and fears; actively listening to the conversation, but also observing the patient with their full senses, capturing body language, facial expression, variation in vocal tone, and so on. Activation of and appropriate application of the "listen and understand" tool enables the nurse to better support patients and relieve their fear of PONV[1].

The second instrument in the nursing toolbox is the "information" tool. An informed patient has a better opportunity to reduce, or possibly eliminate their insecurity and fear surrounding PONV. The nurse serves as the information conduit throughout the surgical/anesthesia continuum, providing patient education regarding preparation, expected experiences and management strategies. This information is critical to strengthening the patient's capacity to physically and psychologically manage all perioperative events they may encounter[1].

The "clinical eye" incorporates the nurse's theoretical and practical skills essential to the individualized assessment, diagnosis and management of each patient encountered. This tool empowers the nurse to synthesize the full patient perspective and tailor a fully engaged, multimodal interventional approach to the prevention and management of PONV/PDNV across the surgical and anesthesia continuum[1].

The final instrument in the nursing toolbox is "availability," which equates to nursing presence, both physical and emotional. Physical presence assures the patient that they are not alone in their experience and that there is a knowledgeable caregiver available to support them. Emotional presence assures the patient of acceptance and understanding, and sometimes provides them with a sense of confidence to face their fears and better manage whatever they may encounter during their surgical and anesthesia experience[1].

The nursing perspective presents with unique challenges and responsibilities across the surgical and anesthesia continuum.

Preadmission testing and preoperative holding

The primary responsibilities of the preadmission testing and preoperative holding nurse are to prepare the patient for surgery through assessment, planning, intervention and education[19]. Assessing the risk of PONV and PDNV is a critical component of preoperative assessment, planning and care. The nurse has multiple responsibilities in the preoperative management of patients at risk for PONV/PDNV. First and foremost, they must serve as the coordinator of care, assuring that patient risk is clearly communicated to all members of the anesthesia and surgical teams. Pre- and intraoperative prophylaxis is essential to the prevention of PONV/PDNV. This prophylaxis will not occur without appropriate risk communication by the preoperative nurse.

Educational intervention is also critical to the prevention and/or management of PONV/PDNV. Patients with a history of protracted PONV/PDNV are often fearful and anxious going into a surgical procedure. Assurance that risk will be communicated and that all resources will be focused on prevention can go a long way in reducing patient anxiety and fear. The patient can also be empowered to act on their own behalf by encouraging them to openly communicate with their anesthesia provider regarding risk. Postoperative education should begin with first contact. Instructing the patient and family in appropriate opioid and antiemetic use may help to assure better symptom management on discharge. A review of common nonpharmacologic management approaches will also provide the patient/family with additional resources to draw upon in PDNV prevention and management. Acupuncture and acupressure are well established as effective interventions in the prevention and management of PONV/PDNV[6,20,21] and should be encouraged as independent patient management strategies across the care continuum.

Intraoperative care

Intraoperative prophylaxis for PONV/PDNV is primarily pharmacologically driven under the direction of the anesthesia team. Nursing communication during hand-off to the intraoperative and postoperative team, however, is critical to assuring that patient risk is communicated. Patient advocacy, to include encouragement of pharmacologic and nonpharmacologic prophylaxis, will help to assure improved outcomes postoperatively.

Postanesthesia care

The primary goal in the immediate postanesthesia period (Phase I) is the safe emergence of the patient from anesthesia and transfer to the next level of inpatient care if appropriate. The later stage of postanesthesia care (Phase II) is focused on the safe transition of the patient to their home environment[19]. The Phase I patient is often unable to advocate for their needs, thus it is critical that the perianesthesia nurse is vigilant to all aspects of patient management, to include the assessment for and management of PONV. Assuring adequate hydration and prudent administration of a multimodal pain management plan, with antiemetics as indicated, are critical to PONV prevention and management. Evidence-based nonpharmacologic interventions, such as acupuncture (including acupressure), should be considered as adjunctive interventions in the management of PONV[6,20,21]. Although a Cochrane Review concluded that the evidence supporting the effectiveness of aromatherapy in the management of PONV/PDNV is inconclusive[22], controlled breathing with or without aromatherapy may be considered a low-risk nursing intervention useful in the management of PONV/PDNV[6,23,24]. Discharge teaching should include an emphasis on home management of PDNV, with an emphasis on the importance of contacting the ambulatory center or surgeon for protracted PDNV. Follow-up phone calls should also capture incidence of PDNV as well as the impact of the symptom on patient recovery and transition to routine daily activities. If early postoperative follow-up calls indicate significant PDNV, continued follow-up at 5–10 days may be indicated to assure that PDNV has been resolved[4,5,9].

Summary

Although PONV/PDNV are considered by many to be the big "little problem"[1,2] it remains a major concern and fear of surgical patients. In addition to being a feared and dreaded experience for the patient, uncontrolled PONV/PDNV is a source of frustration for the anesthesia/surgical team. A collaborative, multidisciplinary multimodal approach to the prevention and/or management of these noxious phenomena is critical to improved healthcare outcomes and patient/family satisfaction.

References

1. Sussanne B, Arwestrom C, Baker A, et al. Nurses' experiences in the relief of postoperative nausea and vomiting. *J Clin Nurs* 2010; 19(13–14):1865–72.
2. Kapur P. The big "little problem". *Anesth Analg* 1991; 73:243–5.
3. Samuels JD. Perioperative nausea and vomiting: much ado about nothing? *Aesthetic Plast Surg* 2013; 37(3):634–5.
4. Odom-Forren J, Hooper V, Moser DK, et al. Postdischarge nausea and vomiting: management strategies and outcomes over 7 days. *J Perianesth Nurs* 2014; 29(4):275–84.
5. Odom-Forren J. Measurement of postdischarge nausea and vomiting for ambulatory surgery patients: a critical review and analysis. *J Perianesth Nurs* 2011; 26(6):372–83.
6. Gan TJ, Diemunsch P, Habib AS, et al. Consensus guidelines for the management of postoperative nausea and vomiting. [Erratum appears in *Anesth Analg* 2014; 118(3):689]. *Anesth Analg* 2014; 118(1):85–113.
7. ASPAN. ASPAN'S Evidence-Based Clinical Practice Guideline for the Prevention and/or Management of PONV/PDNV. *J Perianesth Nurs* 2006; 21(4):230–50.
8. Apfel CC, Philip BK, Cakmakkaya OS, et al. Who is at risk for postdischarge nausea and vomiting after ambulatory surgery? *Anesthesiology* 2012; 117(3):475–86.
9. Odom-Forren J, Jalota L, Moser DK, et al. Incidence and predictors of postdischarge nausea and vomiting in a 7-day population. *J Clin Anesth* 2013; 25(7):551–9.

10. Gundzik K. Nausea and vomiting in the ambulatory surgical setting. *Orthop Nurs* 2008; 27(3):182–8.

11. Lee A, Gin T, Lau AS, et al. A comparison of patients' and health care professionals' preference for symptoms during immediate postoperative recovery and the mnagment of postoperative nausea and vomiting. *Anesth Analg* 2005; 100:87–93.

12. Macario A, Glenn D, Dexter F. What can the postanesthesia care unit manager do to decrease costs in the postanesthesia care unit? *J Perianesth Nurs* 1999; 14:284–93.

13. Gan TJ, Sloan F, Dear Gde I, et al. How much are patients willing to pay to avoid postoperative nausea and vomiting? *Anesth Analg* 2001; 92:393–400.

14. Kerger H, Turan A, Kredel M, et al. Patients' willingness to pay for anti-emetic treatment. *Acta Anaesthesiol Scand* 2007; 51(1):38–43.

15. Diez L. Assessing the willingness of parents to pay for reducing postoperative emesis in children. *Pharmacoeconomics* 1998; 13(5):589–95.

16. Hocking G, Weightman WM, Smith C, et al. Measuring the quality of anaesthesia from a patient's perspective: development, validation, and implementation of a short questionnaire. *Br J Anaesth* 2013; 111(6):979–89.

17. Fetzer SJ, Hand MC, Bouchard PA, et al. Evaluation of the Rhodes Index of Nausea and Vomiting for ambulatory surgery patients. *J Adv Nurs* 2004; 47(1):74–80.

18. Lindley C, Hirsch J, O'Neill C, et al. Quality of life consequences of chemotherapy-induced emesis. *Qual Life Res* 1992; 1(5):331–40.

19. ASPAN. *2015–2017 Perianesthesia Nursing Standards, Practice Recommendations, and Interpretive Statements.* Cherry Hill, NJ: ASPAN; 2014.

20. Cheong KB, Zhang JP, Huang Y, et al. The effectiveness of acupuncture in prevention and treatment of postoperative nausea and vomiting – a systematic review and meta-analysis. *PLoS ONE* 2013; 8(12):e82474.

21. White PF, Zhao M, Tang J, et al. Use of a disposable acupressure device as part of a multimodal antiemetic strategy for reducing postoperative nausea and vomiting. *Anesth Analg* 2012; 115(1):31–7.

22. Hines S, Steels E, Chang A, et al. Aromatherapy for treatment of postoperative nausea and vomiting. *Cochrane Database Syst Rev* 2012; 4:CD007598.

23. Hodge NS, McCarthy MS, Pierce RM. A prospective randomized study of the effectiveness of aromatherapy for relief of postoperative nausea and vomiting. *J Perianesth Nurs* 2014; 29(1):5–11.

24. Sites DS, Johnson NT, Miller JA, et al. Controlled breathing with or without peppermint aromatherapy for postoperative nausea and/or vomiting symptom relief: a randomized controlled trial. *J Perianesth Nurs* 2014; 29(1):12–9.

Chapter 5

Genomics and personalized medicine in postoperative nausea and vomiting management

Keith A. Candiotti, Enisa M.F. Carvalho and Ana C. Mavarez

Introduction

Pharmacogenomics has made significant contributions to several areas of medicine, including psychiatry, where it has been shown to be useful for drug selection[1], and oncology, where it has been shown to be useful in predicting drug efficacy and preventing potentially fatal adverse drug reactions[2]. In the world of anesthesiology, pharmacogenomics has had a limited impact to date. Postoperative nausea and vomiting (PONV) continues to be a problem for many patients after undergoing general anesthesia. The variable course of PONV may arise from a multitude of factors and it has been suggested that genetic factors may play a significant role in the background risk of developing PONV, including resistance to antiemetic prophylaxis and/or therapy[3].

Understanding the factors that contribute to the occurrence of PONV and the variability of responses to antiemetic drugs is critical for the successful management of patients. This chapter will review the current pharmacogenomics literature and how it relates to the development and management of PONV.

PONV risk assessment

The development of PONV is multifactorial in origin and involves numerous receptors and neurotransmitters. PONV risk factors have been described in the literature since the late 1800s[4]. The modern era of PONV risk factor research began in the early 1990s, with the publication of the first studies that attempted to identify PONV risk factors[5,6]. Since that time, various risk factors have been identified: female sex, previous history of PONV and motion sickness (including a family history), nonsmoking, duration of anesthesia, postoperative opioid use, use of general anesthesia with or without nitrous oxide, type of surgery and a younger age[7–10].

Some patients experience PONV whereas others do not, despite undergoing the same surgical procedure and receiving the same doses of opioids[11]. This may be at least partially associated with individual variations in sensitivity to opioids[12]. Genetic variations, of which single-nucleotide polymorphisms (SNPs) play a key role, may be involved in the therapeutic and adverse effects of drugs in surgical patients[13,14].

Most studies continue to pursue an essentially epidemiologic approach, focusing on readily discernible clinical risk factors, whereas genetic and other molecular biological patient characteristics have not been extensively examined in relation to PONV[15,16].

Postoperative Nausea and Vomiting: A Practical Guide, eds. Tong Joo Gan and Ashraf S. Habib. Published by Cambridge University Press.

Genetic factors

Genetic variations can influence a drug's pharmacokinetics by altering the functioning of enzymes responsible for drug metabolism, and hence disposition, as well as the transport of proteins, which influence absorption, distribution and bioavailability. Genetic variation also plays a role in pharmacodynamics: influencing enzymes and receptors that play a major role in drug effect[17]. Evidence now specifically suggests that pharmacogenomics influences perioperative medications from absorption through elimination.

The history of clinical research as it relates to inherited factors involved in the pathogenesis of PONV or motion sickness is relatively new, with the oldest paper in this area being published less than 10 years ago. The most frequently addressed question relates to inherited resistance to antiemetic drugs and to a lesser degree the genetics and risks of developing or not developing PONV[3]. The targets of researchers are the principal receptors, ligands and their associate polymorphisms linked to nausea and/or vomiting sensitivity or pharmacology (Table 5.1).

5-Hydroxytryptamine receptor antagonists

PONV may be successfully prevented or treated by administering 5-hydroxytryptamine type 3 (5-HT_3)-receptor antagonists[18]. This finding, together with the fact that the activation of 5-HT_3 receptors on vagal gastrointestinal afferents or in the central chemoreceptor trigger zone may provoke acute emesis, indicates an involvement of the serotonin system in the pathogenesis of PONV[19,20]. There are several 5-HT_3 receptor genes (5-HT_3 A–E) with high sequence homology[21,22]. In particular, the genes for the subunits 5-HT_3A (*HTR3A*) and 5-HT_3B (*HTR3B*) are located close together on chromosome 11q23.1. The 5-HT_3B subunit is considered to be effective only in conjugation with the 5-HT_3A subunit and may specifically modify its function. Both subunits are coexpressed in diverse cerebral and intestinal regions and appear to form the 5-HT_3 receptor as a heteromeric complex[23–27].

The contribution of *HTR3A* and *HTR3B* polymorphisms, as they relate to nausea and vomiting, has been examined in a cohort of patients undergoing cancer chemotherapy, where it was demonstrated that patients who were homozygous for the 100_02 AAG deletion in the noncoding promoter region of the *HTR3B* gene experienced vomiting more frequently whilst receiving chemotherapy[28,29]. A pilot study investigated both *HTR3A* and *HTR3B* genes for genetic variants in a cohort of postoperative vomiting (POV) patients after general anesthesia. This study identified 16 different variants in the *HTR3A* gene and 19 in the *HTR3B* gene, reflecting a remarkable genetic heterogeneity. The *HTR3A* variant c1377A>G was associated with a significantly higher risk for POV and the *HTR3B* variants c5p+201_+202delCA and c6-137C>T were associated with a lower risk for POV. However, all significant genetic variants were located in noncoding regions of their respective genes. The study concluded that genetic variations in the *HTR3A* and *HTR3B* genes may be associated with the individual risk of developing POV[30].

Additionally, a study addressing the effects of *HTR3A* and *HTR3B* gene polymorphisms on nausea induced by the drug paroxetine in 78 Japanese psychiatric patients[31] demonstrated that the Tyr129Ser polymorphism of the *HTR3B* gene significantly increased the risk of nausea. They also reported that *HTR3A* gene polymorphisms and the *CYP2D6* gene polymorphisms had no significant effect on the incidence of nausea in this cohort.

In 2013, a study investigated whether common genomic variations of the A and B subunits of *HTR3* affect the incidence of POV in a Chinese Han population undergoing gynecological

Table 5.1 Known human genes and their polymorphisms associated with occurrence of PONV, CINV and motion sickness[3][a]

Target protein	Gene symbol	Type of observed polymorphism
Serotonin receptor type 3	$5HT_3$	SNP in *HTR3A*: 1377A>G SNP in *HTR3B*: rs1176744, rs1672717, rs3782025, rs3758987, Tyr129Ser, Ala223Thr, Y129S; -100_-102delAAG deletion, c5+201_+202delCA, c6-137C>T SNP in *HTR3C*: K163 N, A405G SNP in *HTR3D*: rs6443930
Cytochrome P450 2D6 isoform	CYP2D6	SNP: rs16947 (CYP2D6*2), rs35742686 (CYP2D6*3A), rs1135824 or rs35742686 (CYP2D6*3B), rs3892097 (CYP2D6*4), rs5030655 (CYP2D6*6), rs5030867 (CYP2D6*7), rs5030865 (CYP2D6*8), rs5030656 (CYP2D6*9), rs1065852 (CYP2D6*10), rs5030863 (CYP2D6*11) further genotypes listed at http://snpedia.com/index.php/CYP2D6
Muscarinic receptor type 3	CHRM3	SNP: rs685550, rs10802789, rs2165870
Dopamine receptor type 2	DRD2	Taq IA
Morphine opioid receptor	OPRM1	SNP: rs1799971, haplotypes
Transporter adenosine triphosphate-binding cassette subfamily B member 1	ABCB1	SNP: rs1045642, rs2032582 and rs1128503, 3435C>T, 2677G>T/A
Catecol-O-methyltransferase	COMT	SNP: rs4680, rs4633, rs165722
Neurokinin 1 receptor	TACR1	SNP: rs3755468, haplotypes

[a] Taken from reference 3, with permission. CINV, chemotherapy-induced nausea and vomiting; SNP, single-nucleotide polymorphism.

surgery[32]. Five SNPs in *HTR3A* and *HTR3B* were identified and one of these (rs3758987 in *HTR3B*) was statistically associated with an increased risk of vomiting. It was therefore concluded that the *HTR3B* rs3758987 SNP might serve as a predictor of POV.

Cytochromes

The cytochrome P450 (CYP450) family contains the most important phase I drug-metabolizing enzymes. All currently used 5-HT_3 antagonists are metabolized via cytochrome P450 enzymes. CYP2D6 is responsible for the majority of the metabolism of dolasetron and tropisetron[33] and partially responsible for the metabolism of ondansetron, which is also broken down by the enzymes CYP3A4, CYP2E1 and CYP1A2[34]. In contrast, granisetron is primarily metabolized by CYP3A4, with no contribution from CYP2D6[35]. Of the various CYP enzymatic pathways, CYP2D6 has gained much attention in relation to 5-HT_3 antagonists. The variable clinical response seen with the 5-HT_3-receptor antagonists may be explained by polymorphisms of the gene encoding for the CYP2D6 enzyme.

There are over 100 CYP2D6 allelic variants identified; however, there are basically four metabolizer states: poor metabolizers (PM) who have two inactive genes and have no enzymatic activity; intermediate metabolizers (IM) who have less than normal activity, usually one inactive and one low activity gene; extensive metabolizers (EM) who have one to two wild-type genes; and ultrarapid metabolizers (UM) who possess more than two wild-type genes and increased enzymatic activity[36]. UMs have a duplication or amplification of the entire *CYP2D6* gene, resulting in increased enzyme production.

The 5-HT-receptor antagonists have revolutionized PONV. These agents have a high efficacy with a low incidence of adverse effects. Unfortunately, not every patient has a beneficial response when treated. This failure to respond seems in part to be due to interindividual genetic variations in the *CYP2D6* gene or other as-yet-uncharacterized variations[37].

One study demonstrated that patients with three active copies of the *CYP2D6* gene (UMs) who received tropisetron for the treatment of chemotherapy-induced nausea and vomiting (CINV) had a significantly higher mean number of vomiting episodes than EMs or PMs. In addition, the effects for the *CYP2D6* UMs were similar for those treated with tropisetron or ondansetron[38].

Failure to respond to ondansetron prophylaxis was also investigated in a recent study on PONV[37]. Patients who possessed three functional copies of the *CYP2D6* allele were more likely to experience vomiting, but not necessarily nausea, in the postoperative period despite the prophylactic administration of ondansetron. The fact that vomiting, but not nausea, increased significantly is not unexpected because ondansetron has previously been shown to be a better antiemetic than antinausea agent[39]. Similar findings were reported in two additional studies in which the efficacy of granisetron and dolasetron in preventing PONV were investigated[40,41]. Subjects receiving dolasetron, and who were carriers of the duplication of the *CYP2D6* allele, had more frequent vomiting episodes than patients in the granisetron group (granisetron is not metabolized by CYP2D6). Another study in 92 surgical patients indicated that those who possessed three or greater active *CYP2D6* alleles (and were thus classified as UMs) had reduced ondansetron plasma concentrations compared to those subjects that had zero to two active alleles[42]. The involvement of the CYP2D6 system in PONV was further confirmed by a study that presented data from trauma patients where it was noted that patients classified as PM had less PONV compared to patients with the EM genotype [43,44].

CYP450 enzyme synthesis may be stimulated or suppressed by environmental influences. Some experts have speculated that the protective effect of smoking against PONV might be related to the induction of CYP450 enzymes by polycyclic aromatic hydrocarbons[45]. These hydrocarbons are components of the "tar" portion of cigarette smoke. Other clinical characteristics that affect CYP450 enzyme expression, for example, the consumption of alcohol or commonly prescribed medications such as cimetidine, erythromycin or terfenadine, or vegetables like cabbage, brussels sprouts, cauliflower or red peppers, could be investigated as potential PONV risk factors.

Diagnostic tests to identify CYP2D6 isoenzyme activity are currently available for clinical use. The AmpliChip CYP450 (Specialty Laboratories, Valencia, CA, USA) is one such test that has been approved by the US Food and Drug Administration. Studies performed so far suggest that antiemetic treatment for POV could be made more efficacious by selecting a 5-HT_3 antagonist and/or another class of antiemetic drugs that is consistent with the patient's CYP2D6 genotype. Specifically, patients that are UMs might benefit from the use of granisetron or an antiemetic that is not metabolized by CYP2D6. This is currently only a theoretical concept since the cost of running such a test far exceeds the cost of using several different antiemetic drugs at the same time. Overall, the cost-effectiveness of pharmacogenomics has not been evaluated, especially for PONV.

The frequency of CYP2D6 metabolizer states tends to vary by ethnicity. Approximately 5–10% of Caucasians are PMs and completely lack CYP2D6 activity, while approximately 2% of Caucasians are categorized as UMs with more than two active genes as a result of a duplication or even a several-fold amplification of the *CYP2D6* gene. Some Hispanic groups may have an increased frequency of UMs, ranging from approximately 5% to 10%. The highest frequency of UMs appears to exist in ethnic groups originating in parts of Northern Africa and the Middle East. In general, given the low frequency of ultrarapid CY2D6 metabolizers in the general US population, the number needed-to-treat for PONV may be as high as 50[46] (this means that 50 patients would have to be genotyped to prevent one patient from vomiting).

Cholinergic muscarinic receptor type 3 polymorphism

The muscarinic acetylcholine receptors including M_3, encoded by the cholinergic muscarinic receptor type 3 (*CHRM3*) gene, have been associated with the emetic pathway and opioid-induced nausea/vomiting[47]. This is indicated by the fact that M_3 muscarinic antagonists impede motion sickness and opioid-induced nausea/vomiting[48]. The involvement of another SNP, in the promoter region of *CHRM3* (rs2165870), was also recently confirmed to be predictive of PONV susceptibility by both a genome-wide association study in a Caucasian population[49] and a targeted genomic association study in Japanese patients[50].

Dopamine receptor polymorphism

Dopamine receptors, specifically D2 and D3, are known to play a role in nausea and emesis, most likely through inhibition of adenylate cyclase[47], which alters the amount of cyclic adenosine 3′-5′-monophosphate within neurons located in the nucleus of the solitary tract and the area postrema[51]. The competitive antagonism of D2, and possibly D3 receptors, provides an explanation for the antiemetic activity of metoclopramide, droperidol, as well as other D2-receptor antagonists. A study performed in a Japanese population showed that the dopamine type 2 receptor (DRD2) Taq1A polymorphism had a moderate strength of association with the occurrence of early PONV[52].

Mu-opioid receptor

Due to the direct association of opioids with the incidence and severity of PONV in surgical patients, a significant number of previous pharmacogenomics investigations have focused on polymorphisms in the mu-opioid receptor (MOR) gene (*OPRM1*), which serves as the main target of all clinically used opioid agonists. The major target of these investigations has focused on the common, nonsynonymous polymorphism in *OPRM1*–A118G (rs179991). The results and conclusions from the studies published so far remain controversial. Two studies reported a higher incidence of PONV in patients who were homozygous (AA) variants[53]. This trend was confirmed by another study from 2008 in postcesarean section patients, which showed that subjects who carried the AA (wild-type) for A118G had a significantly higher rate of PONV, despite a lower consumption of morphine postoperatively[54].

Other studies have not confirmed an association between the A118G polymorphism and the incidence of PONV[40,41,44]. A Chinese study investigated the association of *OPRM1* A118G and the variability of nausea and vomiting from fentanyl analgesia in patients undergoing a total abdominal hysterectomy or myomectomy. They concluded that *OPRM1* A118G had no effect on the individual frequency of PONV or the side effects of fentanyl in Chinese women undergoing gynecologic surgery[55].

The association of the A118G SNP was also recently questioned in a study that directly investigated whether this polymorphism was protective for PONV associated with intravenous patient-controlled opioid analgesia (IV-PCA)[56]. The study found that A118G was not protective against IV-PCA morphine-induced nausea or vomiting. In a recent meta-analysis, six clinical studies were included with a total of 838 women who received epidural analgesia with fentanyl during labor[57]. The meta-analysis indicated that there were no statistically significant differences between an AA homozygote and a G carrier (AG + GG) as it relates to the incidence of nausea and vomiting.

A Japanese double-blinded study of 85 adult patients scheduled to undergo major elective surgery was performed to determine the genotypes and haplotypes of several SNPs in the *OPRM1* gene and their association with PONV during the early postoperative period for patients receiving fentanyl PCA. One out of the eight investigated SNPs rs9397685, in the intronic part of the *OPRM1* gene, was associated with differences in the occurrence and severity of PONV. Four common haplotypes were identified. PONV severity in patients with the GGGAACGC haplotype was significantly lower than in carriers of other haplotypes[58].

ATP-binding cassette, subfamily B, member 1

The ATP-binding cassette, subfamily B, member 1 (ABCB1) drug transporter (also known as P-glycoprotein or multidrug resistance 1) is a transmembrane efflux pump found in many tissues, including the blood–brain barrier[59]. The ABCB1 protein transporter recognizes a broad range of substrates, including the 5-HT_3-receptor antagonists. A study investigated whether the 2677G>T/A and 3435C>T polymorphisms in the *ABCB1* gene influenced the efficacy of ondansetron in preventing PONV in patients undergoing general anesthesia[60]. The incidence of PONV was lower in patients with the 2677TT variant during the first 2 h after surgery. There were no significant differences in the incidence of PONV between the different genotype groups during the period between 2 and 24 h after surgery. The authors concluded that the *ABCB1* genotypes may be a clinical predictor of responsiveness for ondansetron. Another study investigated the association of several genomic factors, including *ABCB1* polymorphisms with PONV[61]. The homozygous *ABCB1* diplotype (GG-CC) conferred an odds ratio of 0.12 with regard to the need for curative antiemetic treatment with ondansetron for PONV. When the association between the *ABCB1* and mu-opioid genes and adverse opioid drug reactions to oxycodone[62] were evaluated, it was noted that nausea and vomiting were more pronounced in the *ABCB1* wild-type genotype carriers (3435CC and 2677GG) when compared with the variant allele carriers (3435CT, 3435TT, 2677GT and 2677TT).

In 2011, an Indonesian study with cancer patients investigated the use of ondansetron and dexamethasone for the prophylaxis of CINV. Multiple SNPs for *ABCB1* (rs1045642, rs2032582 and rs1128503), 5-HTR3B (rs45460698, rs4938058 and rs7943062) and *CYP2D6* ([rs16947-CYP2D6 2], [rs3892097-CYP2D6 4] and [rs1065852-CYP2D6 10]) were evaluated using Taqman assays. Carriers of the CTG haplotype of the *ABCB1* gene experienced CINV more often than other haplotypes in the delayed phase. No associations were found with the 5-HTR3B receptor haplotypes and *CYP2D6*-predicted phenotypes[63].

A SNP at position 3435 in the gene for the ABCB1 transporter was recently demonstrated to affect the antiemetic efficacy of 5-HT_3-receptor antagonists. Cancer patients undergoing chemotherapy were given prophylactic granisetron, ondansetron or tropisetron, and the incidence of nausea, vomiting and the need for rescue antiemetics was examined. Patients who were homozygous for the *ABCB1* 3435T allele responded better to antiemetic therapy compared with individuals who were heterozygous or homozygous for the *ABCB1* 3435C allele. This difference reached statistical significance in the granisetron-treated group[64]. It is possible that patients with the TT genotype accumulate higher concentrations of 5-HT_3-receptor antagonists in the brain and are better protected from emesis as a result of enhanced activity of the ABCB1 transporter.

Catechol-*O*-methyltransferase

Catechol-*O*-methyltransferase (COMT) is an enzyme that acts as a key modulator of the dopaminergic and adrenergic system. COMT polymorphisms may influence nausea and vomiting as the COMT enzyme modulates neurotransmission by metabolizing the catecholamine dopamine. Blocking dopamine D2 receptors in the area postrema and vomiting center has an antiemetic effect, and enhanced dopaminergic activity in patients receiving COMT inhibitors can lead to increased nausea and vomiting. The SNP rs4680 (G472A) in the COMT gene is a missense variant leading to an amino acid exchange (Val158Met)[65]. In patients with migraines without aura, those with the Met-allele (L allele) had an increased incidence of nausea and vomiting, most likely due to the elevated levels of dopamine[66]. A study investigated whether combined COMT and mu-opioid receptor polymorphisms contribute to the morphine response in postoperative analgesia and PONV[67]. Patients received general anesthesia and were screened for the mu-opioid receptor polymorphism A118G (Asn40Asp) and the COMT G1947A (Val158Met) polymorphism. Heterozygous patients with mu-opioid receptor A118G and COMT G1947A mutations presented nausea scores that were significantly lower when compared with homozygous patients.

Neurokinin type 1 (substance P) receptors

Over 500 patents for neurokinin type 1 (NK_1)-receptor antagonists have been filed during the last 20 years, demonstrating the pharmaceutical industry's interest in these agents[68]. Currently in the US there are two NK_1 receptor antagonists that have been shown to be safe and effective for the prevention of PONV in humans, aprepitant (EMEND)[69] and rolapitant[70].

Several preliminary reports (mostly in the abstract form) have attempted to determine the genetic influence of SNPs in the tachykinin receptor 1 (*TACR1*) gene, which encodes for the NK_1 receptors. In a study addressing lower abdominal surgery, it was observed that the SNP rs3755468 in the *TACR1* gene was associated with an increase in the incidence and severity of PONV in female patients. Female gender and wild-type homozygote carriers of the rs3755468 SNP were identified as independent predictors of severe PONV. The odds ratios for the two factors were 6.95- and 4.83-fold higher, respectively. The rs3755468 SNP in the *TACR1* gene appears to be associated with the gender difference in PONV and is located within the predicted estrogen response element and a DNase I hypersensitivity site[71].

A recent review of multiple trials of NK_1-receptor antagonists for treatment of emesis confirmed their effectiveness but also revealed that use may be associated with increased rates of infection, suggesting that ongoing safety assessment is required[72].

Treatment pharmacogenomics

Genetic variation appears to play a significant role in PONV. While there are obvious environmental factors that contribute to PONV, the role of genetics should not be underestimated.

Additionally, it is important for practitioners to keep in mind that resistance to antiemetics may not be due to a mechanistic drug failure but rather genetic resistance. As a general rule, when managing patients with PONV, it would seem reasonable that if a treatment was not successful in the past or less than acceptable, it should not be repeated. This concept appears to apply to all drugs from a given class. Overall, by keeping in mind that the genetics of a patient may affect the PONV phenotype, caregivers may be able to deliver individualized and more effective care.

Summary

Conflicting results between studies are common, making incorporation of pharmacogenetics into clinical care difficult[73–75]. Insufficient power is also a problem with many genetic association studies, probably due to the expense and the difficulty running these types of trials on a very large scale. Taking into consideration the low cost of PONV prophylaxis versus the high cost of genetic analysis, polymorphism analysis might only be considered for very high-risk patients as a component of combination antiemetic therapy[15,16].

Many preliminary studies are still necessary to help develop the framework for larger trials, allowing both the determination of the genetic variations to be investigated as well as providing data to determine the required number of patients to achieve adequately powered trials. Other barriers to the adoption of genetic testing in clinical care include the practicality of performing tests preoperatively and the absence of peer-reviewed guidelines to facilitate transitioning from the bench to the bedside.

In the near future, pharmacogenetic approaches may be implemented to design personalized perioperative intervention trials to demonstrate clinical and economic outcome benefits over empirical treatment. As each patient has a unique genetic background, anesthetic regimens should be tailored to maximize beneficial effects while minimizing adverse effects and any associated economic burden. In the near future, and currently in some cases, pharmacogenetic information will be part of each patient's medical record. The clinical utility of genotyping in the future will depend on strong evidence of genotype–phenotype associations and reproducible personalized interventions in robust clinical studies.

References

1. de Leon J. Pharmacogenomics: the promise of personalized medicine for CNS disorders. *Neuropsychopharmacology* 2009; 34:159–72.
2. Dawood S, Leyland-Jones B. Pharmacology and pharmacogenetics of chemotherapeutic agents. *Cancer Invest* 2009; 27:482–8.
3. Janicki PK, Sugino S. Genetic factors associated with pharmacotherapy and background sensitivity to postoperative and chemotherapy-induced nausea and vomiting. *Exp Brain Res* 2014; 232(8):2613–25.
4. Raeder J. History of postoperative nausea and vomiting. *Int Anesthesiol Clin* 2003; 41:1–12.
5. Palazzo M, Evans R. Logistic regression analysis of fixed patient factors for postoperative sickness: a model for risk assessment. *Br J Anaesth* 1993; 70:135–40.
6. Cohen MM, Duncan PG, DeBoer DP, et al. The postoperative interview: assessing risk factors for nausea and vomiting. *Anesth Analg* 1994; 78:7–16.
7. Sinclair DR, Chung F, Mezei G. Can postoperative nausea and vomiting be predicted? *Anesthesiology* 1999; 91:109–18.

8. Koivuranta M, Laara E, Snare L, et al. A survey of postoperative nausea and vomiting. *Anaesthesia* 1997; 52:443–449.

9. Eberhart LH, Hogel J, Seeling W, et al. Evaluation of three risk scores to predict postoperative nausea and vomiting. *Acta Anaesthesiol Scand* 2000; 44:480–8.

10. Apfel CC, Kranke P, Eberhart LH, et al. Comparison of predictive models for postoperative nausea and vomiting. *Br J Anaesth* 2002; 88:234–40.

11. Gan TJ. Risk factors for postoperative nausea and vomiting. *Anesth Analg* 2006; 102:1884–98.

12. Ikeda K, Ide S, Han W, et al. How individual sensitivity to opiates can be predicted by gene analyses. *Trends Pharmacol Sci* 2005; 26:311–7.

13. Manolio TA, Brooks LD, Collins FS. A HapMap harvest of insights into the genetics of common disease. *J Clin Invest* 2008; 118:1590–605.

14. Feero WG, Guttmacher AE, Collins FS. Genomic medicine – an updated primer. *N Engl J Med* 2010; 362:2001–11.

15. Gan TJ, Meyer T, Apfel CC, et al. Consensus guidelines for managing postoperative nausea and vomiting. *Anesth Analg* 2003; 97:62–71.

16. Habib AS, Gan TJ. Evidence-based management of postoperative nausea and vomiting: a review. *Can J Anesth* 2004; 51:326–41.

17. Cohen M, Sadhasivam S, Vinks AA. Pharmacogenetics in perioperative medicine. *Curr Opin Anesthesiol* 2012; 25:419–27.

18. Ho KY, Gan TJ. Pharmacology, pharmacogenetics, and clinical efficacy of 5-hydroxytryptamine type 3 receptor antagonists for postoperative nausea and vomiting. *Curr Opin Anaesthesiol* 2006; 19:606–11.

19. Andrews PL. Physiology of nausea and vomiting. *Br J Anaesth* 1992; 69(1):2–19.

20. Miller AD, Leslie RA. The area postrema and vomiting. *Front Neuroendocrinol* 1994; 15:301–20.

21. Miyake A, Mochizuki S, Takemoto Y, et al. Molecular cloning of human 5-hydroxytryptamine3 receptor: heterogeneity in distribution and function among species. *Mol Pharmacol* 1995; 48:407–16.

22. Belelli D, Balcarek JM, Hope AG, et al. Cloning and functional expression of a human 5-hydroxytryptamine type 3AS receptor subunit. *Mol Pharmacol* 1995; 48:1054–62.

23. Davies PA, Pistis M, Hanna MC, et al. The 5-HT3B subunit is a major determinant of serotonin-receptor function. *Nature* 1999; 397:359–63.

24. Dubin AE, Huvar R, D'Andrea MR, et al. The pharmacological and functional characteristics of the serotonin 5-HT(3A) receptor are specifically modified by a 5-HT(3B) receptor subunit. *J Biol Chem* 1999; 274:30799–810.

25. Bruss M, Barann M, Hayer-Zillgen M, et al. Modified 5-HT3A receptor function by co-expression of alternatively spliced human 5-HT3A receptor isoforms. *Naunyn Schmiedebergs Arch Pharmacol* 2000; 362:392–401.

26. Gothert M, Propping P, Bonisch H, et al. Genetic variation in human 5-HT receptors: potential pathogenetic and pharmacological role. *Ann NY Acad Sci* 1998; 861:26–30.

27. Bruss M, Eucker T, Gothert M, et al. Exon–intron organization of the human 5-HT3A receptor gene. *Neuropharmacology* 2000; 39:308–15.

28. Kaiser R, Tremblay PB, Sezer O, et al. Investigation of the association between 5-HT3A receptor gene polymorphisms and efficiency of antiemetic treatment with 5-HT3 receptor antagonists. *Pharmacogenetics* 2004; 14:271–8.

29. Tremblay PB, Kaiser R, Sezer O, et al. Variations in the 5-hydroxytryptamine type 3B receptor gene as predictors of the efficacy of antiemetic treatment in cancer patients. *J Clin Oncol* 2003; 21:2147–55.

30. Rueffert H, Thieme V, Wallenborn J, et al. Do variations in the 5-HT3A and 5-HT3B serotonin receptor genes (HTR3A and

HTR3B) influence the occurrence of postoperative vomiting? *Anesth Analg* 2009; 109:1442–7.

31. Sugai T, Suzuki Y, Sawamura K, et al. The effect of 5-hydroxytryptamine 3A and 3B receptor genes on nausea induced by paroxetine. *Pharmacogenomics J* 2006; 6:351–6.
32. Ma XX, Chen QX, Wu SJ, et al. Polymorphisms of the HTR3B gene are associated with post-surgery emesis in a Chinese Han population. *J Clin Pharm Ther* 2013; 38:150–5.
33. Fischer V, Vickers AE, Heitz F, et al. The polymorphic cytochrome P-450 2D6 is involved in the metabolism of both 5-hydroxytryptamine antagonists, tropisetron and ondansetron. *Drug Metab Dispos* 1994; 22:269–74.
34. Dixon CM, Colthup PV, Serabjit-Singh CJ, et al. Multiple forms of cytochrome P450 are involved in the metabolism of ondansetron in humans. *Drug Metab Dispos* 1995; 23:1225–30.
35. Bloomer JC, Baldwin SJ, Smith GJ, et al. Characterization of the cytochrome P450 enzymes involved in the in vitro metabolism of granisetron. *Br J Clin Pharmacol* 1994; 38:557–66.
36. Candiotti KA. Anesthesia and pharmacogenomics: not ready for prime time. *Anesth Analg* 2009; 109:1377–8.
37. Candiotti KA, Birnbach DJ, Lubarsky DA, et al. The impact of pharmacogenomics on postoperative nausea and vomiting: do CYP2D6 allele copy number and polymorphisms affect the success or failure of ondansetron prophylaxis? *Anesthesiology* 2005; 102:543–9.
38. Kaiser R, Sezer O, Papies A, et al. Patient-tailored antiemetic treatment with 5-hydroxytryptamine type 3 receptor antagonists according to cytochrome P-450 genotypes. *J Clin Oncol* 2002; 20,12:2805–11.
39. McKenzie R, Kovac A, O'Connor T, et al. Comparison of ondansetron versus placebo to prevent postoperative nausea and vomiting in women undergoing ambulatory gynecologic surgery. *Anesthesiology* 1993; 78:21–8.
40. Janicki PK, Schuler HG, Jarzembowski TM, et al. Prevention of postoperative nausea and vomiting with granisetron and dolasetron in relation to CYP2D6 genotype. *Anesth Analg* 2006; 102:1127–33.
41. Janicki PK, Schuler G, Francis D, et al. A genetic association study of the functional A118G polymorphism of the human mu-opioid receptor gene in patients with acute and chronic pain. *Anesth Analg* 2006; 103:1011–7.
42. Stamer U, Rauers N, Eun-Hae L, et al. Ondansetron for the treatment of opioid induced nausea and vomiting: impact of cytochrome polymorphisms. *Eur J Pain* 2009; 13:S193/667.
43. Wesmiller SW, Henker RA, Sereika SM, et al. The association of CYP2D6 genotype and postoperative nausea and vomiting in orthopedic trauma patients. *Biol Res Nurs* 2013; 15:382–9.
44. Wesmiller SW, Bender CM, Sereika SM, et al. Association between serotonin transport polymorphisms and postdischarge nausea and vomiting in women following breast cancer surgery. *Oncol Nurs Forum 2014*; 41(2):195–202.
45. Sweeney BP. Why does smoking protect against PONV? *Br J Anaesth* 2002; 89:810–3.
46. Janicki PK. Cytochrome P450 2D6 metabolism and 5-hydroxytryptamine type 3 receptor antagonists for postoperative nausea and vomiting. *Med Sci Monit* 2005; 11:RA322–328.
47. Sanger GJ, Andrews PL. Treatment of nausea and vomiting: gaps in our knowledge. *Auton Neurosci* 2006; 129:3–16.
48. Pergolizzi JV Jr, Philip BK, Leslie JB, et al. Perspectives on transdermal scopolamine for the treatment of postoperative nausea and vomiting. *J Clin Anesth* 2012; 24:334–5.
49. Janicki PK, Vealey R, Liu J, et al. Genome-wide association study using pooled DNA to identify candidate markers mediating susceptibility to

postoperative nausea and vomiting. *Anesthesiology* 2011; 115:54–64.

50. Hayashi H, Sugino Hayase T, Nawa Y, et al. *CHRM3* gene polymorphysm is associated with postoperative nausea and vomiting in the Japanese population. Annual Meeting of the American Society of Anesthesiology Online Abstracts 2012; A1006. http://www.asaabstracts.com/ (accessed December 23, 2015).

51. Hyde TM, Knable MB, Murray AM. Distribution of dopamine D1–D4 receptor subtypes in human dorsal vagal complex. *Synapse* 1996; 24:224–32.

52. Nakagawa M, Kuri M, Kambara N, et al. Dopamine D2 receptor Taq IA polymorphism is associated with postoperative nausea and vomiting. *J Anesth* 2008; 22:397–403.

53. Chou W, Yang L, Lu H, et al. Association of μ-opioid receptor gene polymorphism (AI18G) with variations in morphine consumption for analgesia after total knee arthroplasty. *Acta Anaestesiol Scand* 2006; 50:787–92.

54. Sia A, Lim Y, Lim E, et al. A118G single nucleotide polymorphism of human mu-opioid receptor gene influences pain perception and patient-controlled intravenous morphine consumption after intrathecal morphine for post cesarean analgesia. *Anesthesiology* 2008; 109:520–6.

55. Zhang W, Yuan JJ, Kan QC, et al. Study of the OPRM1 A118G genetic polymorphism associated with postoperative nausea and vomiting induced by fentanyl intravenous analgesia. *Minerva Anestesiol* 2011; 77:33–9.

56. Chen LK, Chen SS, Huang CH, et al. Polymorphism of μ-opioid receptor gene (OPRM1:c.118A>G) might not protect against or enhance morphine-induced nausea or vomiting. *Pain Res Treat* 2013; 259306. http://dx.doi.org/10.1155/2013/259306

57. Song Z, Du B, Wang K, et al. Effects of OPRM1 A118G polymorphism on epidural analgesia with fentanyl during labor: a meta-analysis. *Genet Test Mol Biomarkers* 2013; 17:743–9.

58. Sugino S, Hayase T, Higuchi M, et al. Associations of μ-opioid receptor gene (OPRM1) haplotypes with postoperative nausea and vomiting (PONV) during intravenous patient-controlled analgesia. Biology and Control of Nausea and Vomiting Online Abstracts 2013; 60. www.researchgate.net/publication/262609924_Association_of_m-opioid_receptor_gene_OPRM1_haplotypes_with_postoperative_nausea_and_vomiting (accessed December 18, 2015).

59. Marzolini C, Paus E, Buclin T, et al. Polymorphisms in human MDR1 (P-glycoprotein): recent advances and clinical relevance. *Clin Pharmacol Ther* 2004; 75:13–33.

60. Choi EM, Lee MG, Lee SH, et al. Association of ABCB1 polymorphisms with the efficacy of ondansetron for postoperative nausea and vomiting. *Anaesthesia* 2010; 65:996–1000.

61. Coulbault L, Beaussier M, Verstuyft C, et al. Environmental and genetic factors associated with morphine response in the postoperative period. *Clin Pharmacol Ther* 2006; 79:316–24.

62. Zwisler S, Enggaard T, Noehr-Jensen L, et al. The antinociceptive effect and adverse drug reactions of oxycodone in human experimental pain in relation to genetic variations in the OPRM1 and ABCB1 genes. *Fundam Clin Pharmacol* 2009; 10:1–8.

63. Perwitasari DA, Wessels JA, van der Straaten RJ, et al. Association of ABCB1, 5-HT3B receptor and CYP2D6 genetic polymorphisms with ondansetron and metoclopramide antiemetic response in Indonesian cancer patients treated with highly emetogenic chemotherapy. *Jpn J Clin Oncol* 2011; 41(10):1168–76.

64. Babaoglu MO, Bayar B, Aynacioglu AS, et al. Association of the ABCB1 3435C>T polymorphism with antiemetic efficacy of 5-hydroxytryptamine type 3 antagonists. *Clin Pharmacol Ther* 2005; 78:619–26.

65. Andersen S, Skorpen F. Variation in the COMT gene: implications for pain perception and pain treatment. *Pharmacogenomics* 2009; 10:669–84.

66. Park JW, Lee KS, Kim JS, et al. Genetic contribution of catechol-O-methyltransferase polymorphism in patients with migraine without aura. *J Clin Neurol* 2007; 3:24–30.

67. Kolesnikov Y, Gabovits B, Levin A, et al. Combined catechol-O-methyltransferase and mu-opioid receptor gene polymorphisms affect morphine postoperative analgesia and central side effects. *Anesth Analg* 2011; 112:448–53.

68. Steinhoff MS, von Mentzer B, Geppetti P, et al. Tachykinins and their receptors: contributions to physiological control and the mechanisms of disease. *Physiol Rev* 2014; 94:265–301.

69. Hargreaves R, Ferreira JC, Hughes D, et al. Development of aprepitant, the first neurokinin-1 receptor antagonist for the prevention of chemotherapy-induced nausea and vomiting. *Ann NY Acad Sci* 2011; 1222:40–48.

70. Gan T, Gu J, Singla N, et al. Rolapitant for the prevention of postoperative nausea and vomiting: a prospective, double-blinded, placebo-controlled randomized trial. *Anesthes Analg* 2011; 112: 804–12.

71. Hayase T, Sugino S, Tachibana S, et al. Haplotypes in human TACR1 gene are associated with postoperative nausea and vomiting. Annual Meeting of the American Society of Anesthesiology Online Abstracts 2012. http://www.asaabstracts.com/ A1003 (accessed December 23, 2015).

72. Dos Santos LV, Souza FH, Brunetto AT, et al. Neurokinin-1 receptor antagonists for chemotherapy-induced nausea and vomiting: a systematic review. *J Natl Cancer Inst* 2012; 104:1280–92.

73. Walter C, Lotsch J. Meta-analysis of the relevance of the OPRM1 118A>G genetic variant for pain treatment. *Pain* 2009; 146:270–275.

74. Wong CA, McCarthy RJ, Blouin J, et al. Observational study of the effect of muopioid receptor genetic polymorphism on intrathecal opioid labor analgesia and postcesarean delivery analgesia. *Int J Obstetr Anesth* 2010; 19:246–53.

75. Jannetto PJ, Bratanow NC. Pain management in the 21st century: utilization of pharmacogenomics and therapeutic drug monitoring. *Expert Opin Drug Metab Toxicol* 2011; 7:745–752.

Chapter 6

Pharmacology of serotonin antagonists

Jacob Nouriel and Gildasio De Oliveira

Serotonin antagonists were the first group of drugs specifically developed to prevent and/or treat nausea and vomiting with the advantage of lacking sedating properties. In this chapter, we will discuss specific drugs and their pharmacologic and clinical properties.

Ondansetron

Ondansetron was the first serotonin antagonist marketed[1]. Ondansetron is available for administration by oral or intravenous (IV) route. The compound is a carbazole derivate, structurally related to serotonin and metoclopramide[2]. The drug is available as a racemic mixture, which contains the S (+) and R (−) stereoisomers. Both isomers display a high affinity for the 5-hydroxytryptamine type 3 (5-HT_3) receptor[3]. However, the agent demonstrates non-5-HT_3 receptor-specific binding: 5-HT1B, 5-HT1C, alpha-1-adrenergic and opioid receptors. Non-5-HT_3 receptor binding accounts for 20% of the total binding. Thus, ondansetron is less selective in receptor binding compared to other 5-HT_3 receptor antagonists; chemical structure and/or metabolism may contribute to this difference in binding affinity. This property may be an asset to ondansetron treatment in view of emesis being due to more than 5-HT_3 receptor activation. In humans, the R-isomer, administered in isolation, presents a better safety profile and antiemetic efficacy compared with the racemic mixture[4,5].

In humans, ondansetron is extensively and rapidly metabolized. Five percent of the parent compound is recovered in urine, and hepatic metabolism accounts for 95% of ondansetron clearance[6]. Hydroxylation at the indole ring followed by conjugation is the major route of metabolism. A minor route of metabolism is *N*-demethylation. Due to first-pass metabolism, drug bioavailability is approximately 56% and the beta elimination is 3.7–4.7 h following oral administration. Multiple cytochrome P450 (CYP450) enzymes are involved in ondansetron metabolism: CYP1A1, CYP1A2, CYP2D6 and the CYP3A subfamily[7]. Patients with genetic polymorphism of the CYP2D6 allele metabolize ondansetron at an ultrarapid rate[8]. As a result, an increased incidence of prophylactic postoperative nausea and vomiting (PONV) therapy failure with ondansetron is found in this patient population[9].

Some of the nonconjugated metabolites possess pharmacologic activity; however, contribution to the biological activity of ondansetron is minimal due to low plasma concentrations. Volume of distribution remains unchanged with increasing age, whereas clearance decreases[6]. Gender differences are slightly present: plasma clearance is slower in females.

Postoperative Nausea and Vomiting: A Practical Guide, eds. Tong Joo Gan and Ashraf S. Habib. Published by Cambridge University Press.

Although the cause for such a difference is unclear, a slower plasma clearance in females may be beneficial, considering the increased likelihood of developing PONV in females[10].

In humans, the predominant route of excretion is via the urine[11]. No effect on ondansetron pharmacokinetics was found in patients with renal impairment[12]. Patients with hepatic insufficiency had significantly decreased clearance at a degree analogous to the extent of hepatic impairment[13]. In children, ondansetron displayed pharmacokinetics similar to adults[14].

Clinical findings of ondansetron in antiemetic treatment for chemotherapy- and radiation-induced emesis were followed by the application of the medication for the treatment of PONV. In a meta-analysis including 7,177 patients receiving ondansetron prophylaxis and 5,712 receiving placebo or no treatment, the investigators found that out of 100 surgical patients receiving adequate prophylactic dose of ondansetron, treatment would prevent 20 episodes of postoperative vomiting[15]. In the prevention of PONV, a 1-mg dose administered intravenously was not significantly different from placebo and increasing the dose beyond 8 mg did not further improve efficacy[16]. In contrast, in a nauseated or vomiting patient, 1 mg IV ondansetron was more efficacious than placebo in preventing further episodes of nausea or vomiting. Nevertheless, the results suggested no evidence of a clinically relevant dose–response between 1 and 8 mg.

A cost-effectiveness analysis demonstrated that prophylaxis with effective doses (i.e., 4 or 8 mg) was less cost-effective and less safe than treatment of PONV with effective doses (i.e., 1 or 4 mg)[17]. The aforementioned results might not be applicable now as ondansetron is currently a generic drug. Prophylactic IV administration at the end of surgery compared to before induction of anesthesia was associated with lower nausea scores, earlier intake of normal food, decreased incidence of frequent emesis (more than two episodes) and increased emesis-free time during the first 24 h postoperatively[18]. Half-life may explain these differences in clinical efficacy for different administration times. These results demonstrate that optimal timing of administration is at the end of surgery.

Minimal adverse effects have been found with ondansetron administration. Of 100 patients receiving prophylactic ondansetron, the incidence of headache was 3%[15]. To a lesser extent, constipation and elevated liver enzymes were also reported. All age groups tolerated ondansetron well, that is, there was no increase in adverse events associated with increased age[19]. Ondansetron did not potentiate general anesthesia-induced respiratory depression[20]. Although extrapyramidal symptoms are generally not considered to be a complication of ondansetron, there are case reports of patients receiving ondansetron and experiencing extrapyramidal reactions and psychiatric symptoms both in the postoperative setting and in patients undergoing chemotherapy[21,22]. The good safety profile of ondansetron may be explained by its highly specific binding to 5-HT_3 receptors. Nonetheless, some studies have demonstrated negative effects of ondansetron on QT interval prolongation, which has led to a warning from the US Food and Drug Administration (FDA) about the use of high-dose ondansetron for chemotherapy-induced nausea and vomiting (CINV).

Drug interactions between ondansetron and other compounds is low. Since the hepatic CYP450 enzyme system is active in ondansetron metabolism, inducers and inhibitors of this system are anticipated to affect ondansetron plasma concentration. Elimination of ondansetron was prolonged in a group of patients taking morphine[20]. This analysis was, however, conducted in a small patient population ($n = 8$).

Dolasetron

Dolasetron mesylate was approved for use for the treatment nausea and vomiting by the FDA in 1997. Unlike ondansetron, which binds to the 5-HT_1B, 5-HT_1C, alpha-adrenergic and opioid receptors, dolasetron is a pure 5-HT_3-receptor antagonist for the treatment of nausea and vomiting. Following dolasetron administration, the enzyme carbonyl reductase converts the drug to its active form, hydrodolasteron. Hydrodolasetron has a much higher affinity for the 5-HT_3 receptor[23]. Despite the brief elimination half-life of dolasetron of 0.13–0.24 h, the active form of the drug, hydrodolasteron, has a half-life of 4–8 h. Thus, the duration of pharmacologic effect seen after the administration of dolasetron is significantly longer than that of ondansetron. On first glance, such properties make dolasetron a more appealing pharmacologic modality for extended treatment of nausea and vomiting.

Metabolism of hydrodolasetron occurs from both conjugation and the CYP450 system. The majority of glucuronide or sulfate conjugated to hydrodolasetron is excreted in the urine[23–35]. However, the well-known genetic variation that occurs in the CYP2D6 component of the CYP450 system means that there will be a wide variation in the rates of metabolism of hydrodolasetron ranging from ultrarapid metabolizers (UM) to poor metabolizers (PM). Thus, the efficacy of this drug, like any other pharmacologic agent dependent on the cytochrome P450 system, may be widely disparate.

The high bioavailability of oral administration of dolasetron makes it an attractive option for patients who can tolerate the oral administration of the drug despite their underlying nausea and vomiting[2]. The previous use of intravenously administered dolasetron was suspended by the FDA in 2010 secondary to the risk of hemodynamically unstable tachyarrhythmias. The prolongation of the QTc interval on the electrocardiogram (ECG) seen with dolasetron is noted to be less than the QTc prolongation observed with ondansetron. Potassium channel blockade and subsequently delayed repolarization of the myocardium may be a significant contributor of such arrhythmogenic effects. Dolasetron does slow cardiac depolarization by blocking fast sodium channels[26]. This can also lead to changes in heart rate, PR interval length, QRS duration and QTc prolongation. Patients who receive dolasetron should receive a screening ECG to assess for the presence of QTc prolongation, thereby identifying the patients at highest risk of such phenomena.

The dose of dolasetron administered for control of nausea and vomiting in clinical trials has ranged from 12.5 to 200 mg[2,27]. The use of the medication at doses of 12.5–25 mg in postoperative gynecology patients was shown to achieve significant suppression of nausea and vomiting[2]. Higher doses of the drug have a clinical ceiling effect. Given the increased risk of side effects with higher plasma levels of the drug (i.e., tachyarrhythmias), the minimum effective dose for clinical control of the patient's symptoms should be targeted. The utilization of a 50-mg dose of dolasetron was shown to be as effective as 4 mg of ondansetron in the prevention of nausea and vomiting[2]. Clearly, dolasetron use for the prevention of nausea and vomiting has been shown to be noninferior to ondansetron[28,29].

Despite the large amount of experience with dolasetron, which was approved for use over 15 years ago, its use is significantly limited by its arrhythmogenic side-effect profile, necessitating oral use. Additionally, newer 5-HT_3 antagonists that have a greater duration of action, such as palonosetron, make the use of dolasetron inferior to those agents and to intravenously administered ondansetron.

Granisetron

The empirical formula of granisetron is $C_{18}H_{24}N_{4O}$*HCl; it is an indazole. Granisetron is available for administration by way of mouth or IV route. For IV administration, 0.35–3.0 mg is the recommended dose for the prevention of PONV. This administration may occur before induction of anesthesia or at the end of surgery[30]. Granisetron exhibits little or no affinity for serotonin receptors other than 5-HT_3. Further, suggestive of the affinity of granisetron for the 5-HT_3 serotonin receptor, increasing concentrations of the natural ligand will not displace the antagonist[31,32]. Compared to ondansetron, granisetron is more selective for the serotonin 5-HT_3 receptor. However, in a meta-analysis comparing the efficacy of ondansetron and granisetron in the treatment of CINV, the authors concluded that the compounds have similar antiemetic efficacy[33]. The same conclusion was found in a separate meta-analysis comparing all four serotonin antagonists in the treatment for CINV[34]. This meta-analysis reached an additional conclusion that granisetron demonstrated greater efficacy than tropisetron in the treatment for CINV.

Ondansetron and granisetron exhibit similar clinical antiemetic efficacy. For patients at high risk of PONV, combination therapy is recommended. Granisetron and promethazine coadministration was more effective than promethazine alone in the prevention of PONV in females undergoing outpatient laparoscopies[35,36]. Prophylactic granisetron 1 mg IV was ineffective in the prevention of intraoperative nausea and vomiting during elective cesarean delivery under spinal anesthesia[37]. Granisetron treatment for CINV was significantly affected by genetic polymorphism for the gene for adenosine triphosphate-binding cassette subfamily B member 1 (ABCB1), a transmembrane efflux pump[35,38]. Individuals with the TT genotype for the nucleotide at position 3435 of the gene for the ABCB1 protein transporter displayed better control of emesis than individuals who had the heterozygous or homozygous CC genotype[39]. A possible explanation is that the antiemetic agents accumulate to a higher concentration in the brain in individuals with the TT genotype due to enhanced activity of the ABCB1 transporter than individuals with the heterozygous or homozygous CC genotype[39].

Granisetron metabolism in the liver is rapid. Following incubation of granisetron with human liver microsomes, *N*-demethylation or hydroxylation metabolites via the CYP system were identified as major products, with the hydroxyl product predominating. Ketoconazole is a CYP3A inhibitor. The inhibition of granisetron metabolism by chemical inhibitors suggests that CYP3A is responsible for the metabolism of granisetron[40]. Metabolism by way of CYP3A isoenzyme is unique to granisetron compared to other serotonin antagonists. No inhibition of other CYP activities was found in the presence of granisetron.

Granisetron has an elimination half-life between 5 and 8 h. Its prolonged duration of action is an attractive property of this drug. However, because multiple factors besides serotonin contribute to PONV, granisetron's high selectivity for serotonin receptors may make this drug less attractive when compared to a less-selective drug such as ondansetron. Within 24 h of drug administration, 12% of granisetron dose is found excreted unchanged in the urine[40]. Because granisetron is metabolized primarily by the CYP3A subfamily, patients who are CYP2D6 UM do not experience a change in the clinical efficacy of granisetron. Accordingly, granisetron may be appropriate with the concomitant administration of drugs, which may have inhibitory or induced effects on the CYP2D6 isoenzyme. The incidence of side effects did not differ between granisetron treatment and placebo groups in an analysis of pediatric patients in the postoperative setting[41].

Adverse drug interactions have not been observed when granisetron is concomitantly administered with benzodiazepines, antipsychotics, anti-ulcer medications and chemotherapeutic agents. The effects of a selective serotonin re-uptake inhibitor would be expected to be reduced in the presence of granisetron due to the latter's prolonged antagonism at 5-HT_3 receptors[42,43].

Tropisetron

Tropisetron has not been approved by the FDA. However, it is available internationally. In addition to antagonizing 5-HT_3 receptors, tropisetron is also an alpha-7-nicotinic receptor agonist[44]. In addition to its use for the treatment of nausea and vomiting, the drug has also been used experimentally for the treatment of pain secondary to fibromyalgia. When compared to ondansetron, which has a beta half-life of 3–5 h, tropisetron has a beta elimination half-life of 6 h leading to a longer duration of action[45].

Metabolism of tropisetron occurs via the CYP2D6 isoenzyme component of the hepatic cytochrome P450 system. Following its oxidative hydroxylation by this system, the metabolite is made soluble by conjugation with glucuronide and sulfate moieties. Thus, tropisetron and its respective metabolites undergo renal excretion[46,47]. The contrast in the metabolism of tropisetron when compared to ondansetron is an important consideration clinically. Patients who experience genetic variation of the CYP2D6 and are UM experienced more CINV when compared to UM who received ondansetron[48].

Diagnostic tests are now available to identify genetic variation in CYP2D6 activity, and such information may be particularly useful in utilizing drugs such as tropisetron for the treatment of nausea and vomiting. However, the cost-effectiveness of genetically targeted drug therapy remains an unknown variable that warrants future investigation. Nonetheless, the largely CYP2D6 metabolism pathway of tropisetron warrants concern for interactions with other pharmacologic agents that also rely heavily on CYP2D6 metabolism. Agents such as doxorubicin, tamoxifen, amiodarone, cimetidine, ranitidine and tricyclic antidepressants are additional pharmacologic agents that are metabolized by this pathway and may compete with tropisetron metabolism via the CYP2D6 pathway.

Dosing of IV tropisetron has varied between 2 and 5 mg[30,49–51]. Whilst some studies have shown a significant clinical benefit of using higher doses, other studies have demonstrated the appearance of a ceiling effect, much like that noted with other 5-HT_3 antagonists. Perhaps, such variable results are related to the different emetogenic potential of different surgical procedures, and stratification of at-risk patients would be useful in determining which patients may benefit from a higher dosing regimen. Because of the advantageous duration of action of tropisetron, it has been used for once-daily dosing in the treatment of nausea and vomiting.

Palonosetron

Palonosetron is a new generation 5-HT_3 antagonist approved for the prevention and treatment of PONV. It has been described as a "second generation" 5-HT_3 antagonist since it has greater receptor-binding properties, which results in a much longer half-life than the previously described drugs[52].

The pharmacokinetic properties of the drug have been studied in healthy human volunteers[52]. The drug is vastly distributed in tissues and is moderately bound to plasma proteins. The metabolism of palonosetron is primarily hepatic by the CYP450 enzyme system.

Currently, it remains to be determined if the metabolism of palonosentron is altered in UM. Renal clearance of palonosetron is small when compared to the total excretion of the drug, which is responsible for the long half-life of approximately 40 h[53]. Palonosetron binds tightly to the 5-HT_3 receptors resulting in a drug potency of 100 times greater than ondansetron. The strong receptor binding of the drug is responsible for the long half-life of palonosetron.

The efficacy of palonosetron has been evaluated in randomized clinical trials. Kovac et al. concluded that, after studying female patients undergoing gynecological or breast surgery, a single 0.075-mg IV dose of palonosetron decreased the severity of nausea and delayed the time to emesis and treatment failure, but that lower doses were not as effective[54]. This finding has been recently confirmed by a different group of investigators in patients undergoing elective general surgery[55]. Moon et al. demonstrated in patients undergoing thyroidectomy that palonosetron was more efficacious than ondasentron to reduce nausea and vomiting 2–24 h after the surgery[56].

Ramosetron

Ramosetron hydrochloride (ramosetron), a tetra-hydrobenzimidazole derivative, is also a 5-HT_3 receptor antagonist used for PONV prophylaxis and treatment. However, ramosetron is currently only licenced for use in Japan and selected Southeast Asian countries. Ramosetron also competitively blocks serotonin-mediated contraction of the colon, and this pharmacologic property confers the drug an application in improving diarrhea-predominant inflammatory bowel syndrome[57].

Initial studies demonstrated some benefits of ramosetron in reducing PONV when compared to ondansetron[58]. Nevertheless, a recent meta-analysis including 12 studies and 1,372 patients did not demonstrate any benefit of ramosetron when compared to ondansetron[59].

References

1. Scuderi PE. Pharmacology of serotonin antagonists. In: Gan TJ, ed. *Post-Operative Nausea and Vomiting*. Pennsylvania: Lippincott Williams & Wilkins, 2003; 41–66.
2. Gyermek L. 5-HT(3) receptors: pharmacologic and therapeutic aspects. *J Clin Pharmacol* 1995; (35): 637–40.
3. Kilpatrick GJ, Jones BJ, Tyers MB. Indentification and distribution of 5-HT3 receptors in rat brain using radioligand bind. *Nature* 1987; 330: 746–8.
4. Garud KL, Godbole S, Mankar S, et al. Efficacy and safety of R(+) ondansetron solution in the treatment of nausea and vomiting in children: results of an open-label, non-comparative, prospective clinical study. *Indian Med Gazette* 2006; 140: 112–14.
5. Shinde J, Mandora VP, Joshi PK, et al. Efficacy and safety of R-ondansetron 4 mg versus racemic ondansetron 8 mg: results of a randomized, double blind, multicentric clinical trial. *Indian Med Gazette* 2005; 139: 444–7.
6. Pritchard JF. Ondansetron metabolism and pharmacokinetics. *Semin Oncol* 1992; 19(4 Suppl 10): 9–15.
7. Dixon CM, Colthup PV, Serabjit-Singh CJ, et al. Multiple forms of cytochrome P450 are involved in the metabolism of ondansetron in humans. *Drug Metab Dispos* 1995; 23(11): 1225–30.
8. Kaiser R, Sezer O, Papies A, et al. Patient-tailored antiemetic treatment with

5-hydroxytryptamine type 3 receptor antagonists according to cytochrome P-450 2D6 genotypes. *J Clin Oncol* 2002; 20(12): 2805–11.

9. Candiotti KA, Birnbach DJ, Lubarsky DA, et al. The impact of pharmacogenomics on postoperative nausea and vomiting: do CYP2D6 allele copy number and polymorphisms affect the success or failure of ondansetron prophylaxis? *Anesthesiology* 2005; 102(3): 543–9.
10. Gan TJ. Risk factors for postoperative nausea and vomiting. *Anesth Analg* 2006; 102(6): 1884–98.
11. Saynor DA, Dixon CM. The metabolism of ondansetron. *Eur J Clin Oncol* 1989; 25(1): S75–S77.
12. Amantea MA, Yarboro C, Forrest A, et al. Population pharmacokinetics of intravenous and oral ondansetron in patients with systemic lupus erythematosus (SLE). *J Clin Pharmacol* 1993; 33: 1004.
13. Figg WD, Dukes GE, Pritchard F, et al. Pharmacokinetics of ondansetron in patients with hepatic insufficiency. *J Clin Pharmacol* 1996; 36: 206–25.
14. Sphar-Schopfer IA, Lerman J, Sikich N, et al. Pharmacokinetics of intravenous ondansetron in health children undergoing ear, nose, and throat surgery. *Clin Pharmacol Ther* 1995; 58: 316–21.
15. Tramer MR, Reynolds DJM, Moore RA, et al. Efficacy, dose–response, and safety of ondansetron in prevention of postoperative nausea and vomiting. *Anesthesiology* 1997; 87: 1277–89.
16. Tramer MR, Moore RA, Reynolds DJM, et al. A quantitative systematic review of ondansetron in treatment of established postoperative nausea and vomiting. *BMJ* 1997; 314: 1088–92.
17. Tramer MR, Phillips C, Reynolds DJM, et al. Cost-effectiveness of ondansetron for postoperative nausea and vomiting. *Anesthesia* 1999; 54: 226–34.
18. Tang J, Wang B, White PF, et al. The effect of timing of ondansetron administration on its efficacy, cost-effectiveness, and cost–benefit as a prophylatic antiemetic in the ambulatory setting. *Anesth Analg* 1998; 86: 274–82.
19. Bryson JC. Clinical safety of ondansetron. *Semin Oncol* 1992; 19(6 Suppl 15): 26–32.
20. Baber N, Palmer JL, Frazer NM, et al. Clinical pharmacology of ondansetron in postoperative nausea and vomiting. *Eur J Anesthesiol Suppl* 1992; 6: 11–8.
21. Tolan MM, Fuhrman TM, Tsueda K, et al. Perioperative extrapyramidal reactions associated with ondansetron [Letter]. *Anesthesiology* 1990; 90: 340–1.
22. Halperin JR, Murphy B. Extrapyramidal reaction to ondansetron [Letter]. *Cancer* 2010; 69(5): 1275.
23. Gregory RE, Ettinger DS. 5-HT3 receptor antagonists for the prevention of chemotherapy-induced nausea and vomiting. *Drugs* 1998; 55: 173–89.
24. Balfour JA, Goa KL. Dolasetron: a review of its pharmacology and therapeutic potential in the management of nausea and vomiting induced by chemotherapy, radiotherapy, or surgery. *Drugs* 1998; 54: 273–98.
25. Janicki, PK. Cytochrome P450 2DB metabolism and 5-hydroxytryptamine type 3 receptor antagonists for postoperative nausea and vomiting. *Med Sci Monit* 2005; 11: RA322–238.
26. Benedict CR, Arbogast R, Martin L, et al. Single-blind study of the effects of intravenous dolasetron mesylate versus ondansetron on electrocardiographic parameters in normal volunteers. *J Cardiovasc Pharmacol* 2006; 28: 53–9.
27. Kuryshev Ya, Brown AM, Wang L, et al. Interactions of the 5-hydroxytryptamine 3 antagonist class of antiemetic drugs within human cardiac ion channels. *J Pharmacol Exp Ther* 2000; 295: 614–20.
28. Keefe DL. The cardiotoxic potential of the 5-HT(3) receptor antagonist antiemetics: is there cause for concern? *Oncologist* 2002; 7: 65–72.
29. Grote TH, Pineda LF, Figlin RA, et al. Oral dolasetron mesylate in patients receiving moderately emetogenic platinum-containing chemotherapy. Oral Dolasetron

Dose Response Study Group. *Cancer J Sci Am* 1997; 3: 45–51.

30. Gan TJ, Diemunsch P, Habib AS et al. Consensus guidelines for the management of postoperative nausea and vomiting. *Anesth Analg* 2014; 118: 85–113.

31. Newberry NR, Watkins CJ, Sprosen TS, et al. BRL 46460 potently antagonizes neural responses activated by 5-HT3 receptors. *Neuropharmacology* 1993; 32: 729–35.

32. Gregory RE, Ettinger DS. 5-HT3 receptor antagonists for the prevention of chemotherapy-induced nausea and vomiting. A comparison of their pharmacology and clinical effect. *Drugs* 1998; 55: 173–89.

33. del Giglio A, Soares HP, Caparroz C, et al. Granisetron is equivalent to ondansetron for prophylaxis of chemotherapy-induced nausea and vomiting: results of a meta-analysis of randomized controlled trials. *Cancer* 2000; 89(11): 2301–2308.

34. Jordan K, Hinke A, Grothey A, et al. A meta-analysis comparing the efficacy of four 5-HT3-receptor antagonists for acute chemotherapy-induced emesis. *Support Care Cancer* 2007; 15(9): 1023–33.

35. White PF, Tang J, Hamza MA, et al. The use of oral granisetron versus intravenous ondansetron for antiemetic prophylaxis in patients undergoing laparoscopic surgery: the effect on emetic symptoms and quality of recovery. *Anesth Analg* 2006; 102: 679–83.

36. Gan TJ, Candiotti KA, Klein SM, et al. Double-blind comparison of granisetron, promethazine, or a combination of both for the prevention of postoperative nausea and vomiting in females undergoing outpatient laparoscopies. *Can J Anaesth* 2009; 56(11): 829–36.

37. Balki M, Kasodekar S, Dhumne S, et al. Granisetron does not prevent post delivery nausea and vomiting during elective cesarean delivery under spinal anesthesia. *Anesth Analg* 2007; 104: 679–683.

38. Babaoglu Mo, Bayar B, Aynacioglu AS, et al. Association of the ABCB1 3435C>T polymorphism with antiemetic efficacy of 5-hydroxytryptamine type 3 antagonists. *Clin Pharmacol Ther* 2005; 78: 619–26.

39. Bloomer JC, Baldwin SJ, Smith GJ, et al. Characterisation of the cytochrome P450 enzymes involved in the in vitro metabolism of granisetron. *Br J Clin Pharmacol* 1994; 38: 557–66.

40. Roche. Prescribing Information: *Kytril* (granisetron hydrochloride) injection premixed. Research Triangle Park, NC: Roche, 2006.

41. Janicki PK, Schuler HG, Jarzembowski Tm, et al. Prevention of post-operative nausea and vomiting with granisetron and dolasetron in relation to CYP2D6 genotype. *Aneth Analg* 2006; 102:1127–33.

42. Cieslak GD, Watch MF, Phillips MB, et al. The dose–response relation and cost-effectiveness of granisetron for the prophylaxis of pediatric postoperative emesis. *Anesthesiology* 1996; 85(5): 1076–85.

43. Cooper Sm, Arnold BDC, Rapeport WG. Inhibition of 5-HT induced axon-reflex flares by BRL 43694, a novel 5-HT3 receptor antagonist. *Br J Clin Pharamcol* 1988; 25: 106P–7P.

44. Macor JE, Gurley D, Lanthorn T, et al. The 5-HT3 antagonist tropisetron (ICS 205–930) is a potent and selective alpha7 nicotinic receptor partial agonist. *Bioorg Med Chem Lett* 2001; 11: 319–21.

45. Kees F, Farber L, Bucher M, et al. Pharmacokinetics of therapeutic doses of tropisetron in health volunteers. *Br J Clin Pharmacol* 2001; 52:705–7.

46. Fischer V, Baldeck JP, Tse FL. Pharmacokinetics and metabolism of the 5-hydroxytryptamine antagonist tropisetron after single oral doses in humans. *Drug Metab Dispos* 1992; 20:603–7.

47. Vickers AE, Fischer V, Connors MS, et al. Biotransformation of the antiemetic 5-HT3 antagonist tropisetron in liver and kidney slices of human, rat and dog with a comparison to in vivo. *Eur J Drug Metabo Pharmacokinet* 1996; 21: 43–50.

48. Kaiser R, Sezer O, Papies A, et al. Patient-tailored antiemetic treatment with

5-hydroxytryptamine type 3 receptor antagonists according to cytochrome P-450 2D6 genotypes. *J Clin Oncol* 2002; 20: 2805–11.

49. Zomers PJW, Langenber CJM, de Bruijn KM. Tropisetron for postoperative nausea and vomiting in patients after gynaecological surgery. *Br J Anesth* 1993; 71: 667–80.

50. Alon E, Kocian R, Nett OR, et al. Tropisetron for the prevention of postoperative nausea and vomiting in women undergoing gynecologic surgery. *Anesth Analg* 1996; 82: 238–41.

51. Capouet V, De Pauw C, Vernet B, et al. Single dose i.v. tropisetron in the prevention of postoperative nausea and vomiting after gynaecological surgery. *Br J Anesth* 1996; 76: 54–60.

52. Stoltz R, Cyong JC, Shah A, et al. Pharmacokinetic and safety evaluation of palonosetron, a 5-hydroxytryptamine-3 receptor antagonist, in U.S. and Japanese healthy subjects. *J Clin Pharmacol* 2004; 44: 520–31.

53. Stoltz R, Parisi S, Shah A, et al. Pharmacokinetics, metabolism and excretion of intravenous [14C]-palonosetron in healthy human volunteers. *Biopharm Drug Dispos* 2004; 25: 329–37.

54. Kovac AL, Eberhart L, Kotarski J, et al. Palonosetron 04-07 Study Group. A randomized, double-blind study to evaluate the efficacy and safety of three different doses of palonosetron versus placebo in preventing postoperative nausea and vomiting over a 72-hour period. *Anesth Analg* 2008; 107: 439–44.

55. Chun HR, Jeon IS, Park SY, et al. Efficacy of palonosetron for the prevention of postoperative nausea and vomiting: a randomized, double-blinded, placebo-controlled trial. *Br J Anaesth* 2014; 112: 485–90.

56. Moon YE, Joo J, Kim JE, et al. Anti-emetic effect of ondansetron and palonosetron in thyroidectomy: a prospective, randomized, double-blind study. *Br J Anaesth* 2012; 108: 417–22.

57. Hirata T, Funatsu T, Keto Y, et al. Pharmacological profile of ramosetron, a novel therapeutic agent for IBS. *Inflammopharmacology* 2007; 15: 5–9.

58. Hahm TS, Ko JS, Choi SJ, et al. Comparison of the prophylactic anti-emetic efficacy of ramosetron and ondansetron in patients at high-risk for postoperative nausea and vomiting after total knee replacement. *Anaesthesia* 2010; 65: 500–4.

59. Mihara T, Tojo K, Uchimoto K, et al. Reevaluation of the effectiveness of ramosetron for preventing postoperative nausea and vomiting: a systematic review and meta-analysis. *Anesth Analg* 2013; 117: 329–39.

Chapter 7

Pharmacology of histamine, muscarine and dopamine antagonists

Tricia A. Meyer and Russell K. McAllister

Multiple receptors are involved in the transmission of impulses to the vomiting center. This chapter will focus on the medications that interact at the histamine, muscarine and dopamine receptors, and will examine the efficacy of these medications alone, or in combination with other drug classes, for the prophylaxis and treatment of postoperative nausea and vomiting (PONV) (Table 7.1). Most of the available medications that act at these receptors are well-established, older drugs. However, some may be older drugs that have found a new use, such as haloperidol, or have a different delivery system, such as transdermal scopolamine[1,2].

Histamine antagonists

Histamine antagonists, or antihistamines, competitively inhibit the effects of histamine at the H_1 receptors. Antihistamine agents can be classified chemically as ethylenediamines, ethanolamine, alkylamines, phenothiazines or piperazine derivatives. Antihistamines can be clinically divided into first and second generations, with sedation being prominent in first-generation medications due to the central anticholinergic effects. For the same reason, these agents typically have antiemetic and antimotion sickness properties. Meclizine and dimenhydrinate are commonly used for motion sickness. Diphenhydramine, cyclizine and promethazine have also been used to treat the symptoms of nausea and vomiting due to motion sickness. Hydroxyzine also has antiemetic properties[3–9]. Based on the antiemetic activity of the antihistamines and the evidence that motion sickness is a strong predictor of PONV, many of the histamine antagonists have been used and/or evaluated for management of PONV[1,10]. Second-generation antihistamines have not been found to have significant antiemetic properties[3].

Dimenhydrinate

Dimenhydrinate is an ethanolamine derivative and contains a diphenhydramine moiety, which is likely the source of its antiemetic effects. The drug is typically prescribed to treat motion sickness and its related nausea, vomiting and dizziness. The exact mechanism is unknown although the action is presumed to inhibit vestibular stimulation. The drug also inhibits the acetylcholine receptor. Dimenhydrinate is available as a tablet (50 mg) and a solution (12.5 mg/5 mL) as over-the-counter formulations[4]. Dimenhydrinate injectable 50 mg/mL is also available and used for many of the same symptoms and can be given by the

Postoperative Nausea and Vomiting: A Practical Guide, eds. Tong Joo Gan and Ashraf S. Habib. Published by Cambridge University Press.

Table 7.1 Dosages of histamine, muscarine and dopamine antagonists for management of PONV in adults

Class	Agent	Usual PONV dosage/route
Antihistamines	Dimenhydrinate	1–2 mg/kg or 50–100 mg IM, IV
	Diphenhydramine	12.5–50 mg IM, IV
	Meclizine	25–50 mg PO
	Cyclizine[a]	25–50 mg IM, IV
	Hydroxyzine	25–50 mg IM
Phenothiazines	Promethazine[b]	6.25–12.5 mg IV 12.5–25 mg IM
	Perphenazine	2–4 mg PO 2.5–5 mg IM[c]; 1 mg IV[c]
	Prochlorperazine	5–10 mg IM, IV
Butyrophenones	Droperidol	0.625–1.25 mg IV
	Haloperidol	0.5–2 mg IM, IV
Benzamides	Metoclopramide	10–20 mg IM, IV
Anticholinergics	Transdermal scopolamine	1.5 mg transdermal

IM, intramuscular; IV, intravenous; PO, oral.
[a] Not available in USA. [b]Also classified as an antihistamine. [c]Not available in parenteral form in USA.

intravenous (IV; diluted over a period of 2 min) or intramuscular (IM) route[4]. Small amounts of the drug are excreted in breast milk so nursing mothers should use appropriate caution[2,4,11].

The most frequent adverse reaction to dimenhydrinate is drowsiness. Symptoms of dizziness, dry mouth, nose and throat, blurred vision, difficult or painful urination, headache, anorexia, nervousness, restlessness or insomnia (particularly in pediatric patients), skin rash, thickening of bronchial secretions, tachycardia, epigastric distress, lassitude, excitation and nausea have been reported. This drug may be potentially inappropriate for use in geriatric patients. Common off-label uses of dimenhydrinate include treatment of Meniere's disease and nausea/vomiting related to pregnancy or anesthesia[2,4,11].

An inpatient, placebo-controlled study of females undergoing laparoscopic cholecystectomy, thyroid resection or knee arthroscopy found that 62 mg of dimenhydrinate IV given at induction with three additional doses over 48 h effectively decreased the incidence of PONV (38.8% versus 15.1%) and was associated with little to no significant side effects. Severe PONV was also reduced from 39.4% to 14.9%[12].

Prophylactic administration of dimenhydrinate 50 mg IV was found to be as effective as ondansetron 4 mg for prevention of PONV in patients undergoing elective laparoscopic cholecystectomy. The need for rescue antiemetics was 34% in the ondansetron group and 29% in the dimenhydrinate group[13].

Conversely, another study comparing dimenhydrinate 0.3 mg/kg and metoclopramide 0.3 mg/kg found both agents were ineffective for PONV prevention when given alone. However, the combination of both medications reduced the incidence of PONV compared with placebo[14].

Dimenhydrinate and promethazine were evaluated in patients initially receiving either prophylactic administration of droperidol 0.625 mg to 1.25 mg or ondansetron 4 mg. In patients who failed prophylaxis, rescue with dimenhydrinate 25–50 mg or promethazine 6.25–25 mg was more effective than a repeat (rescue) dose of the original prophylactic drug (droperidol or ondansetron)[15].

A meta-analysis of 18 trials including over 3,000 patients showed dimenhydrinate to be effective as a prophylactic antiemetic for patients at moderate-to-high risk for PONV with side effects similar to the placebo group. More research is needed to determine the most appropriate dose, timing and frequency for dimenhydrinate in the management of PONV[16]. The Society for Ambulatory Anesthesia guidelines for PONV concluded that dimenhydrinate, in placebo-controlled trials, has similar efficacy to the 5-HT_3 receptor antagonists, dexamethasone and droperidol[10].

Diphenhydramine

Diphenhydramine is a first-generation antihistamine and an ethanolamine derivative that acts at the H_1 receptors at the nucleus tractus solitarius and acetylcholine receptors in the vestibular apparatus. The antiemetic properties are thought to be a result of suppression of motion-enhanced vestibular neuronal firing, leading to its effectiveness in treating vertigo, motion sickness and PONV in high-risk patients, such as those having middle ear surgery or those with a history of motion sickness. Like other H_1 receptor antagonists, diphenhydramine can also be used to manage a multitude of other symptoms (urticaria, rhinitis, conjunctivitis, vertigo, insomnia or dyskinesia), that can be associated with other disease processes[3,5].

A study of 200 women who had total abdominal hysterectomies and utilized morphine patient-controlled analgesia regimens found that metoclopramide and diphenhydramine used in combination provided significantly better prevention of nausea and vomiting in the postoperative phase than either drug alone when added to patient-controlled morphine analgesia[17]. For every mg of morphine, metoclopramide 0.5 mg or diphenhydramine 0.6 mg or the combination of both were used.

Meclizine

Meclizine is a piperazine derivative antihistamine commonly used for prevention of motion sickness by depressing the labyrinth excitability and conduction in vestibular-cerebellar pathways. The antiemetic action is a result of the anticholinergic and central nervous system (CNS) depressant effects. The onset of action is 1 h with a duration of 24 h. Meclizine should be used with caution in patients with asthma, glaucoma (narrow angle), prostatic hyperplasia and pyloric/duodenal obstruction. Meclizine and dimenhydrinate are considered to have equal efficacy for motion sickness, although meclizine has less associated drowsiness and a longer duration of action[18]. Additionally, caution should be used in elderly patients. Meclizine is available in oral dosage form of 25 and 50 mg[6,10,11].

Few studies exist for use of meclizine as a single agent for treatment of PONV. However, a placebo-controlled study of 77 patients at high risk for PONV (four out of five major risk factors: general anesthesia, female, nonsmoker, motion sickness history and PONV history) showed that, when combined with ondansetron at surgical closure, preoperatively administered meclizine 50 mg effectively reduced PONV, as well as postdischarge nausea and vomiting, more than ondansetron alone[19].

Hydroxyzine

Hydroxyzine is piperazine derivative antihistamine. Hydroxyzine has antihistamine, analgesic, bronchodilation and antiemetic properties[1]. The drug competes with the histamine H_1 receptor site on effector cells in the gastrointestinal tract, blood vessels and respiratory tract. The antiemetic dose is 25–100 mg intramuscularly. The drug is a vesicant and IV administration is contraindicated, which limits some of its usefulness in the postoperative phase where IV administration is the preferred route. Hydroxyzine should be used with caution in the presence of glaucoma (narrow angle), prostatic hyperplasia/urinary stricture and respiratory disease. CNS depression can be a significant side effect. Therefore, care should be used in the elderly. Hydroxyzine may enhance the analgesic effects of opioids[1,7]. Limited studies on hydroxyzine's effectiveness for prevention of PONV exist. However, a study evaluated 150 patients who received droperidol 2.5 mg IM or hydroxyzine 100 mg IM at induction of anesthesia, and the hydroxyzine group were found to have less PONV than patients receiving droperidol 2.5 mg[20].

Cyclizine

Cyclizine is a piperazine derivative and a first-generation histamine antagonist, which is not available in the USA. Although the exact mechanism is unknown, it likely has a direct central effect on the labyrinthine apparatus and the chemoreceptor trigger zone (CTZ). Cyclizine is most commonly used for prophylaxis and treatment of nausea, vomiting and vertigo associated with motion sickness. Due to the anticholinergic effect, elderly patients should receive the lowest effective dose. Excess sedation is the most frequent side effect of this drug[1,8].

In a study in adults, cyclizine 50 mg was shown to have a similar efficacy to ondansetron 4 mg[21]. A trend was seen with the patients who received the cyclizine of having a longer mean time to eye opening, but it did not influence discharge times. However, in children, ondansetron 0.1 mg/kg significantly reduced vomiting events compared to cyclizine 20 mg[22]. Interestingly, in a Cochrane review of 737 studies, cyclizine was listed as one of the eight antiemetics that reliably prevented PONV[23].

Dopamine antagonists

Phenothiazines are used for the prevention and treatment of nausea and vomiting caused by various etiologies including PONV. Phenothiazine antiemetics act primarily via central dopamine (D_2) receptor blockade[1]. However, for nausea and vomiting in pregnancy, these drugs are either contraindicated or have not been proven safe and should only be used if the potential benefit justifies the risks to the fetus. Phenothiazines have numerous side effects; the very young and the very old appear to be most sensitive to those side effects[24]. Common phenothiazines used for PONV include prochlorperazine and promethazine. Phenothiazines are available as oral, parenteral and rectal formulations. These drugs may cause extrapyramidal symptoms such as dystonia, tardive dyskinesia and akathisia[1,2,9,24–26].

Promethazine

Promethazine is a histamine antagonist and a phenothiazine derivative with significant antidopaminergic and anticholinergic activity. The antimotion sickness action may be due to

Table 7.2 FDA recommendations for IV use of promethazine[29]

• Deep IM injection is the preferred way to administer promethazine hydrochloride injection, USP products
• Intra-arterial and subcutaneous administration of promethazine are contraindicated
• The 50 mg/mL promethazine hydrochloride injection, USP product is for deep IM injection only
• The 25 mg/mL promethazine hydrochloride injection, USP product may be administered by deep IM injection or IV injection
• If IV administration of promethazine is required, the maximum recommended concentration is 25 mg per mL and the maximum recommended rate of administration is 25 mg per min through the tubing of an IV infusion set known to be functioning properly
• Be alert for signs and symptoms of potential tissue injury including burning or pain at the site of injection, phlebitis, swelling and blistering
• Injections should be stopped immediately if a patient complains of pain during injection
• Inform patients that side effects may occur immediately while receiving the injection or may develop hours to days after an injection

IM, intramuscular; IV, intravenous.

the central anticholinergic effect on the vestibular apparatus, the integrative vomiting center and the medullary CTZ. Promethazine is more effective for motion sickness than the other phenothiazines[1,9], The onset of action is 3–5 min for IV administration and 20 min when given IM. Duration of action is 4–6 h but effects of the drug may last as long as 12 h[1,9,27].

Promethazine is available as an oral solution and tablets. Suppositories of various dosage strengths are also marketed. Injectable promethazine in 25 mg/mL (IV or IM) and 50 mg/mL (IM only) are the parenteral dosage forms. Because promethazine is a vesicant, deep IM injection is the preferred route of administration since severe tissue injury can occur following IV administration. The concern is an inadvertent intra-arterial needle placement or perivascular extravasation that may result in an ischemic injury. If the IV route must be used, the package insert calls for several safety strategies (Table 7.2). The US Food and Drug Administration (FDA) also issued a boxed warning against the use of promethazine in children <2 years of age due to postmarketing cases of sedation and respiratory depression. For the same reason, the FDA also recommends using caution when administering the drug to all pediatric patients. Similarly, the elderly can be particularly susceptible to these sedating effects. Due to the anticholinergic effects, extrapyramidal symptoms and neuroleptic malignant syndrome may occur. The medication should be avoided or used with caution in the presence of narrow angle glaucoma, Parkinson's disease, Myasthenia gravis, patients with seizures, respiratory and cardiovascular disease[1,3,9,24,27]. The adult antiemetic dose is 12.5–25 mg every 4–6 h, regardless of the route of administration. However, newer studies indicate a lower dose of 6.25 mg for PONV is effective and may cause less sedation compared to higher doses[9,27,28].

In a double-blind randomized placebo-controlled study of adult patients undergoing middle ear surgery, promethazine (12.5 mg) combined with ondansetron (2 mg) significantly reduced the incidence and severity of nausea, vomiting and PONV during the first 24 h postoperatively when compared to placebo or monotherapy[30].

A retrospective database analysis of patients undergoing general anesthesia who received ondansetron 4 mg prophylactically showed that doses of 6.25 mg, 12.5 mg and 25 mg all had similar efficacy and were all more effective for PONV rescue than a second dose of ondansetron. The 6.25 mg promethazine dose was as effective as the 12.5 and 25 mg doses[28].

Perphenazine

Perphenazine is a phenothiazine with a mechanism of action that includes blockade of postsynaptic mesolimbic dopaminergic receptors in the brain, blockade of alpha-adrenergic effect and depression of the release of hypothalamic and hypophyseal hormones. The drug is used for psychotic disorders and severe nausea and vomiting in adults. The drug is available as oral tablets[26]. Dosing for severe nausea and vomiting is 8–16 mg daily in divided doses; however, doses as high as 24 mg (maximum) have been used. Caution should be used in the geriatric population since the FDA has placed a boxed warning of increased mortality in elderly patients with dementia-related psychosis with the use of perphenazine[24,26].

A quantitative systematic review included 11 randomized controlled trials with 2,081 participants, receiving prophylactic perphenazine or another drug or placebo. Perphenazine doses were 2.5 mg and 5 mg or a weight-based calculation of 0.11 mg/kg. The children's dose was weight adjusted at 0.07 mg/kg. The doses were given orally, IM or IV (injectable form no longer available in USA). The authors concluded that perphenazine was well tolerated and is an effective medication for PONV prevention. The conclusion stated that further data are needed to determine the most appropriate dose, timing and route; however, the authors suggested 5 mg as the most efficacious dose[31].

Prochlorperazine

Prochlorperazine is a piperazine phenothiazine antipsychotic that blocks postsynaptic mesolimbic dopaminergic receptors, including the CTZ. The drug has a strong alpha-adrenergic and anticholinergic blocking effect. Prochlorperazine has strong antiemetic activity with a faster onset of action and less sedation than promethazine. The antiemetic doses are 5–10 mg IM or IV 15–30 min prior to induction of anesthesia or 5–10 mg every 3–4 h IM postsurgery. The IV dose should be given slowly to not exceed 5 mg/min or as an IV infusion. The maximum dose is 40 mg/day. The IM onset of action is 10–20 min and the peak antiemetic effect of IV administration is 30–60 min. Some of the side effects include anticholinergic effects, altered cardiac conduction, extrapyramidal symptoms, sedation and blood dyscrasias. A boxed warning is included in the labeling of increased mortality for patients with dementia and any use in the elderly may not be appropriate. Clinicians should use caution in patients with cardiovascular disease, narrow angle glaucoma, Parkinson's disease, seizure disorders, hepatic and/or renal impairment and Reye's syndrome[1,11,24].

A double-blind randomized trial compared ondansetron (4 mg IV) with prochlorperazine (10 mg IM) given at surgical closure for the prevention of PONV in 78 patients undergoing orthopedic procedures. Prochlorperazine was significantly more effective in preventing nausea and was associated with a lower incidence of severe nausea as compared with ondansetron. The reduction in mean number of emetic episodes did not reach statistical significance[32].

Droperidol

Droperidol is a butyrophenone antipsychotic, frequently referred to as a first-generation antipsychotic[33]. Droperidol exerts its antiemetic effect through the blockade of dopamine receptors in the CTZ. It also has alpha-adrenergic blockade activity, which may lead to vasodilation, orthostatic hypotension and reflex tachycardia. Droperidol also possesses low-level anticholinergic effects[33]. It can be administered intravascularly or intramuscularly in doses of 0.625–1.25 mg and can be repeated every 6 h as needed. The onset of action is 3–10 min with a peak effect at 30 min and an action of 2–4 h that can be prolonged up to 12 h in rare instances. Droperidol is excreted in the urine and feces and is known to cross the blood–brain barrier and the placenta. Its excretion in breast milk is not known and caution should be used in nursing mothers[33].

Droperidol 1.25 mg was found to have similar efficacy for PONV prophylaxis to ondansetron 4 mg and dexamethasone 4 mg, with each reducing PONV by about 25%[34]. The number needed-to-treat for prevention of early PONV for droperidol 75 μg/kg was found to be 5.3 if given at induction and 2.4 if given at the end of surgery or in the recovery room[35]. The combination of droperidol with ondansetron was found to be more effective than either drug alone and the QT prolongation was found to be equal to either drug used alone[36].

The use of droperidol as an antiemetic has been controversial since it was discovered to have an association with the development of life-threatening arrhythmias, most notably torsade de pointes. Due to this risk, the FDA issued a black box warning that patients should be evaluated for the presence of prolonged QT interval (QTc greater than 440 ms in males and 450 ms in females) prior to the use of droperidol. It is contraindicated if prolonged QT intervals exist. In addition, it is recommended that 2–3 h of continuous electrocardiogram monitoring be completed after administration of droperidol. Since this FDA warning, droperidol use for PONV prophylaxis in the USA has dropped significantly; however, it continues to be used routinely for PONV prophylaxis in the majority of European countries[37].

Numerous investigators have attempted to show that droperidol's black box warning is excessive and unnecessary. Droperidol was found in one study of 85 patients to have equal incidence of QTc prolongation as ondansetron[38]. Another study showed that there was an indistinguishable QTc prolongation caused by both saline and droperidol when given before general anesthesia[39]. A large study of over 20,000 patients given over 35,000 doses of droperidol 0.625 mg revealed that none of the patients developed polymorphic ventricular tachycardia. Interestingly, over 500 of those patients had known prolonged QT intervals. This suggests that the association of prolonged QT intervals, low-dose droperidol, and ventricular tachycardia, if it exists at all, is likely a very rare phenomenon[40].

As with other drugs in the same class, extrapyramidal symptoms may rarely occur[35]. Because of its antidopaminergic effects, droperidol should be used with caution in patients with Parkinson's disease. Moreover, droperidol has sedating properties and should be used with caution in susceptible patient populations[33].

Haloperidol

Haloperidol is a butyrophenone antipsychotic, similar in activity to droperidol. It blocks dopaminergic D_1 and D_2 receptors in the brain[41]. Typically, haloperidol is used to treat psychiatric disorders; however, following droperidol's FDA black box warning, its use has been explored as an alternative for PONV. Interestingly, haloperidol is approved for oral or IM use, but IV administration is not an FDA approved route of administration. Haloperidol has an onset of 30–60 min, a half-life of 18 h, and is eliminated in urine and feces. It is excreted in breast milk and not recommended for nursing mothers[41].

Haloperidol at low doses (0.5–2 mg IV or IM) has shown antiemetic effects with a number needed-to-treat of between 4 and 6[42]. At low doses, sedation does not occur and arrhythmias have not been reported. Although haloperidol carries a risk of QT prolongation, the risk was found to be equal to ondansetron and placebo in a study of 93 patients[43], However, given the potential for arrhythmias, haloperidol is not recommended as a first-line therapy[10]. Low-dose haloperidol (1 mg) was found to be as effective as 0.625 mg of droperidol for PONV[44]. Another randomized, placebo-controlled study of 244 patients in a mixed surgical population found the same low dose of haloperidol to be comparable to ondansetron 4 mg for the prevention of PONV[45]. Efficacy of haloperidol can be increased by combining it with other agents, such as 5-HT_3 receptor antagonists[46].

The side-effect profile for haloperidol is similar to droperidol, although at low doses, the risk of sedation, extrapyramidal effects and cardiac arrhythmias are thought to be very low. However, it must be remembered that the FDA has warned that elderly patients with dementia-related psychosis who are treated with antipsychotic drugs are at an increased risk of death, although the cause and effect are not understood[41].

Metoclopramide

Metoclopramide blocks dopamine receptors and also, in high doses, blocks serotonin receptors in the CTZ as well as accelerating gastric emptying and increasing lower esophageal sphincter tone. In IV form, its onset occurs in 1–3 min with a duration of 2 h. It is excreted mostly in the urine but also enters breast milk, so caution should be used in nursing mothers[47].

Metoclopramide is considered a weak antiemetic. At low doses of 10 mg, metoclopramide has been shown to be ineffective for reducing the incidence of PONV[48]. However, a large study of over 3,000 patients showed that, combined with dexamethasone 8 mg, metoclopramide in doses of 25 and 50 mg had a similar effect on early PONV to ondansetron 4 mg[49].

Due to its dopamine blocking effects, metoclopramide can lead to extrapyramidal effects or tardive dyskinesia with a number needed-to-harm of 140[49]. For the same reason, it should be avoided in patients with Parkinson's disease. It can also lead to paradoxical worsening of hypertension in patients with pheochromocytoma. Because of its effect on gastric motility, it should be avoided in patients with intestinal obstruction.

Muscarinic antagonists

Transdermal scopolamine is a centrally acting anticholinergic agent that was initially developed for the treatment of motion sickness but was approved in 2001 by the FDA for the treatment of PONV. It blocks the action of acetylcholine in smooth muscle, secretory glands, and CNS regions of the parasympathetic nervous system. Scopolamine also antagonizes histamine and serotonin[50]. Onset of action in the transdermal form can take 6–8 h, so it is typically placed the evening prior to surgery or 2–4 h prior to surgery. It can also be applied up to the time of surgery and may still be somewhat effective if the length of surgery is prolonged. Scopolamine is metabolized in the urine and excreted in the urine and feces. It is also excreted in breast milk, so caution must be used if scopolamine is administered to nursing mothers[50]. Transdermal scopolamine is typically available in a 1.5 mg patch and is programmed to deliver this dose over 72 h[50].

Transdermal scopolamine can be used as a single agent for PONV prophylaxis and has been shown to be as effective as ondansetron or droperidol[51,52]. It can also be combined with other agents to reduce the incidence of PONV more than single agents alone[53].

The typical anticholinergic side effects of scopolamine are generally mild when delivered transdermally. The most common symptoms include visual disturbances (typically worse at 24–48 h), dry mouth and dizziness[53]. Patients and providers must be educated to wash their hands thoroughly after handling the patch and to avoid eye contact, since it has been reported to cause unilateral mydriasis, which can cloud the clinical picture, particularly in patients who may have other factors that could lead to anisocoria[54].

References

1. Kovac A. Prevention and treatment of postoperative nausea and vomiting. *Drugs* 2000; 59: 213–43.
2. Golembiewski J, Tokumara S. Pharmacological prophylaxis and management of adult postoperative/postdischarge nausea and vomiting. *J Perianesth Nurs* 2006; 21: 385–97.
3. McEvoy GK, Snow ED, eds. *AHFS: Drug Information*. Bethesda, MD: American Society of Health-System Pharmacists, 2013; 1–14.
4. Wolters Kluwer. *Lexicomp* Online: Dimenhydrinate, 2014. http://online.lexi.com/lco/action/search?q=dimenhydrinate&t=name. (Accessed October 25, 2014.)
5. Wolters Kluwer. *Lexicomp* Online: Diphenhydramine. 2014. http://online.lexi.com/lco/action/search?q=diphenhydramine&t=name. (Accessed October 25, 2014.)
6. Wolters Kluwer. *Lexicomp* Online: Meclizine, 2014 http://online.lexi.com/lco/action/search?q=meclizine&t=name. (Accessed October 25, 2014.)
7. Wolters Kluwer. *Lexicomp* Online: Hydroxyzine, 2014. http://online.lexi.com/lco/action/search?q=hydroxyzine&t=name. (Accessed October 25, 2014.)
8. Wolters Kluwer. *Lexicomp* Online: Cyclizine, 2014. http://online.lexi.com/lco/action/search?q=cyclizine&t=name. (Accessed October 25, 2014.)
9. Wolters Kluwer. *Lexicomp* Online: Promethazine, 2014. http://online.lexi.com/lco/action/search?q=promethazine&t=name. (Accessed October 25, 2014.)
10. Gan TJ, Diemunsch P, Habib A, et al. Consensus guidelines for the management of postoperative nausea and vomiting. *Anesth Analg* 2014; 118: 85–113.
11. McEvoy GK, Snow ED, eds. *AHFS: Drug Information*. Bethesda, MD: American Society of Health-System Pharmacists, 2013; 2942–5.
12. Eberhart LH, Seeling W, Bopp TI, et al. Dimenhydrinate for prevention of post-operative nausea and vomiting in female in-patients. *Eur J Anaesthesiol* 1999; 16: 284–9.
13. Kothari SN, Boyd WC, Bottcher ML, et al. Antiemetic efficacy of prophylactic dimenhydrinate (Dramamine) vs. ondansetron (Zofran): a randomized, prospective trial inpatients undergoing laparoscopic cholecystectomy. *Surg Endosc* 2000; 14: 926–9.
14. Eberhart LH, Seeling W, Ulrich B, et al. Dimenhydrinate and metoclopramide alone or in combination for prophylaxis of PONV. *J Clin Anesth* 2000; 47: 780–5.
15. Habib A, Gan TJ. The effectiveness of rescue antiemetics after failure of prophylaxis with ondansetron or droperidol: a preliminary report. *J Clin Anesth* 2005; 17: 62–5.
16. Kranke P, Morin AM, Roewer N, et al. Dimenhydrinate for prophylaxis of postoperative nausea and vomiting: a meta-analysis of randomized controlled trials. *Acta Anaesthesiol Scand* 2002; 46: 238–44.

17. Lu CW, Jean WH, Wu CC, et al. Antiemetic efficacy of metoclopramide and diphenhydramine added to patient-controlled morphine analgesia: a randomised controlled trial. *Eur J Anaesthesiol* 2010; 27: 1052–7.

18. Priesol AJ, Deschler DG, Park L. Motion sickness. http://www.uptodate.com/contents/search?source=USER_PREF&search (Accessed October 27, 2014.)

19. Forrester CM, Benfield DA, Matern CE, et al. Meclizine in combination with ondansetron for prevention of postoperative nausea and vomiting in high risk population. *AANA* 2007; 75: 27–33.

20. McKenzie R, Wadhwa RK, Uy NT, et al. Antiemetic effectiveness of intramuscular hydroxyzine compare with intramuscular droperidol. *Anesth Analg* 1981; 60: 783–8.

21. Grimsehl K, Whiteside JB, Mackenzie N. Comparison of cyclizine and ondansetron for the prevention of postoperative nausea and vomiting in laparoscopic day-case gynaecological surgery. *Anaesthesia* 2002: 57: 61–5.

22. O'Brien CM, Titley G, Whitehouse P. A comparison of cylcizine, ondansetron and placebo as prophylaxis against postoperative nausea and vomiting in children. *Anaesthesia* 2003; 58: 707–11.

23. Carlisle J, Stevenson CA. Drugs for preventing postoperative nausea and vomiting. *Cochrane Database Syst Rev* 2006; 19: CD004125.

24. McEvoy GK, Snow ED (eds). *AHFS: Drug Information*. Bethesda, MD: American Society of Health-System Pharmacists; 2013: 2528–45.

25. Wolters Kluwer. *Lexicomp* Online: Prochlorperazine, 2014. http://online.lexi.com/lco/action/search?t=name&q=Prochlorperazine (Accessed October 25, 2014.)

26. Wolters Kluwer. *Lexicomp* Online: Perphenazine, 2014. http://online.lexi.com/lco/action/search?t=name&q=Perphenazine. (Accessed October 25, 2014.)

27. McEvoy GK, Snow ED, (eds). *AHFS: Drug Information*. Bethesda, MD, American Society of Health-System Pharmacists, 2013; 2631–3.

28. Habib AS, Reuveni J, Taguchi A, et al. A comparison of ondansetron with promethazine for treating postoperative nausea and vomiting in patients who received prophylaxis with ondansetron: a retrospective database analysis. *Anesth Analg* 2007; 104: 548–51.

29. US Food and Drug Administration. Information for Healthcare Professionals: Intravenous Promethazine and Severe Tissue Injury, Including Gangrene. http://www.fda.gov/Drugs/DrugSafety/PostmarketDrugSafetyInformationforPatientsandProviders/DrugSafetyInformationforHeathcareProfessionals/ucm182169.htm# (Accessed November 4, 2014.)

30. Khalil S, Philbrook L, Rabb M, et al. Ondansetron/promethazine combination or promethazine for the prevention alone reduces nausea and vomiting after middle ear surgery. *J Clin Anesth* 1999; 11: 596–600.

31. Schnabel A, Eberhart LH, Muellenbach R, et al. Efficacy of perphenazine to prevent postoperative nausea and vomiting: a quantitative systematic review. *Eur J Anesthesiol* 2010; 27: 1044–51.

32. Chen JJ, Frame DG, White TJ. Efficacy of ondansetron and prochlorperazine for the prevention of postoperative nausea and vomiting after total hip replacement or total knee replacement procedures: a randomized, double-blind, comparative trial. *Arch Intern Med* 1998; 158: 2124–8.

33. Wolters Kluwer. *Lexicomp* Online: Droperidol, 2014. http://online.lexi.com/lco/action/search?q=droperidol&t=name. (Accessed October 25, 2014.)

34. Apfel CC, Korttila K, Abdalla M, et al. A factorial trial of six interventions for the prevention of postoperative nausea and vomiting. *N Engl J Med* 2004; 350: 2441–51.

35. Henzi I, Sonderegger J, Tramèr MR. Efficacy, dose–response, and adverse effects of droperidol for prevention of postoperative nausea and vomiting. *Can J Anaesth* 2000; 47: 537–51.

36. Chan MT, Choi KC, Gin T, et al. The additive interactions between ondansetron and droperidol for preventing postoperative nausea and vomiting. *Anesth Analg* 2006; 103: 1155–62.

37. Schaub I, Lysakowski C, Elia N, et al. Low-dose droperidol (≤1 mg or ≤15 μg kg-1) for the prevention of postoperative nausea and vomiting in adults: quantitative systematic review of randomised controlled trials. *Eur J Anaesthesiol* 2012; 29(6): 286–94.

38. Charbit B, Albaladejo P, Funck-Brentano C, et al. Prolongation of QTc interval after postoperative nausea and vomiting treatment by droperidol or ondansetron. *Anesthesiology* 2005; 102: 1094–100.

39. White PF, Song D, Abrao J, et al. Effect of low-dose droperidol on the QT interval during and after general anesthesia: a placebo-controlled study. *Anesthesiology* 2005; 102: 1101–5.

40. Nuttall GA, Malone AM, Michels CA, et al. Does low-dose droperidol increase the risk of polymorphic ventricular tachycardia or death in the surgical patient? *Anesthesiology* 2013; 118: 382–6.

41. Wolters Kluwer. *Lexicomp* Online: Haloperidol, 2014. http://online.lexi.com/lco/action/search?q=haloperidol&t=name. (Accessed October 25, 2014.)

42. Büttner M, Walder B, von Elm E, et al. Is low-dose haloperidol a useful antiemetic?: A meta-analysis of published and unpublished randomized trials. *Anesthesiology* 2004; 101: 1454–63.

43. Aouad MT, Siddik-Sayyid SM, Taha SK, et al. Haloperidol vs. ondansetron for the prevention of postoperative nausea and vomiting following gynaecological surgery. *Eur J Anaesthesiol* 2007; 24: 171–8.

44. Wang TF, Liu YH, Chu CC, et al. Low-dose haloperidol prevents post-operative nausea and vomiting after ambulatory laparoscopic surgery. *Acta Anaesthesiol Scand* 2008; 52: 280–4.

45. Rosow CE, Haspel KL, Smith SE, et al. Haloperidol versus ondansetron for prophylaxis of postoperative nausea and vomiting. *Anesth Analg* 2008; 106: 1407–9.

46. Feng PH, Chu KS, Lu IC, et al. Haloperidol plus ondansetron prevents postoperative nausea and vomiting in patients undergoing laparoscopic cholecystectomy. *Acta Anaesthesiol Taiwan* 2009; 47(1): 3–9.

47. Wolters Kluwer. *Lexicomp* Online: Metoclopramide. 2014. http://online.lexi.com/lco/action/search?q=metocl&t=name. (Accessed October 25, 2014.)

48. Henzi I, Walder B, Tramèr MR. Metoclopramide in the prevention of postoperative nausea and vomiting: a quantitative systematic review of randomized, placebo-controlled studies. *Br J Anaesth* 1999; 83: 761–71.

49. Wallenborn J, Gelbrich G, Bulst D, et al. Prevention of postoperative nausea and vomiting by metoclopramide combined with dexamethasone: randomised double blind multicentre trial. *BMJ* 2006; 12: 324.

50. Wolters Kluwer. *Lexicomp* Online: Scopolamine. 2014. http://online.lexi.com/lco/action/doc/retrieve/docid/patch_f/1801741. (Accessed October 25, 2014.)

51. Bailey PL, Streisand JB, Pace NL et al. Transdermal scopolamine reduces nausea and vomiting after outpatient laparoscopy. *Anesthesiology* 1990; 72: 977–80.

52. White PF, Tang J, Song D, et al. Transdermal scopolamine: an alternative to ondansetron and droperidol for the prevention of postoperative and postdischarge emetic symptoms. *Anesth Analg* 2007; 104: 92–6.

53. Apfel CC, Zhang K, George E, et al. Transdermal scopolamine for the prevention of postoperative nausea and vomiting: a systematic review and meta-analysis. *Clin Ther* 2010; 32: 1987–2002.

54. Lee DT, Jenkins NL, Anastasopulos AJ. Transdermal scopolamine and perioperative anisocoria in craniofacial surgery: a report of 3 patients. *J Craniofac Surg* 2013; 24: 470–2.

Chapter 8

Pharmacology of neurokinin antagonists and novel antiemetics

Linda M.L. Lai, William K.K. Wu and Matthew T.V. Chan

In 1931, von Euler and Gaddum identified a mysterious protein from the extract of horse brain that would produce rapid smooth muscle contraction in isolated intestine[1]. The extract was stored as dried powder and was conveniently referred as substance P (for "powder"). Animal research has since found that substance P was concentrated in the vomiting center of the brain[2–4]. When substance P was given intravenously or applied topically to the area posterma, the animals reacted with profuse vomiting and retching[5]. In contrast, as endogenous substance P was depleted by the administration of resiniferatoxin, there was marked reduction in vomiting even in the presence of potent emetogenic stimuli[6]. These findings suggested that pharmacologic modulation of the interaction between substance P and its receptor, neurokinin type 1 (NK_1), would be helpful in managing vomiting. The purpose of this chapter is to outline the development and current research progress of NK_1-receptor antagonists for the management of postoperative nausea and vomiting (PONV). In addition, we also discuss the pharmacology of an emerging antiemetic for PONV – amisulpride.

Substance P and the NK_1 receptor

Substance P is an 11-amino acid neuropeptide[7,8] and is the first and the most notable member of the tachykinin family. The other members in the family include neurokinin A, neurokinin B, neuropeptide K, neuropeptide γ, hemokinin-1 and endokinin A–D[9]. These molecules bind to three neurokinin receptors (NK_1, NK_2 and NK_3), encoded by the tachykinin receptor (*Tacr)* genes[9,10]. It is known that substance P binds preferentially to the NK_1 receptor. Therefore, the bulk of research has focused on the NK_1 receptor (Table 8.1) [9,11,12].

NK_1 receptor is a G-protein coupled receptor that contains seven membrane-spanning domains with three extracellular and three intracellular loops. It is widely expressed in the central and enteric nervous systems[9,13]. After binding to the NK_1 receptor, substance P activates a number of signaling pathways[9]. This includes mobilization of intracellular calcium stores through the phospholipase C pathway, activation of adenylate cyclase and the formation of cyclic adenosine 3′-5′-monophosphate resulting in the stimulation of protein kinase A and activation of phospholipase A_2, generating arachidonic acid and other pro-inflammatory mediators. Recent studies suggested that the receptor interaction also activates Rho-associated protein kinases, leading to the production of microparticles, derived

Postoperative Nausea and Vomiting: A Practical Guide, eds. Tong Joo Gan and Ashraf S. Habib. Published by Cambridge University Press.

Table 8.1 NK receptor subtypes

Receptor	Encoding gene	Distribution	Ligand binding affinity
Neurokinin-1 (NK_1)	*Tacr1*	CNS and peripheral tissues (e.g., GI tract, urinary bladder and lung)	SP >> NKA > NKB
Neurokinin-2 (NK_2)	*Tacr2*	Smooth muscles in GI tract, bronchial tree and urinary bladder. Little expression in the CNS	NKA > NKB > SP
Neurokinin-3 (NK_3)	*Tacr3*	CNS, rarely found in peripheral tissue	NKB > NKA > SP

CNS, central nervous system; GI, gastrointestinal; SP, substance P; NKA, neurokinin A; NKB, neurokinin B; *Tacr*, tachykinin receptor gene.

from membrane blebbing for intercellular communication[14]. Substance P has also been shown to transactivate epidermal growth factor receptor, which leads to mitogenesis and proliferation[15]. With the extensive postreceptor signaling, it is not surprising to note that receptor interaction produces a wide range of effects, including neuronal excitation, inflammation, cell proliferation and migration[9]. In this respect, substance P has been implicated in nausea and vomiting, asthma, chronic pain disorders, pruritus, psychosis and affective disorders, malignancy and inflammatory bowel disease[9,11].

Development of NK_1-receptor antagonists

Given the therapeutic potentials, a number of NK_1-receptor antagonists have been produced since the early 1980s. By substituting L-amino acids with their D-forms, Engberg and co-workers produced the first synthetic analogue of substance P that blocked the interaction with its receptor in a competitive fashion[16]. Others have developed peptidomimetic molecules with side-chains that contain part of the amino acid sequence for substance P[12]. These compounds were potent inhibitors of NK_1 receptor in cellular experiments. However, the peptides were too bulky to pass through the blood–brain barrier and were excluded from further development[17].

In order to increase central nervous system penetration, smaller compounds were developed (Figure 8.1). To date, over 500 patents for non-peptide NK_1-receptor antagonist have been filed[18,19]. Naturally, only a handful of these compounds were eventually tested in clinical context. The first non-peptide NK_1-receptor antagonist (CP96345) was produced by Pfizer in 1991 following an extensive search in their chemical library[20]. This compound contained a rigid quinuclidine scaffold that conferred stereochemical properties. Together with the benzhydryl group and an *o*-methoxybenzylamine moiety, they provided the binding elements for the NK_1 receptor. Subsequent modifications by replacing the quinuclidine scaffold with a piperidine ring and substituting the benzhydryl moiety with a phenyl group, resulted in a compound (CP99994) with higher receptor affinity and more potent inhibition[21]. Clinical utility of these two compounds were, however, limited because they interacted with calcium channels leading to undesirable cardiovascular effects, such as hypotension and bradycardia[12,22].

Using CP96345 and CP99994 as templates for drug design, Merck synthesized the first commercially available NK_1 antagonist – aprepitant[23,24]. In this drug, the piperidine ring was replaced by a morpholine ring to improve oral absorption, and an electron-withdrawing group was attached to the piperidine nitrogen to avoid calcium-channel activation. Finally,

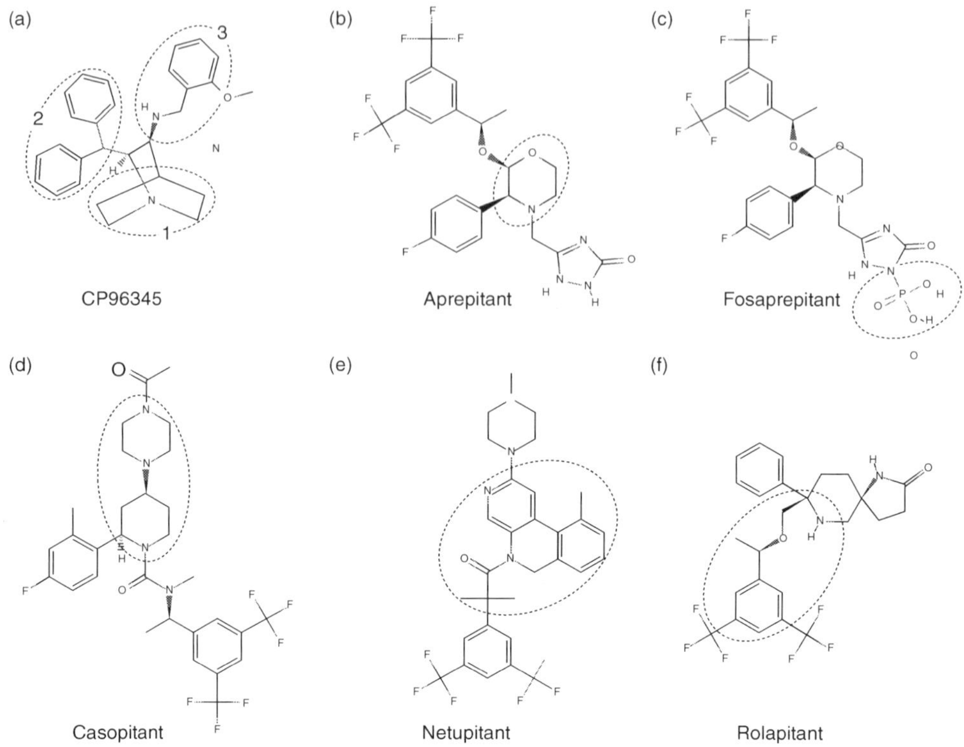

Figure 8.1 Structures of neurokinin-1 (NK_1)-receptor antagonists according to the PubChem database. (a) CP96345 (PubChem CID 104943). The binding elements for NK_1 receptor are shown in dotted circles: (1) quinuclidine group; (2) benzhydryl group; and (3) *o*-methoxybenzylamine group. (b) Aprepitant (PubChem CID 151165) with the morpholine ring highlighted. (c) Fosaprepitant (PubChem CID 219090) with the phosphate group on the oxotriazolyl ring shown. (d) Casopitant (PubChem CID 9917021) with the phenylpiperazine ring shown. (e) Netupitant (PubChem CID 6451149) showing the aryl-isoxazol group. (f) Rolapitant (PubChem CID 10311306) with the phenylglycinol group highlighted. (National Center for Biotechnology Information http://pubchem.ncbi.nlm.nih.gov/ accessed July 10, 2015.)

metabolic stability was achieved by methylation of alpha-carbon and fluorination of the aromatic ring. Recently, a water-soluble prodrug of aprepitant was produced (fosaprepitant) by phosphorylation of the oxotriazolyl ring and has been given intravenously[25].

In parallel, several pharmaceutical companies were interested in developing NK_1-receptor antagonists for a variety of indications. GlaxoSmithKline found that molecules with phenylpiperazine rings bound to the NK_1 receptor readily[26]. Among these compounds, casopitant was the most active. The drug was tested in a series of phase III clinical trials for preventing nausea and vomiting after chemotherapy and surgery. However, further development was discontinued in 2009 because substantial work was needed to fulfill regulatory requirements. Netupitant was developed by Roche, which was modified from aryl-isoxazoles and recently approved for the prevention of chemotherapy-induced nausea and vomiting (CINV)[27]. Rolapitant was developed by Schering-Plough, which is a phenylglycinol derivative and is currently under evaluation by a number of regulatory authorities[28].

Effects of NK_1-receptor antagonists

NK_1 receptor blockade demonstrates profound anti-inflammatory effects in cellular experiments[9]. Depending on the sites of action, NK_1-receptor antagonists produce diverse effects in different organ systems. Table 8.2 shows a summary of the therapeutic effects of NK_1-receptor antagonists observed in preclinical studies.

These therapeutic effects can be summarized as follows:

(1) Centrally and peripherally acting NK_1 antagonists were effective in attenuating nociceptive responses in different experimental pain models, particularly those related to nerve injury and tissue inflammation, among different species (e.g., gerbils, rats and guinea pigs)[29,30].
(2) In dogs and ferrets, NK_1-receptor antagonists were highly effective against all forms of emetic stimuli[31,32].
(3) Dual selective NK_1/NK_2 receptor antagonist (DNK333) reduced airway responsiveness to allergen challenge in guinea pig[33].
(4) DNK333 attenuated gut secretion and motility, but did not affect normal gut peristalsis[34,35].
(5) NK_1-receptor antagonist reduced scratching behavior in a mouse model of dermatitis[36].
(6) NK_1-receptor antagonist (TAK637) reduced detrusor hyperreflexia in a guinea pig model of capsaicin-induced bladder contraction[37].
(7) NK_1 antagonists produced anxiolytic-like effect in cats[38] and attenuated vocalization due to maternal separation in guinea pigs; these data suggested a potential antidepressant effect[39].
(8) Intraperitoneal aprepitant reduced fibrous adhesions following experimental laparotomy in rats[40].
(9) NK_1 antagonists (SR140333) reduced leukocyte recruitment and prevented lung injury in a Swiss mouse model of polymicrobial sepsis[41].
(10) In cellular experiments, NK_1-receptor antagonist (L733060) suppressed proliferation of colonic carcinoma[42].

Despite the benefits shown in cell and animal experiments, replication of these findings in adequately designed clinical trials has been largely disappointing. Currently, apart from the management of nausea and vomiting, there is a lack of clinical evidence to show that NK_1 antagonists could be used to alleviate pruritus, bronchial hypersensitivity[43] or symptoms associated with irritable bowel syndrome and overactive bladder[34,44]. There is also a lack of efficacy for NK_1 antagonists to reduce pain[45]. In a small trial of 78 patients having third molar extraction, an infusion of CP99994 (750 µg/kg) prior to surgery produced limited analgesia that lasted <90 min. More importantly, pain relief was inferior to oral ibuprofen 600 mg[46]. In another study evaluating the effects of aprepitant on PONV in 60 women having gynecologic laparoscopic surgery, consumption of postoperative analgesics was reduced by half in patients receiving aprepitant, but there was no difference in pain score between groups[47]. Other studies have also failed to demonstrate useful analgesia with NK_1 antagonists in migraine[48,49] and pain associated with osteoarthritis and diabetic neuropathy[43,50,51]. Similarly, NK_1 antagonists did not appear to relieve symptoms of major depression or other

Table 8.2 Effects of NK_1-receptor antagonism in preclinical studies and clinical trials

Effects	Preclinical study	Clinical trials
Analgesia	++	–
Antiemetic	+++	+++
Reduce bronchial hypersensitivity	++	–
Reduce gut hypermotility	++	±
Antipruritic	+	?
Reduce detrusor hyperreflexia	++	±
Reduce postoperative fibrous adhesion	++	±
Antidepressant	++	±
Antisepsis	++	?
Antineoplastic	++	?

+++, marked effect; ++, moderate effect; –, no effect; ±, equivocal data; ?, no clinical trial has been performed.

affective and addictive disorders[52]. There is currently no study evaluating the effects of NK_1-receptor antagonists in sepsis or cancer growth.

It is unclear why human studies have failed to confirm the findings in preclinical experiments. Investigators have speculated that differences in receptor function and distribution among species may have contributed to the discrepancy[9,45,53]. Nevertheless, the lack of effect of NK_1-receptor antagonists for other indications in humans added to the safety profile of these compounds for PONV.

NK_1-receptor antagonists for managing nausea and vomiting

Currently, clinical application of NK_1-receptor antagonists is largely limited to the management of nausea and vomiting. In particular, research has focused on the use of these compounds to control CINV and those following anesthesia and surgery.

Chemotherapy-induced nausea and vomiting

In an early trial, a single dose of fosaprepitant (60 or 100 mg) given intravenously was found to be ineffective to prevent acute (<24 h) vomiting following cisplatin treatment, but the control for delayed (day 2–7) nausea and vomiting was superior in the fosaprepitant group compared with ondansetron[54]. Subsequent trials, however, showed that the addition of NK_1-receptor antagonists (vofopitant[55], CP122721[56], ezlopitant[57], aprepitant[58–64] and casopitant[65–68]) to ondansetron or granisetron ($5\text{-}HT_3$ antagonists) and dexamethasone (i.e., triple therapy) increased the complete response rate (defined as no vomiting and no need for rescue antiemetic) from 42–61% to 51–86% (relative increase of 18–47%) in both acute and delayed phases. These data demonstrated that multimodal therapy using a combination of antiemetics is required when dealing with intense emetogenic stimuli. Based on this idea, a longer-acting NK_1-receptor antagonist (netupitant) is currently marketed as a combination pill, which included another long-acting $5\text{-}HT_3$-receptor antagonist (palonosetron) in a fixed-dose ratio. In a series of phase III studies, NEPA (netupitant 300 mg and palonosetron 0.5 mg) was highly effective and prevented vomiting in 98.5% of patients receiving cisplatin chemotherapy in the acute phase and 91.9% in the subsequent 4 days[69]. In another trial, NEPA with dexamethasone was compared with palonosetron and dexamethasone in patients having moderately emetogenic chemotherapy. The complete response rate was increased from 66.6% to 74.3%[70]. Finally, in patients having repeated cycles of chemotherapy, prophylaxis with NEPA and dexamethasone performed similarly to that of aprepitant regimen with an overall complete response rate >76%[71]. The current guidelines from the European Society of Medical Oncology and the Multinational Association of Supportive Care in Cancer recommend the addition of an NK_1-receptor antagonist to a $5\text{-}HT_3$-receptor antagonist and dexamethasone for the prophylaxis of nausea and vomiting after highly emetogenic chemotherapy[72]. At present, aprepitant, fosaprepitant and NEPA are approved for managing CINV.

Postoperative nausea and vomiting

Building on the success of NK_1-receptor antagonists in CINV, investigators moved quickly to evaluate the impact of these drugs in preventing PONV. The first clinical study was a small randomized trial in 36 women having major gynecologic surgery. Intravenous vofopitant (GR205171) 25 mg compared with placebo reduced the incidence of vomiting, severity of nausea and the requirement for rescue antiemetic[73]. In another study using CP122721 100–200 mg orally in women having abdominal hysterectomy (n = 243), the effect was striking. During the entire 72-h study period, the incidence of vomiting and retching was reduced from 80% in the placebo group to 46% in patients receiving CP122721, with a number needed-to-treat of 3 (95% confidence intervals (CI), 1.9–6.9)[74]. The drug also compared favorably with ondansetron. Over the first day after surgery, the incidence of vomiting in CP122721 group was 11.1% and was significantly lower than that in the ondansetron group (46.2%, $P = 0.002$). Unfortunately, both drugs were not further developed for commercialization.

Two larger-scale, multicenter parallel studies evaluated the efficacy of aprepitant for the prevention of PONV in patients having major abdominal surgery[75,76]. Based on an identical protocol, the two trials compared aprepitant 40 and 125 mg with ondansetron 4 mg as active control. Both trials reported a profound reduction in postoperative vomiting (POV) after aprepitant treatment compared with ondansetron (11.6% versus 27.6%; odds ratio (OR), 0.34; 95% CI, 0.26–0.45; $P < 0.001$)[77]. However, the effect of aprepitant on postoperative nausea was less obvious. Sixty-two percent of patients in the aprepitant group reported nausea in the first day after surgery and 79% of these patients had significant nausea with a visual nausea score >4 out of 10. Aprepitant (40 mg) seemed to produce a similar effect compared with aprepitant 125 mg (Figure 8.2) [76], but it is unclear whether bigger doses of aprepitant would produce better protection. Further dose–response studies may be required to define the optimal dose of aprepitant for preventing PONV. When compared with ondansetron, there was only a marginal effect for aprepitant to prevent nausea (OR, 0.81; 95% CI, 0.65–1.00; $P = 0.05$)[75–77]. The preferential effect of aprepitant on POV was again demonstrated in subsequent trials of patients having craniotomy[78,79], ambulatory procedures[80], gynecologic[81,82], rhinolaryngologic[83] and bariatric surgery[84]. Overall, the number of patients needed to be treated with aprepitant, instead of $5\text{-}HT_3$-receptor antagonists, in order to avoid an episode of POV was 6 (95% CI, 4.9–7.6). In contrast, the corresponding number for avoiding nausea was 12 (95% CI, 7.2–23.8).

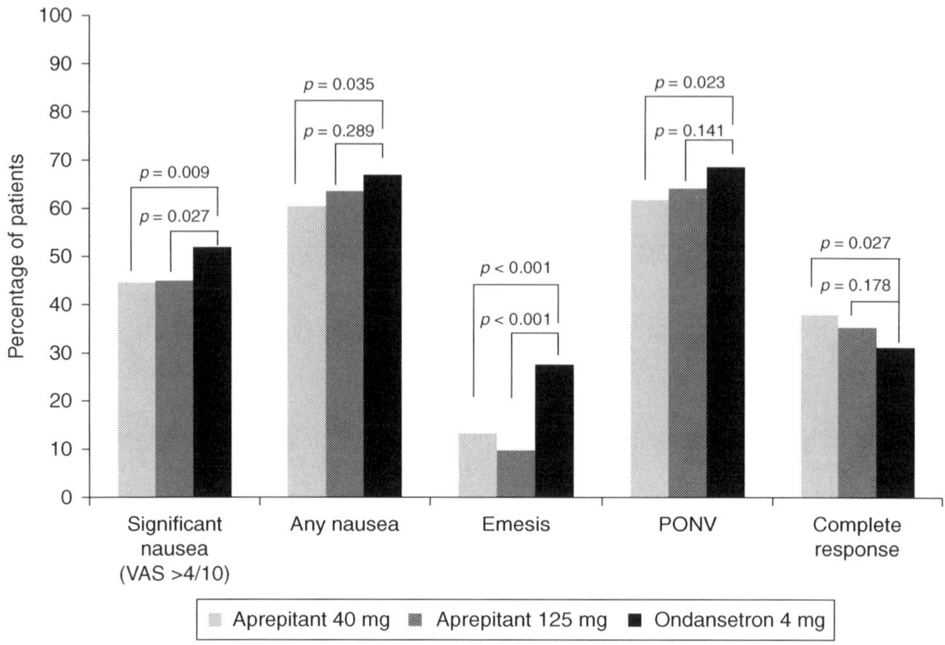

Figure 8.2 Percentage of patients reporting significant nausea, vomiting, postoperative nausea and vomiting (PONV) and complete response in trials comparing aprepitant 40 mg ($n = 541$) and 125 mg ($n = 532$), and ondansetron 4 mg ($n = 526$). VAS, visual analog scale.

Similar results were reported for casopitant. In 1,700 women at high risk of PONV, the incidence of POV was reduced from 28% in the ondansetron group to 8.8% in those receiving casopitant 50–150 mg (OR 0.25; 95% CI, 0.17–0.35; $P < 0.001$)[85,86]. The impact of casopitant on nausea remained suboptimal. Finally, in 619 patients having open abdominal surgery, rolapitant (a longer-acting NK_1-receptor antagonist) at doses of 70 or 200 mg prevented PONV between 24–120 h after surgery compared with ondansetron (25.6% versus 38.5%, $P = 0.03$)[87]. In both groups, >83% reported nausea during the study period.

Current data suggest that NK_1-receptor antagonists are potent antiemetics that could reduce the incidence of POV to ≤10%, even in patients at high risk of PONV. However, their effect on postoperative nausea is limited. Interestingly, vofopitant is also ineffective in motion sickness, a condition where nausea is a prominent feature[88]. Currently, only aprepitant is approved for the prevention of PONV.

Pharmacokinetics of NK_1-receptor antagonists

The pharmacokinetic parameters of NK_1-receptor antagonists are shown in Table 8.3.

Aprepitant

Aprepitant is a highly lipophilic base with a pKa value of 9.7 (at pH 2–12). Given the lipophilicity, aprepitant cannot be dissolved in aqueous solution for intravenous (IV) injection. For the same reason, gut absorption of the drug is highly dependent on dietary fat.

Table 8.3 Pharmacokinetic parameters of NK_1-receptor antagonists

	Aprepitant	Fosaprepitant	Casopitant	Netupitant	Rolapitant
Bioavailability	60–65%	–	83%	High	High
Time to peak absorption (h)	3–4	–	0.5–1.5	5	2–3
Protein binding	>95%	–	>99%	99%	NA
Volume of distribution (L/kg)	1	0.1	3–4	30–40	NA
Elimination half-life	9–13 h	2.3 min	8–15 h	96 h	180 h
Clearance (mL/min)	60–90	~60	200	300	NA
Metabolism pathway	Liver, oxidation by CYP3A4 to weakly active metabolites	Blood and tissue by ubiquitous phosphatase, convert to aprepitant	Liver, oxidation and *N*-dealkylation by CYP3A4 to inactive metabolites	Liver, oxidation by CYP3A4, metabolites capable to bind to NK_1 receptor	Liver, oxidation by CYP3A4 to inactive metabolites
Dose reported for prevention of nausea and vomiting					
PONV	40 mg orally, 3 h prior to surgery	No data	50 mg orally, 1 h prior to surgery or 30 mg IVI at induction of anesthesia	No data	50–200 mg, 0.5 h prior to surgery
CINV	125 mg before and 80 mg daily for day 1 and 2	115 mg produce similar effect as oral aprepitant 125 mg	150 mg orally before and 50 mg daily for day 1 and 2	300 mg orally before chemotherapy	200 mg orally before chemotherapy

CYP, cytochrome; CINV, chemotherapy-induced nausea and vomiting; IVI, intravenous infusion; NA, not available; PONV, postoperative nausea and vomiting.

In order to increase bioavailability, current formulation reduces particle size to nanoscale (<150 nm)[89]. The nanoparticles increase surface exposure by 3–4-fold and oral bioavailability to about 60–65%. Drug absorption of the nanoparticle is independent of food intake. In previous studies, peak plasma concentrations were achieved at 3 and 4 h following oral administration of aprepitant 40 and 125 mg, respectively, and the corresponding plasma concentrations were 700 ng/mL and 1400 ng/mL[90,91]. At these plasma concentrations, NK_1 receptors in the brain were estimated to be >99% occupied.

Aprepitant is largely bound to plasma proteins (>95%) with a steady-state volume of distribution of about 1 L/kg[91]. Aprepitant is largely metabolized by microsomes (CYP3A4 isoenzyme) in the liver, where it is oxidized at the morpholine ring to produce a number of inactive metabolites. Plasma clearance is in the range of 60–90 mL/min, resulting in a terminal half-life of 9–13 h[91]. Renal impairment has no apparent effect on drug elimination. No study has evaluated the effect of liver failure on the metabolism of aprepitant.

Aprepitant is a substrate as well as a mild-to-moderate inhibitor of CYP3A4. There have been concerns that aprepitant may alter the pharmacokinetics of concomitantly administered drugs that are metabolized by CYP3A4, and hence resulting in adverse drug interactions. CYP3A4 inhibition appears to affect CYP3A4 in the gut more than that in the liver. In this respect, bioavailability of orally administered midazolam was substantially increased (3.3-fold) by coadministration of aprepitant for 5 days[92]. In contrast, plasma midazolam concentration was modestly increased by 25% when the drug was given intravenously[93]. Currently, the only notable interaction for aprepitant is coadministration of dexamethasone or methylprednisolone. When aprepitant was given for 3 days according to standard regimen for CINV, plasma concentrations of the two corticosteroids were increased by greater than twofold[94]. Currently, no study has evaluated the clinical relevance of this drug interaction. Nevertheless, it is recommended that the dosage of coadministered dexamethasone or methylprednisolone should be halved[95]. Aprepitant also induces CYP2D6 and may decrease the effects of warfarin and oral contraceptive drugs. Therefore, monitoring of anticoagulation effect has been recommended[96]. Aprepitant has no apparent effect on 5-HT_3 receptor antagonists[95]. It should be noted that all these drug interaction studies were performed in subjects receiving multiple and large doses of aprepitant. A single dose of aprepitant 40 mg given before surgery for preventing PONV is unlikely to produce significant drug interaction.

Fosaprepitant

Fosaprepitant is a water-soluble *N*-phosphoryl derivative of aprepitant[25]. As a prodrug, fosaprepitant is rapidly converted to its parent compound by ubiquitous phosphatases after IV administration. In volunteers receiving fosaprepitant 115 mg, the elimination half-life of fosaprepitant was 2.3 min, so that all drug was cleared from plasma within 30 min of injection[97]. There is hardly any tissue distribution and the volume of distribution is estimated to be about 5 L[97,98]. Fosaprepitant is capable of binding to NK_1 receptors but with much lower affinity (binding affinity (IC_{50}) values for aprepitant and fosaprepitant of 0.09 and 1.2 nM, respectively)[25]. Therefore, the effect of fosaprepitant can be attributed entirely to aprepitant.

Casopitant

Casopitant is a substituted piperazine derivative. It has been formulated as a powder and in film-coated tablets for oral administration, and has been dissolved in sodium citrate buffer for IV injection. After oral ingestion, casopitant is rapidly absorbed with a bioavailability in excess of 83% and is not affected by dietary factors. Peak plasma concentration is reached in 30–90 min[99]. Casopitant crosses the blood–brain barrier freely. In volunteers receiving multiple doses of oral casopitant, a steady-state plasma concentration >20 ng/mL was associated with an NK_1 receptor occupancy of >95%[100]. It should be noted that a single dose of casopitant of 50 mg produced a peak plasma concentration >100 ng/mL. Casopitant is highly bound to plasma proteins (>99%) with a volume of distribution of 2–3 L/kg. It is primarily metabolized (oxidation and *N*-dealkylation) in the liver by CYP3A4 to produce a large number of inactive metabolites. The total clearance is about 200 mL/min[101]. The terminal half-life varies between 8.8 and 15.1 h. Casopitant is a mild-to-moderate inhibitor of CYP3A4, and therefore shares the same concerns of potential drug interactions with aprepitant. Current data suggest that a single dose of casopitant has little effect on the pharmacokinetics of coadministered 5-HT_3 receptor antagonists, dexamethasone and midazolam[99].

Netupitant

Netupitant is a long-acting NK_1-receptor antagonist (elimination half-life of 96 h). It is a lipophilic molecule, currently formulated as a combination pill with another long-acting 5-HT_3 receptor antagonist – palonosetron (half-life of 44 h). Following oral administration, absorption is almost complete, producing peak plasma concentration at about 5 h. Netupitant is highly bound to plasma proteins (99%), with a volume of distribution of 30–40 L/kg. It is metabolized in the liver by CYP3A4. In contrast to the other NK_1-receptor antagonists, the resulting metabolites were capable of binding to NK_1 receptors. Current data show that netupitant has no effect on the pharmacokinetics of palonosetron, but the dosage of dexamethasone should be reduced[102].

Rolapitant

This is a very long-acting NK_1-receptor antagonist, with an elimination half-life of 180 h. It is rapidly absorbed with the peak plasma concentration occurring at 2–3 h after oral administration. Rolapitant is metabolized in the liver but does not inhibit liver enzymes, including CYP3A4. Therefore, risk of drug interaction is considered low.

Taken together, NK_1-receptor antagonists appear to be very safe. Reported adverse events in clinical trials were similar to those in the control groups (usually ondansetron)[103]. The most common side effects were headache and constipation.

Novel antiemetic: the antipsychotic amisulpride

Several antipsychotics have been tried in the management of nausea and vomiting. Amisulpride, a second-generation antipsychotic, has emerged as a novel antiemetic for managing PONV. As a substituted benzamide, amisulpride preferentially blocks dopamine (D_2 and D_3) receptors. At therapeutic dosage for treatment of psychosis (400–1,200 mg/day), there is no interaction with adrenergic, 5-HT and cholinergic receptors[104]. Consequently, the risk of extrapyramidal movement, sedation and cardiac arrhythmia with prolonged QTc intervals were lower compared with first-generation agents such as haloperidol[105].

The efficacy of amisulpride to prevent PONV has been studied in a recently published randomized controlled trial[106]. In this trial, 215 patients at risk of PONV were randomized to receive placebo or IV amisulpride 1, 5 or 20 mg. Interestingly, only amisulpride 1 or 5 mg reduced the risk of PONV during the first 24 h after surgery. The numbers needed-to-treat were 5 (95% CI, 2.7–21.6) for PONV and 5 (95% CI, 2.4–15.8) for nausea. These are encouraging data and further trials are required to define the role of low-dose amisulpride as an antiemetic after surgery.

Summary

In summary, current data confirm that NK_1 antagonists are potent antiemetics that could reduce the risk of POV substantially. These compounds are safe. However, their effect on postoperative nausea remains limited. The emerging novel antiemetic agent amisulpride may also be useful to prevent PONV, but further data are needed.

References

1. von Euler US, Gaddum JH. An unidentified depressor substance in certain tissue extracts. *J Physiol* 1931; 72: 74–87.
2. Newton BW, Maley B, Traurig H. The distribution of substance P, enkephalin, and serotonin immunoreactivities in the area postrema of the rat and cat. *J Comp Neurol* 1985; 234: 87–104.
3. Baude A, Lanoir J, Vernier P, Puizillout JJ. Substance P-immunoreactivity in the dorsal medial region of the medulla in the cat: effects of nodosectomy. *J Chem Neuroanat* 1989; 2: 67–81.
4. Armstrong DM, Pickel VM, Reis DJ. Electron microscopic immunocytochemical localization of substance P in the area postrema of rat. *Brain Res* 1982; 243: 141–6.
5. Carpenter DO, Briggs DB, Strominger N. Peptide-induced emesis in dogs. *Behav Brain Res* 1984; 11: 277–81.
6. Andrews PL, Bhandari P. Resinferatoxin, an ultrapotent capsaicin analogue, has anti-emetic properties in the ferret. *Neuropharmacology* 1993; 32: 799–806.
7. Tregear GW, Niall HD, Potts JT Jr, et al. Synthesis of substance P. *Nat New Biol* 1971; 232: 87–9.
8. Chang MM, Leeman SE, Niall HD. Amino-acid sequence of substance P. *Nat New Biol* 1971; 232: 86–7.
9. Steinhoff MS, von Mentzer B, Geppetti P, et al. Tachykinins and their receptors: contributions to physiological control and the mechanisms of disease. *Physiol Rev* 2014; 94: 265–301.
10. Almeida TA, Rojo J, Nieto PM, et al. Tachykinins and tachykinin receptors: structure and activity relationships. *Curr Med Chem* 2004; 11: 2045–81.
11. Quartara L, Maggi CA. The tachykinin NK1 receptor. Part II: Distribution and pathophysiological roles. *Neuropeptides* 1998; 32: 1–49.
12. Quartara L, Maggi CA. The tachykinin NK1 receptor. Part I: ligands and mechanisms of cellular activation. *Neuropeptides* 1997; 31: 537–63.
13. Shimizu Y, Matsuyama H, Shiina T, et al. Tachykinins and their functions in the gastrointestinal tract. *Cell Mol Life Sci* 2008; 65: 295–311.
14. Chen P, Douglas SD, Meshki J, et al. Neurokinin 1 receptor mediates membrane blebbing and sheer stress-induced microparticle formation in HEK293 cells. *PLoS ONE* 2012; 7: e45322.
15. Koon HW, Zhao D, Na X, et al. Metalloproteinases and transforming growth factor-alpha mediate substance P-induced mitogen-activated protein kinase activation and proliferation in human colonocytes. *J Biol Chem* 2004; 279: 45519–27.
16. Engberg G, Svensson TH, Rosell S, et al. A synthetic peptide as an antagonist of substance P. *Nature* 1981; 293: 222–3.
17. Lee CM, Campbell NJ, Williams BJ, et al. Multiple tachykinin binding-sites in peripheral-tissues and in brain. *Eur J Pharmacol* 1986; 130: 209–217.
18. Rojas C, Raje M, Tsukamoto T, et al. Molecular mechanisms of 5-HT3 and NK1 receptor antagonists in prevention of emesis. *Eur J Pharmacol* 2014; 722: 26–37.
19. Huang SC, Korlipara VL. Neurokinin-1 receptor antagonists: a comprehensive patent survey. *Expert Opin Ther Pat* 2010; 20: 1019–45.
20. Snider RM, Constantine JW, Lowe JA, et al. A potent nonpeptide antagonist of the substance P (NK1) receptor. *Science* 1991; 251: 435–7.
21. Desai MC, Lefkowitz SL, Thadeio PF, et al. Discovery of a potent substance P antagonist: recognition of the key molecular determinant. *J Med Chem* 1992; 35: 4911–3.
22. Schmidt AW, McLean S, Heym J. The substance P receptor antagonist CP-96,345 interacts with Ca^{2+} channels. *Eur J Pharmacol* 1992; 219: 491–2.

23. Hargreaves R, Ferreira JC, Hughes D, et al. Development of aprepitant, the first neurokinin-1 receptor antagonist for the prevention of chemotherapy-induced nausea and vomiting. *Ann N Y Acad Sci* 2011; 1222: 40–8.
24. Hale JJ, Mills SG, MacCoss M, et al. 2(S)-((3,5-Bis(trifluoromethyl)benzyl) oxy)-3(S)-phenyl-4-((3-oxo-1,2,4-triazol- 5-yl)methyl)morpholine (1): A potent, orally active, morpholine-based human neurokinin-1 receptor antagonist. *J Med Chem* 1996; 39: 1760–2.
25. Hale JJ, Mills SG, MacCoss M, et al. Phosphorylated morpholine acetal human neurokinin-1 receptor antagonists as water-soluble prodrugs. *J Med Chem* 2000; 43: 1234–41.
26. Di Fabio R, Alvaro G, Griffante C, et al. Discovery and biological characterization of (2R,4S)-1′-acetyl-N-{(1R)-1-[3,5-bis(trifluoromethyl) phenyl]ethyl}-2-(4-fluoro-2-methylphenyl)-N-methyl-4,4′-bipiperidine-1-carboxamide as a new potent and selective neurokinin 1 (NK1) receptor antagonist clinical candidate. *J Med Chem* 2011; 54: 1071–9.
27. Rizzi A, Campi B, Camarda V, et al. In vitro and in vivo pharmacological characterization of the novel NK1 receptor selective antagonist Netupitant. *Peptides* 2012; 37: 86–97.
28. Duffy RA, Morgan C, Naylor R, et al. Rolapitant (SCH 619734): a potent, selective and orally active neurokinin NK1 receptor antagonist with centrally mediated antiemetic effects in ferrets. *Pharmacol Biochem Behav* 2012; 102: 95–100.
29. Rupniak NM, Hill RG. Neurokinin antagonists. In *Novel aspects of pain management: opioids and beyond*. Sawynok J, Cowan A (eds). New York: Wiley-Liss, 1999; 135–55.
30. De Koninck Y, Henry JL. Substance P-mediated slow excitatory postsynaptic potential elicited in dorsal horn neurons in vivo by noxious stimulation. *Proc Natl Acad Sci U S A* 1991; 88: 11344–8.
31. Rupniak NM, Kramer MS. Discovery of the antidepressant and anti-emetic efficacy of substance P receptor (NK1) antagonists. *Trends Pharmacol Sci* 1999; 20: 485–90.
32. Watson JW, Gonsalves SF, Fossa AA, et al. The anti-emetic effects of CP-99,994 in the ferret and the dog: role of the NK1 receptor. *Br J Pharmacol* 1995; 115: 84–94.
33. Lewis CA, El-Hashim AZ, Gerspacher M, et al. The airways pharmacology of DNK333, a potent, selective, non-peptide dual NK1/NK2 receptor antagonist. *Drug Develop Res* 2004; 63: 161–173.
34. Zakko S, Barton G, Weber E, et al. Randomised clinical trial: the clinical effects of a novel neurokinin receptor antagonist, DNK333, in women with diarrhoea-predominant irritable bowel syndrome. *Aliment Pharmacol Ther* 2011; 33: 1311–21.
35. Tough IR, Lewis CA, Fozard J, et al. Dual and selective antagonism of neurokinin NK(1) and NK(2) receptor-mediated responses in human colon mucosa. *Naunyn Schmiedebergs Arch Pharmacol* 2003; 367: 104–8.
36. Ohmura T, Hayashi T, Satoh Y, et al. Involvement of substance P in scratching behaviour in an atopic dermatitis model. *Eur J Pharmacol* 2004; 491: 191–4.
37. Doi T, Kamo I, Imai S, et al. Effects of TAK-637, a tachykinin receptor antagonist, on the micturition reflex in guinea pigs. *Eur J Pharmacol* 2000; 395: 241–6.
38. Shaikh MB, Steinberg A, Siegel A. Evidence that substance P is utilized in medial amygdaloid facilitation of defensive rage behavior in the cat. *Brain Res* 1993; 625: 283–94.
39. Kramer MS, Cutler N, Feighner J, et al. Distinct mechanism for antidepressant activity by blockade of central substance P receptors. *Science* 1998; 281: 1640–5.
40. Lim R, Morrill JM, Prushik SG, et al. An FDA approved neurokinin-1 receptor antagonist is effective in reducing intraabdominal adhesions when administered intraperitoneally, but not orally. *J Gastrointest Surg* 2008; 12: 1754–61.

41. Hegde A, Zhang H, Moochhala SM, et al. Neurokinin-1 receptor antagonist treatment protects mice against lung injury in polymicrobial sepsis. *J Leukoc Biol* 2007; 82: 678–85.

42. Gillespie E, Leeman SE, Watts LA, et al. Truncated neurokinin-1 receptor is increased in colonic epithelial cells from patients with colitis-associated cancer. *Proc Natl Acad Sci U S A* 2011; 108: 17420–5.

43. Fahy JV, Wong HH, Geppetti P, et al. Effect of an NK1 receptor antagonist (CP-99,994) on hypertonic saline-induced bronchoconstriction and cough in male asthmatic subjects. *Am J Respir Crit Care Med* 1995; 152: 879–84.

44. Frenkl TL, Zhu H, Reiss T, et al. A multicenter, double-blind, randomized, placebo controlled trial of a neurokinin-1 receptor antagonist for overactive bladder. *J Urol* 2010; 184: 616–22.

45. Hill R. NK(1) (substance P) receptor antagonists – why are they not analgesic in humans? *Trends Pharmacol Sci* 2000; 21: 244–6.

46. Dionne RA, Max MB, Gordon SM, et al. The substance P receptor antagonist CP-99,994 reduces acute postoperative pain. *Clin Pharmacol Ther* 1998; 64: 562–8.

47. Kakuta N, Tsutsumi YM, Horikawa YT, et al. Neurokinin-1 receptor antagonism, aprepitant, effectively diminishes post-operative nausea and vomiting while increasing analgesic tolerance in laparoscopic gynecological procedures. *J Med Invest* 2011; 58: 246–51.

48. Goldstein DJ, Wang O, Saper JR, et al. Ineffectiveness of neurokinin-1 antagonist in acute migraine: a crossover study. *Cephalalgia* 1997; 17: 785–90.

49. Diener HC; RPR100893 Study Group. RPR100893, a substance-P antagonist, is not effective in the treatment of migraine attacks. *Cephalalgia* 2003; 23: 183–5.

50. Goldstein DJ, Wang O, Gitter BD, et al. Dose–response study of the analgesic effect of lanepitant in patients with painful diabetic neuropathy. *Clin Neuropharmacol* 2001; 24: 16–22.

51. Sindrup SH, Graf A, Sfikas N. The NK1-receptor antagonist TKA731 in painful diabetic neuropathy: a randomised, controlled trial. *Eur J Pain* 2006; 10: 567–71.

52. Keller M, Montgomery S, Ball W, et al. Lack of efficacy of the substance P (neurokinin$_1$ receptor) antagonist aprepitant in the treatment of major depressive disorder. *Biol Psychiatry* 2006; 59: 216–23.

53. Urban LA, Fox AJ. NK(1) receptor antagonists – are they really without effect in the pain clinic. *Trends Pharmacol Sci* 2000; 21: 462–4.

54. Cocquyt V, Van Belle S, Reinhardt RR, et al. Comparison of L-758,298, a prodrug for the selective neurokinin-1 antagonist, L-754,030, with ondansetron for the prevention of cisplatin-induced emesis. *Eur J Cancer* 2001; 37: 835–42.

55. Fumoleau P, Graham E, Giovanni M. Control of acute cisplatin-induced emesis and nausea with the NK1 receptor antagonist GR205171 in combination with ondansetron. *Proc Annu Meet Am Soc Clin Oncol* 1998; 17: 58a 255.

56. Kris MG, Radford JE, Pizzo BA, et al. Use of an NK1 receptor antagonist to prevent delayed emesis after cisplatin. *J Natl Cancer Inst* 1997; 89: 817–818.

57. Hesketh PJ, Gralla RJ, Webb RT, et al. Randomized phase II study of the neurokinin 1 receptor antagonist CJ-11,974 in the control of cisplatin-induced emesis. *J Clin Oncol* 1999; 17: 338–43.

58. Warr DG, Hesketh PJ, Gralla RJ, et al. Efficacy and tolerability of aprepitant for the prevention of chemotherapy-induced nausea and vomiting in patients with breast cancer after moderately emetogenic chemotherapy. *J Clin Oncol* 2005; 23: 2822–30.

59. Schmoll HJ, Aapro MS, Poli-Bigelli S, et al. Comparison of an aprepitant regimen with a multiple-day ondansetron regimen, both with dexamethasone, for antiemetic efficacy in high-dose cisplatin treatment. *Ann Oncol* 2006; 17: 1000–6.

60. Poli-Bigelli S, Rodrigues-Pereira J, Carides AD, et al. Aprepitant Protocol 054 Study Group. Addition of the neurokinin 1 receptor antagonist aprepitant to standard antiemetic therapy improves control of chemotherapy-induced nausea and vomiting. Results from a randomized, double-blind, placebo-controlled trial in Latin America. *Cancer* 2003; 97: 3090–8.

61. Hesketh PJ, Grunberg SM, Gralla RJ, et al. Aprepitant Protocol 052 Study Group. The oral neurokinin-1 antagonist aprepitant for the prevention of chemotherapy-induced nausea and vomiting: a multinational, randomized, double-blind, placebo-controlled trial in patients receiving high-dose cisplatin – the Aprepitant Protocol 052 Study Group. *J Clin Oncol* 2003; 21: 4112–9.

62. Herrstedt J, Muss HB, Warr DG, et al. Aprepitant Moderately Emetogenic Chemotherapy Study Group. Efficacy and tolerability of aprepitant for the prevention of chemotherapy-induced nausea and emesis over multiple cycles of moderately emetogenic chemotherapy. *Cancer* 2005; 104: 1548–55.

63. de Wit R, Herrstedt J, Rapoport B, et al. The oral NK_1 antagonist, aprepitant, given with standard antiemetics provides protection against nausea and vomiting over multiple cycles of cisplatin-based chemotherapy: a combined analysis of two randomised, placebo-controlled phase III clinical trials. *Eur J Cancer* 2004; 40: 403–10.

64. Chawla SP, Grunberg SM, Gralla RJ, et al. Establishing the dose of the oral NK1 antagonist aprepitant for the prevention of chemotherapy-induced nausea and vomiting. *Cancer* 2003; 97: 2290–300.

65. Grunberg SM, Rolski J, Strausz J, et al. Efficacy and safety of casopitant mesylate, a neurokinin 1 (NK1)-receptor antagonist, in prevention of chemotherapy-induced nausea and vomiting in patients receiving cisplatin-based highly emetogenic chemotherapy: a randomised, double-blind, placebo-controlled trial. *Lancet Oncol* 2009; 10: 549–58.

66. Herrstedt J, Apornwirat W, Shaharyar A, et al. Phase III trial of casopitant, a novel neurokinin-1 receptor antagonist, for the prevention of nausea and vomiting in patients receiving moderately emetogenic chemotherapy. *J Clin Oncol* 2009; 27: 5363–9.

67. Arpornwirat W, Albert I, Hansen VL, et al. Phase 2 trial results with the novel neurokinin-1 receptor antagonist casopitant in combination with ondansetron and dexamethasone for the prevention of chemotherapy-induced nausea and vomiting in cancer patients receiving moderately emetogenic chemotherapy. *Cancer* 2009; 115: 5807–16.

68. Gridelli C, Haiderali AM, Russo MW, et al. Casopitant improves the quality of life in patients receiving highly emetogenic chemotherapy. *Support Care Cancer* 2010; 18: 1437–44.

69. Hesketh PJ, Rossi G, Rizzi G, et al. Efficacy and safety of NEPA, an oral combination of netupitant and palonosetron, for prevention of chemotherapy-induced nausea and vomiting following highly emetogenic chemotherapy: a randomized dose-ranging pivotal study. *Ann Oncol* 2014; 25: 1340–6.

70. Aapro M, Rugo H, Rossi G, et al. A randomized phase III study evaluating the efficacy and safety of NEPA, a fixed-dose combination of netupitant and palonosetron, for prevention of chemotherapy-induced nausea and vomiting following moderately emetogenic chemotherapy. *Ann Oncol* 2014; 25: 1328–33.

71. Gralla RJ, Bosnjak SM, Hontsa A, et al. A phase III study evaluating the safety and efficacy of NEPA, a fixed-dose combination of netupitant and palonosetron, for prevention of chemotherapy-induced nausea and vomiting over repeated cycles of chemotherapy. *Ann Oncol* 2014; 25: 1333–9.

72. Roila F, Herrstedt J, Aapro M, et al. ESMO/MASCC Guidelines Working Group. Guideline update for MASCC and ESMO in the prevention of

chemotherapy- and radiotherapy-induced nausea and vomiting: results of the Perugia consensus conference. *Ann Oncol* 2010; 21 Suppl 5: v232–43.

73. Diemunsch P, Schoeffler P, Bryssine B, et al. Antiemetic activity of the NK_1 receptor antagonist GR205171 in the treatment of established postoperative nausea and vomiting after major gynaecological surgery. *Br J Anaesth* 1999; 82: 274–6.

74. Gesztesi Z, Scuderi PE, White PF, et al. Substance P (Neurokinin-1) antagonist prevents postoperative vomiting after abdominal hysterectomy procedures. *Anesthesiology* 2000; 93: 931–7.

75. Gan TJ, Apfel CC, Kovac A, et al. Aprepitant-PONV Study Group. A randomized, double-blind comparison of the NK1 antagonist, aprepitant, versus ondansetron for the prevention of postoperative nausea and vomiting. *Anesth Analg* 2007; 104: 1082–9.

76. Diemunsch P, Gan TJ, Philip BK, et al. Aprepitant-PONV Protocol International Study Group. Single-dose aprepitant vs ondansetron for the prevention of postoperative nausea and vomiting: a randomized, double-blind phase III trial in patients undergoing open abdominal surgery. *Br J Anaesth* 2007; 99: 202–11.

77. Diemunsch P, Apfel C, Gan TJ, et al. Preventing postoperative nausea and vomiting: post hoc analysis of pooled data from two randomized active-controlled trials of aprepitant. *Curr Med Res Opin* 2007; 23: 2559–65.

78. Habib AS, Keifer JC, Borel CO, et al. A comparison of the combination of aprepitant and dexamethasone versus the combination of ondansetron and dexamethasone for the prevention of postoperative nausea and vomiting in patients undergoing craniotomy. *Anesth Analg* 2011; 112: 813–8.

79. Tsutsumi YM, Kakuta N, Soga T, et al. The effects of intravenous fosaprepitant and ondansetron for the prevention of postoperative nausea and vomiting in neurosurgery patients: a prospective, randomized, double-blinded study. *Biomed Res Int* 2014; 2014: 307025.

80. Vallejo MC, Phelps AL, Ibinson JW, et al. Aprepitant plus ondansetron compared with ondansetron alone in reducing postoperative nausea and vomiting in ambulatory patients undergoing plastic surgery. *Plast Reconstr Surg* 2012; 129: 519–26.

81. Moon HY, Baek CW, Choi GJ, et al. Palonosetron and aprepitant for the prevention of postoperative nausea and vomiting in patients indicated for laparoscopic gynaecologic surgery: a double-blind randomised trial. *BMC Anesthesiol* 2014; 14: 68.

82. Lee SJ, Lee SM, Kim SI, et al. The effect of aprepitant for the prevention of postoperative nausea and vomiting in patients undergoing gynecologic surgery with intravenous patient controlled analgesia using fentanyl: aprepitant plus ramosetron vs ramosetron alone. *Korean J Anesthesiol* 2012; 63: 221–6.

83. Lim CS, Ko YK, Kim YH, et al. Efficacy of the oral neurokinin-1 receptor antagonist aprepitant administered with ondansetron for the prevention of postoperative nausea and vomiting. *Korean J Anesthesiol* 2013; 64: 212–7.

84. Sinha AC, Singh PM, Williams NW, et al. Aprepitant's prophylactic efficacy in decreasing postoperative nausea and vomiting in morbidly obese patients undergoing bariatric surgery. *Obes Surg* 2014; 24: 225–31.

85. Altorjay A, Melson T, Chinachoit T, et al. Casopitant and ondansetron for postoperative nausea and vomiting prevention in women at high risk for emesis: a phase 3 study. *Arch Surg* 2011; 146: 201–6.

86. Singla NK, Singla SK, Chung F, et al. Phase II study to evaluate the safety and efficacy of the oral neurokinin-1 receptor antagonist casopitant (GW679769) administered with ondansetron for the prevention of postoperative and postdischarge nausea and vomiting in high-risk patients. *Anesthesiology* 2010; 113: 74–82.

87. Gan TJ, Gu J, Singla N, et al. Rolapitant Investigation Group. Rolapitant for the prevention of postoperative nausea and vomiting: a prospective, double-blinded, placebo-controlled randomized trial. *Anesth Analg* 2011; 112: 804–12.

88. Reid K, Palmer JL, Wright RJ, et al. Comparison of the neurokinin-1 antagonist GR205171, alone and in combination with the 5-HT3 antagonist ondansetron, hyoscine and placebo in the prevention of motion-induced nausea in man. *Br J Clin Pharmacol* 2000; 50: 61–4.

89. Olver I, Shelukar S, Thompson KC. Nanomedicines in the treatment of emesis during chemotherapy: focus on aprepitant. *Int J Nanomedicine* 2007; 2: 13–8.

90. Van Laere K, De Hoon J, Bormans G, et al. Equivalent dynamic human brain NK1-receptor occupancy following single-dose i.v. fosaprepitant vs. oral aprepitant as assessed by PET imaging. *Clin Pharmacol Ther* 2012; 92: 243–50.

91. Curran MP, Robinson DM. Aprepitant: a review of its use in the prevention of nausea and vomiting. *Drugs* 2009; 69: 1853–78.

92. Majumdar AK, McCrea JB, Panebianco DL, et al. Effects of aprepitant on cytochrome P450 3A4 activity using midazolam as a probe. *Clin Pharmacol Ther* 2003; 74: 150–6.

93. Shadle CR, Lee Y, Majumdar AK, et al. Evaluation of potential inductive effects of aprepitant on cytochrome P450 3A4 and 2C9 activity. *J Clin Pharmacol* 2004; 44: 215–23.

94. McCrea JB, Majumdar AK, Goldberg MR, et al. Effects of the neurokinin1 receptor antagonist aprepitant on the pharmacokinetics of dexamethasone and methylprednisolone. *Clin Pharmacol Ther* 2003; 74: 17–24.

95. Aapro MS, Walko CM. Aprepitant: drug–drug interactions in perspective. *Ann Oncol* 2010; 21: 2316–23.

96. Depre M, Van Hecken A, Oeyen M, et al. Effect of aprepitant on the pharmacokinetics and pharmacodynamics of warfarin. *Eur J Clin Pharmacol* 2005; 61: 341–6.

97. Lasseter KC, Gambale J, Jin B, et al. Tolerability of fosaprepitant and bioequivalency to aprepitant in healthy subjects. *J Clin Pharmacol* 2007; 47: 834–40.

98. Colon-Gonzalez F, Kraft WK. Pharmacokinetic evaluation of fosaprepitant dimeglumine. *Expert Opin Drug Metab Toxicol* 2010; 6: 1277–86.

99. Ruhlmann C, Herrstedt J. Casopitant: a novel NK_1-receptor antagonist in the prevention of chemotherapy-induced nausea and vomiting. *Ther Clin Risk Manag* 2009; 5: 375–84.

100. Zamuner S, Rabiner EA, Fernandes SA, et al. A pharmacokinetic PET study of NK_1 receptor occupancy. *Eur J Nucl Med Mol Imaging* 2012; 39: 226–35.

101. Pellegatti M, Bordini E, Fizzotti P, et al. Disposition and metabolism of radiolabeled casopitant in humans. *Drug Metab Dispos* 2009; 37: 1635–45.

102. Lanzarotti C, Rossi G. Effect of netupitant, a highly selective NK_1 receptor antagonist, on the pharmacokinetics of midazolam, erythromycin, and dexamethasone. *Support Care Cancer* 2013; 21: 2783–91.

103. Munoz M, Covenas R. Safety of neurokinin-1 receptor antagonists. *Expert Opin Drug Saf* 2013; 12: 673–85.

104. Coulouvrat C, Dondey-Nouvel L. Safety of amisulpride (Solian): a review of 11 clinical studies. *Int Clin Psychopharmacol* 1999; 14: 209–18.

105. Leucht S, Cipriani A, Spineli L, et al. Comparative efficacy and tolerability of 15 antipsychotic drugs in schizophrenia: a multiple-treatments meta-analysis. *Lancet* 2013; 382: 951–62.

106. Kranke P, Eberhart L, Motsch J, et al. I.V. APD421 (amisulpride) prevents postoperative nausea and vomiting: a randomized, double-blind, placebo-controlled, multicentre trial. *Br J Anaesth* 2013; 111: 938–45.

Chapter 9

Propofol and other sedatives as antiemetics

Aaron Skolnik and Tong Joo Gan

Anesthesia providers have an extensive list of medications from which to choose when administering sedation to their patients. Examples of such sedative agents include propofol, benzodiazepines and alpha-2 adrenergic receptor agonists such as clonidine and dexmedetomidine. Although these sedative medications act through unique mechanisms, they all produce sedation, and all have been demonstrated to be effective in reducing the incidence of postoperative nausea and vomiting (PONV). In this chapter, we will review the mechanisms and antiemetic effects of propofol, benzodiazepines (e.g., lorazepam and midazolam) and alpha-2 adrenergic receptor agonists, while giving special attention to propofol, perhaps the sedative best-characterized in terms of its property of preventing PONV.

Propofol

Mechanism of action

Propofol (Diprivan; AstraZeneca Pharmaceuticals, Wilmington, DE, USA) is an alkylphenol hypnotic agent commonly regarded as the intravenous (IV) anesthetic associated with a low incidence of PONV. Its mechanism of action is still unclear, although it appears to enhance gamma-aminobutyric acid (GABA) receptor function, thereby inhibiting synaptic transmission in the brain's vomiting center, a collection of structures in the medulla located near the fourth ventricle[1].

Most of the commonly used antiemetics exert their effect in the area postrema (also known as the chemoreceptor trigger zone) of the medulla where dopamine, serotonin, histamine, muscarine and neurokinin receptors can be found. It is unknown whether propofol has a direct or an indirect effect on these receptors[2].

In order to investigate propofol's interaction with dopamine, Hvarfner et al. administered apomorphine, a dopamine agonist, to healthy volunteers until vomiting was induced[3]. The authors found that a nonsedating bolus of propofol did not alter the patients' sensitivity to apomorphine compared with the saline control. They concluded that a nonsedative dose of propofol has no effect on vomiting induced by apomorphine, suggesting that propofol does not have a direct antidopaminergic effect.

To further examine the mechanism of action of propofol, Cechetto et al. performed immunohistochemical analyses of serotonin in the area postrema of rats' brains[4]. They demonstrated that a propofol infusion significantly decreased the serotonergic activity

Postoperative Nausea and Vomiting: A Practical Guide, eds. Tong Joo Gan and Ashraf S. Habib. Published by Cambridge University Press.

(17% ± 6%) (mean ± standard error of the mean) in the area postrema. Additionally, the serotonergic inhibition was antagonized by bicuculline, an inhibitor at the GABA receptor. The authors suggested that propofol reduces serotonin secretion by promoting GABA function, possibly via GABA-mediated effects on serotonin receptors located in the area postrema.

A brief history of propofol and antiemesis

In 1981, Briggs et al. reported that the recovery period after propofol anesthesia was "characterized by lack of emetic sequelae." The group was credited with the earliest observation of propofol's antiemetic effect[5].

As propofol appeared to decrease the incidence of PONV, interest grew in the use of single doses of propofol as prophylaxis for emesis. In 1988, McCollum et al. reported that repeated doses of propofol for anesthesia during gynecologic surgery resulted in a significantly lower incidence of PONV than with methohexital, suggesting that propofol has an intrinsic antiemetic effect[6].

Two years later, Campbell and Thomas completed the first prospective study investigating the use of propofol as an antiemetic[7]. Fifty-three women undergoing laparoscopic gynecologic surgery received either saline placebo or a single subhypnotic dose of propofol prior to emergence. The authors reported no difference in the incidence of PONV between the treatment and control groups.

Many of these early single-dose studies were limited by the fact that the effective antiemetic doses of propofol had not yet been established. In 1997, Gan et al. reported the results of the first dose–response study on the antiemetic effect of propofol[8]. Patients who exhibited nausea, retching or vomiting during recovery in the postanesthesia care unit (PACU) received propofol via a target-controlled continuous infusion device. The computer-guided infusion increased the dose of propofol in a stepwise fashion (from a 200 ng/mL targeted plasma concentration) until the patient reported resolution of the nausea. The authors found that the median plasma concentration of propofol associated with a successful antiemetic response was 343 ng/mL, a level that can be achieved quickly with a 10-mg bolus of propofol followed by an infusion at the rate of 10 μg/kg/min. This dose, referred to as the "subhypnotic dose," is below the concentrations typically associated with the sedative/hypnotic effects of propofol (800–1500 ng/mL) and total intravenous anesthesia (TIVA) with propofol (3–4 mcg/mL).

Antiemetic efficacy of propofol

Intraoperative propofol versus ondansetron in breast surgery

Gan et al. evaluated the efficacy of ondansetron versus intraoperative propofol administered in various regimens[9]. Eighty-nine patients scheduled for breast surgery were randomized to one of four groups. Group O received ondansetron 4 mg, while Group PI received propofol for induction, isoflurane, nitrous oxide–oxygen and fentanyl. Group PIP was administered propofol for induction, isoflurane, nitrous oxide–oxygen and fentanyl. Thirty minutes prior to skin closure, the isoflurane was discontinued and propofol was administered for maintenance of anesthesia. Group PP received propofol for induction and maintenance of anesthesia, nitrous oxide–oxygen and fentanyl. The authors found that propofol, when used for both induction and maintenance of anesthesia (Group PP), was significantly more effective than ondansetron in decreasing the incidence of vomiting as well as the use of rescue

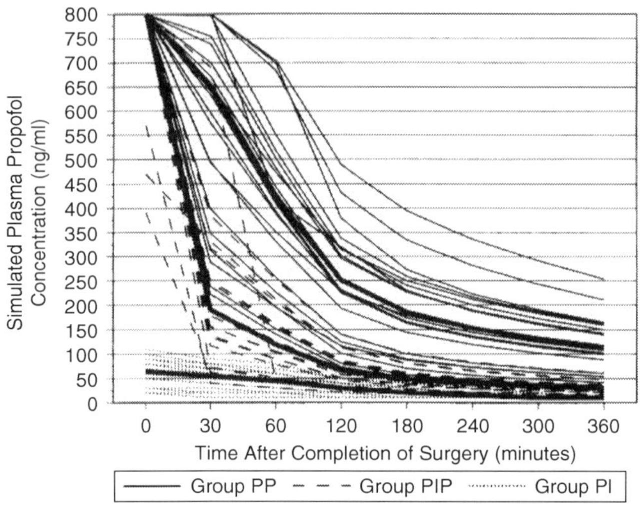

Figure 9.1 Simulated plasma concentrations of propofol during the first 6 h postoperatively. Propofol administered as an induction agent (PI); propofol administered for induction and at the end of surgery (PIP); propofol used for both induction and maintenance of anesthesia (PP). The bold lines indicate median concentrations for each group.

antiemetics in the first 6 h postoperatively. However, propofol administered as an induction agent (Group PI) or for induction and at the end of surgery (Group PIP) was not as effective in the prevention of PONV. Finally, the investigators used the pharmacokinetic parameters of propofol previously reported by Gepts et al. to simulate their dosing regimen[10]. The results of the simulated data (Figure 9.1) demonstrated higher plasma concentrations of propofol in Group PP at all times during the first 6 h postoperatively compared with those of Groups PI and PIP ($P < 0.01$; analysis of variance)[9].

Propofol versus thiopental in middle ear surgery

In a double-blind, randomized trial, Honkavaara et al. compared the antiemetic efficacy of thiopental (1.0 mg/kg) versus propofol (0.5 mg/kg) administered at the end of middle ear surgery, a procedure often associated with emetic sequelae[11]. The subhypnotic dose of propofol provided superior prophylaxis against retching and vomiting during the first 6 postoperative hours. The authors noted, however, that the incidence of nausea was not significantly reduced by propofol when compared with thiopental.

Propofol versus inhaled anesthetics

In a systematic review of the literature, Gupta et al. compared postanesthesia recovery from either propofol, isoflurane, desflurane or sevoflurane[12]. The authors reported that a propofol infusion was associated with a lower incidence of PONV and postdischarge nausea and vomiting (PDNV) over inhaled anesthetics, with a number needed-to-treat (NNT) of 8.6 and 11.2 and an NNT of 12.5 and 10.3 for PONV and PDNV, respectively.

Visser et al. conducted a randomized trial involving over 2,000 surgical patients randomized to receive anesthesia with either isoflurane–nitrous oxide or TIVA with propofol. TIVA with propofol resulted in a statistically significant reduction of PONV compared with isoflurane–nitrous oxide anesthesia, with an NNT of 6[13].

As experience with the administration of TIVA has grown and costs have declined, the use of TIVA with propofol has become increasingly popular, particulary for use in outpatient procedures. However, recent financial analyses suggest that the routine use of TIVA for prophylaxis against PONV is not cost-effective[13]. Therefore, it would be reasonable to reserve the use of propofol TIVA for patients who are at the highest risk for experiencing PONV. Gan recommends considering TIVA with propofol in patients with at least four of the following PONV risk factors: female gender, nonsmoker status, history of PONV or motion sickness, or use of postoperative opioid medications[14]. Additionally, patients undergoing laparoscopy, laparotomy, major breast surgery, otolaryngologic surgery, craniotomy, plastic surgery or strabismus surgery are at increased risk for PONV[14].

Patient-controlled propofol for PONV

Gan et al. evaluated the efficacy of patient-controlled (on-demand) subhypnotic doses of propofol for the direct treatment of PONV[15]. Patients undergoing ambulatory surgery who experienced significant nausea (defined as a nausea score of at least 5 on an 11-point nausea verbal rating scale) or emesis and who requested an antiemetic within 1 h of entry to the PACU were randomized to receive either propofol 20 or 40 mg, or intralipid as a placebo. The authors found that patients receiving 20 mg of propofol experienced a 25% lower incidence of nausea, and patients receiving 40 mg of propofol experienced a 29% lower incidence of nausea compared with the placebo group (20 mg dose versus placebo, $P = 0.03$; 40 mg dose versus placebo, $P = 0.006$). Additionally, the time to discharge from the PACU was significantly shorter in the groups receiving propofol compared with the placebo group (20 mg propofol, 131 ± 35 [mean ± standard deviation] min; 40 mg propofol, 141 ± 34 min; placebo, 191 ± 92 min; $P = 0.005$). Because the authors found no difference in efficacy between the two doses of propofol, they recommended the lower 20-mg demand dose of propofol in order to avoid the side effects that are possible with a higher dose.

Benzodiazepines

Benzodiazepines, such as midazolam and lorazepam, have sedative, anxiolytic and amnestic properties as a result of their ability to enhance the effect of the neurotransmitter gamma-aminobutyric acid (GABA). Benzodiazepines have been demonstrated, in both pediatric and adult populations, to decrease the anxiety often associated with anesthesia and surgery, thereby decreasing the incidence of PONV[16].

Midazolam versus placebo in children undergoing tonsillectomy

In a double-blind study, Splinter et al. assessed the antiemetic effect of midazolam in pediatric patients undergoing tonsillectomy[17]. The children ($n = 215$) were administered either placebo or midazolam 75 μg/kg IV after induction of anesthesia with nitrous oxide and halothane. The administration of midazolam was associated with a lower incidence of vomiting when compared with placebo (42% versus 57%, respectively; $P < 0.02$). Additionally, the placebo group experienced a higher incidence of unscheduled admissions to the hospital secondary to nausea and vomiting (9% versus 2%, respectively; $P < 0.05$). It was concluded that IV midazolam administered intraoperatively reduces vomiting after tonsillectomy in children.

Midazolam versus propofol during cesarean section

Tarhan et al. compared the effects of subhypnotic doses of midazolam and propofol on peripartum nausea and vomiting during cesarean deliveries under spinal anesthesia[18].

Parturients received, at random, either IV placebo (normal saline), a propofol infusion (1.0 mg/kg/h), or a midazolam infusion (1.0 mg/h) once the umbilical cord was clamped. The researchers found that the incidence of nausea and vomiting was significantly lower in patients who received propofol or midazolam compared with those in the control group, leading to the conclusion that midazolam is as effective as propofol in reducing the incidence of nausea and vomiting in women undergoing cesarean section.

Midazolam versus metoclopramide during cesarean section

Shahriari et al. compared the prophylactic antiemetic efficacy of a bolus dose of midazolam versus metoclopramide during cesarean delivery under spinal anesthesia[19]. In this study, 80 parturients were randomly allocated to receive midazolam (2 mg) or metoclopramide (10 mg) immediately preceding skin incision. The incidence of nausea and vomiting was lower in the midazolam group compared with those receiving metoclopramide (15% versus 52%, respectively). However, sedation scores within the first three postoperative hours were significantly higher in patients receiving midazolam. Additionally, there were incidences of respiratory depression (respiratory rate <10 breaths per minute) observed in 17 patients who had received midazolam; no respiratory depression was observed in those receiving metoclopramide. Given these findings, the authors emphasized the need for additional studies to further evaluate the safety of midazolam in cesarean deliveries.

Midazolam versus ondansetron in adults

Lee et al. compared the efficacy of midazolam with ondansetron in preventing PONV in 90 patients scheduled for either hysteroscopy or ureteroscopy[20]. IV midazolam (2 mg) or ondansetron (4 mg) was administered 30 min prior to the conclusion of the procedure. The percentages of patients who experienced PONV during the first 24 h postoperatively were not significantly different between the midazolam and ondansetron groups (30% and 27%, respectively), suggesting antiemetic prophylaxis with ondansetron was not superior to midazolam in these procedures.

Lorazepam versus droperidol in children

In a double-blind study, Khalil et al. compared the efficacy of lorazepam versus droperidol in reducing emetic symptoms of children (1–13 years of age) undergoing strabismus correction surgery[21]. The children were randomly allocated to receive IV droperidol (75 μg/kg), IV lorazepam (10 μg/kg) or placebo. They reported that lorazepam and droperidol resulted in a lower incidence of postoperative vomiting (POV) compared with placebo ($P < 0.024$), with no difference between lorazepam and droperidol.

Alpha-2 adrenergic agonists (clonidine and dexmedetomidine)

Clonidine, a centrally acting agonist of alpha-2 adrenergic receptors, is commonly used to reduce blood pressure by decreasing peripheral vascular resistance. Clonidine binding to its receptors inhibits the release of norepinephrine, which decreases sympathetic tone[22]. Although clonidine has been historically prescribed for its antihypertensive properties, other uses have been described more recently. New studies have demonstrated the efficacy of clonidine in treating postoperative, neuropathic and cancer-associated pain[23].

Clonidine is also effective as a preanesthetic medication in the adult and pediatric populations. Clonidine has been shown to blunt the sympathetic response to anesthesia, decrease intraoperative anesthetic requirements, provide preoperative sedation, stabilize perioperative hemodynamics, and even prevent POV[24].

Some clinical trials in adults have suggested that oral clonidine is effective in reducing the incidence of PONV. However, there are conflicting results in the literature regarding clonidine's antiemetic efficacy[25–27].

Clonidine versus placebo in adults undergoing ear surgery

Taheri et al. evaluated the effect of oral clonidine on PONV in adult patients undergoing outpatient ear surgery[25]. In a double-blind study, 60 adults were randomized to receive either clonidine or placebo. A complete response (no PONV and no need for rescue antiemetic medication) during the first 24 h postoperatively was 33% with placebo and 67% with clonidine ($P = 0.01$). The authors concluded that oral premedication with clonidine reduces the incidence of PONV in adults undergoing outpatient ear surgery.

Clonidine versus placebo in children undergoing appendectomy

Investigations of clonidine's antiemetic efficacy in children have, however, yielded mixed results. In a randomized, double-blind clinical trial by Alizadeh et al.[26], 60 children scheduled for appendectomy were randomized to receive either 4 μg/kg clonidine in apple juice or only apple juice 1 h prior to being transported to the operating room. Children who received clonidine experienced statistically significantly less episodes of PONV than did children in the control group ($P < 0.001$). Additionally, the number of children who received rescue antiemetic medication was also significantly lower in the treatment group ($P < 0.001$). The authors concluded that oral clonidine at a dose of 4 μg/kg administered preoperatively is associated with a reduced incidence of POV in children undergoing appendectomy.

Clonidine versus placebo in children receiving strabismus correction surgery

Gulhas et al. similarly assessed the efficacy of oral clonidine on PONV in children undergoing strabismus surgery[27]. In this double-blind study, 80 children were randomized to receive either clonidine (4 μg/kg) in apple juice or apple juice only. There were no statistically significant differences between the clonidine and control groups in terms of the number of children with complete response (21 versus 18), vomiting (19 versus 22) or need for rescue antiemetic medication (9 versus 12), respectively, during the first 48 postoperative hours.

Dexmedetomidine added to a balanced anesthesia regimen

Dexmedetomidine, another alpha-2 adrenergic agonist, has been commonly used for sedation in intensive care patients and, more recently, in nonintubated patients undergoing surgery. Massad et al. studied the antiemetic effect of adding dexmedetomidine to a balanced anesthetic technique during laparoscopic gynecologic surgery[28]. Eighty-one female patients were randomized to receive either an infusion of dexmedetomidine or

0.9% saline. The anesthetic technique was the same for both groups: induction of anesthesia was achieved with IV propofol (2 mg/kg) and fentanyl (1 μg/kg), whilst IV rocuronium (0.6 mg/kg) was used to facilitate intubation and sevoflurane (0.5–2.0% end tidal concentration) was used for maintenance of anesthesia. The authors reported that during the first 24 h postoperatively, patients receiving dexmedetomidine experienced significantly less PONV than those in the placebo group (31.0% versus 59.0%, respectively; $P = 0.04$). Additionally, significantly less intraoperative fentanyl and sevoflurane were required in the group receiving dexmedetomidine. The authors concluded that the administration of dexmedetomidine as part of a balanced anesthesia regimen reduces the incidence of PONV, either directly or by decreasing the requirement for anesthetic drugs that are known to be emetogenic.

Summary

In summary, various sedative agents such as propofol, benzodiazepines, clonidine and dexmedetomidine have been shown to be effective in the prevention of PONV through various mechanisms. Propofol, while not directly antidopaminergic, appears to exert its antiemetic effects through the stimulation of GABA receptors and a reduction in the secretion of serotonin. It is recommended that propofol TIVA be administered to patients at high risk for PONV. Additionally, there has been encouraging data to suggest the efficacy of patient-controlled subhypnotic doses of propofol for the direct treatment of nausea and vomiting. Similarly, benzodiazepines such as midazolam and lorazepam enhance the effect of GABA and have been shown to prevent PONV, possibly by decreasing the anxiety commonly experienced by patients undergoing surgery. Finally, clonidine and dexmedetomidine are alpha-2 adrenergic agonists that are associated with a decreased incidence of PONV. The mechanism of this effect remains unclear, although it may be related to a reduced requirement for anesthetics known to cause nausea and vomiting. As clinical trials involving the aforementioned medications proceed, we hope to further elucidate and appreciate the beneficial antiemetic effects that these sedative agents offer.

References

1. Vuyk J, Sitsen E, Reekers M. Intravenous anesthetics. In: Miller RD, ed. *Miller's Anesthesia*, 8th ed. Philadelphia: Elsevier/Saunders; 2015:821–63.
2. DeBalli P. The use of propofol as an antiemetic. *Int Anesthesiol Clin* 2003; 41(4):67–77.
3. Hvarfner A, Hammas B, Thorn SE, et al. The influence of propofol on vomiting induced by apomorphine. *Anesth Analg* 1995; 80:967–9.
4. Cechetto DF, Diab T, Gibson CJ, et al. The effects of propofol in the area postrema of rats. *Anesth Analg* 2001; 92:934–42.
5. Briggs LP, Clarke RS, Dundee JW, et al. Use of diisopropyl phenol as main agent for short procedures. *Br J Anesth* 1981; 53:1197–202.
6. McCollum JS, Milligan KR, Dundee JW. The antiemetic action of propofol. *Anesthesia* 1988; 43:239–40.
7. Campbell NN, Thomas AD. Does propofol have an antiemetic effect? A prospective study of the antiemetic effect of propofol following laparoscopy. *Anesth Intensive Care* 1991; 19:385–7.
8. Gan TJ, Glass PS, Howell ST, et al. Determination of plasma concentrations of propofol associated with 50% reduction in postoperative nausea. *Anesthesiology* 1997; 87:779–84.

9. Gan TJ, Ginsberg B, Grant AP, et al. Double-blind, randomized comparison of ondansetron and intraoperative propofol to prevent postoperative nausea and vomiting. *Anesthesiology* 1996; 85(5):1036–42.

10. Gepts E, Camu F, Cockshott, ID, et al. Disposition of propofol administered as constant rate intravenous infusions in humans. *Anesth Analg* 1987; 66:1256–63.

11. Honkavaara P, Saarnivaara L. Comparison of subhypnotic doses of thiopentone vs propofol on the incidence of postoperative nausea and vomiting following middle ear surgery. *Acta Anesthesiol Scand* 1998; 42(2):211–5.

12. Gupta A, Stierer T, Zuckerman R, et al. Comparison of recovery profile after ambulatory anesthesia with propofol, isoflurane, sevoflurane and desflurane: a systematic review. *Anesth Analg* 2004; 98(3):632–41.

13. Visser K, Hassink EA, Bonsel GJ, et al. Randomized controlled trial of total intravenous anesthesia with propofol versus inhalation anesthesia with isoflurane-nitrous oxide: postoperative nausea with vomiting and economic analysis. *Anesthesiology* 2001; 95(3):616–26.

14. Gan TJ. Postoperative nausea and vomiting – can it be eliminated? *JAMA* 2002; 287:1233–6.

15. Gan TJ, El-Molem H, Ray J, et al. Patient-controlled antiemesis: a randomized, double-blind comparison of two doses of propofol versus placebo. *Anesthesiology* 1999; 90(6):1564–70.

16. Giacalone VF. Antianxiety/sedative drugs: the benzodiazepines. *Clin Podiatr Med Surg* 1992; 9:465–79.

17. Splinter WM, MacNeill HB, Menard EA. Midazolam reduces vomiting after tonsillectomy in children. *Can J Anesth* 1995; 42:201–3.

18. Tarhan O, Canbay O, Celebi N, et al. Subhypnotic doses of midazolam prevent nausea and vomiting during spinal anesthesia for cesarean section. *Minerva Anesthesiol* 2007; 73(12):629–33.

19. Shahriari A, Khooshideh M, Heidari MH. Prevention of nausea and vomiting in caesarean section under spinal anesthesia with midazolam or metoclopramide? *JPMA* 2009; 59(11):756–9.

20. Lee Y, Wang JJ, Yang YL, et al. Midazolam vs ondansetron for preventing postoperative nausea and vomiting: a randomised controlled trial. *Anesthesia* 2007; 62(1):18–22.

21. Khalil SN, Berry JM, Howard G, et al. The antiemetic effect of lorazepam after outpatient strabismus surgery in children. *Anesthesiology* 1992; 77:915–9.

22. Eisenach JC, De Kock M, Klimscha W. α 2-Adrenergic agonists for regional anesthesia: a clinical review of clonidine (1984–1995). *Anesthesiology* 1996; 85:655–74.

23. Chan AK, Cheung CW, Chong YK. Alpha-2 agonists in acute pain management. *Expert Opin Pharmacother* 2010; 11:2849–68.

24. Nishina K, Mikawa K, Shiga M, Obara H. Clonidine in paediatric anesthesia. *Paediatr Anaesth* 1999; 9:187–202.

25. Taheri A, Javadimanesh MA, Ashraf H. The effect of oral clonidine premedication on nausea and vomiting after ear surgery. *MEJ Anesth* 2010; 20(5):691–4.

26. Alizadeh R, Mireskandari S, Azarshahin M. Oral clonidine premedication reduces nausea and vomiting in children after appendectomy. *Iran J Pediatr* 2012; 22(3):399–403.

27. Gulhas N, Turkoz A, Durmus M, et al. Oral clonidine premedication does not reduce postoperative vomiting in children undergoing strabismus surgery. *Acta Anesthesiol Scand* 2003; 47(1):90–3.

28. Massad IM, Mohsen WA, Basha AS, et al. A balanced anesthesia with dexmedetomidine decreases postoperative nausea and vomiting after laparoscopic surgery. *Saudi Med J* 2009; 30(12):1537–41.

Chapter 10

Nonpharmacologic management of postoperative nausea and vomiting

Anna Lee and Tony Gin

Postoperative nausea and vomiting (PONV) are common and unpleasant complications following surgery and anesthesia. In patients at high risk (≥80%) for PONV, the latest Consensus Guidelines for the Management of PONV recommend that nonpharmacologic therapies be considered as adjuncts to pharmacologic therapy[1]. This chapter reviews the current evidence for the use of common nonpharmacologic therapies for the management of PONV, such as acupuncture-related techniques stimulating the wrist pericardium meridian point 6 (PC6) acupoint, ginger (*Zingiber officinale)* and aromatherapy.

We performed a systematic search of randomized controlled trials (RCTs) and systematic reviews published within the last decade using the Cochrane Controlled Trials Register at the Cochrane Library and MEDLINE (the date of the last search was December 31, 2014). Where appropriate, we updated published systematic reviews with RCTs that were published after the reported date of electronic search of the literature. The primary outcomes for prevention of PONV were incidences of postoperative nausea and postoperative vomiting (POV) as separate entities and the need for rescue antiemetics. The primary outcome for PONV treatment was the need for rescue antiemetic.

We defined the overall quality of evidence using the Grading of Recommendations Assessment, Development and Evaluation (GRADE) approach, which considered the study design, risk of bias in individual trials according to the Cochrane Handbook for Systematic Reviews of Intervention[2] and the potential for publication bias, precision of pooled estimates, consistency of results across studies, suitability of the individual study populations, interventions, and outcome assessments in directly addressing the clinical question and magnitude of effect[3]. For classifying the quality of the evidence, the four levels were: high, moderate, low and very low[4].

Acupoint PC6 stimulation

Most nonpharmacologic studies for managing PONV have focused on the stimulation of the wrist at the "PC6 acupuncture point" to reduce nausea and vomiting. The PC6 acupoint lies between the tendons of the palmaris longus and flexor carpi radialis muscles, 4 cm proximal to the wrist crease (Figure 10.1)[5].

According to Traditional Chinese Medicine (TCM) theory, surgery interrupts the balanced state of the human body by disturbing the movement of both *qi* (energy flow) and blood, leading to stomach *qi* going upward to cause nausea and vomiting[6]. By regulating

Postoperative Nausea and Vomiting: A Practical Guide, eds. Tong Joo Gan and Ashraf S. Habib. Published by Cambridge University Press.

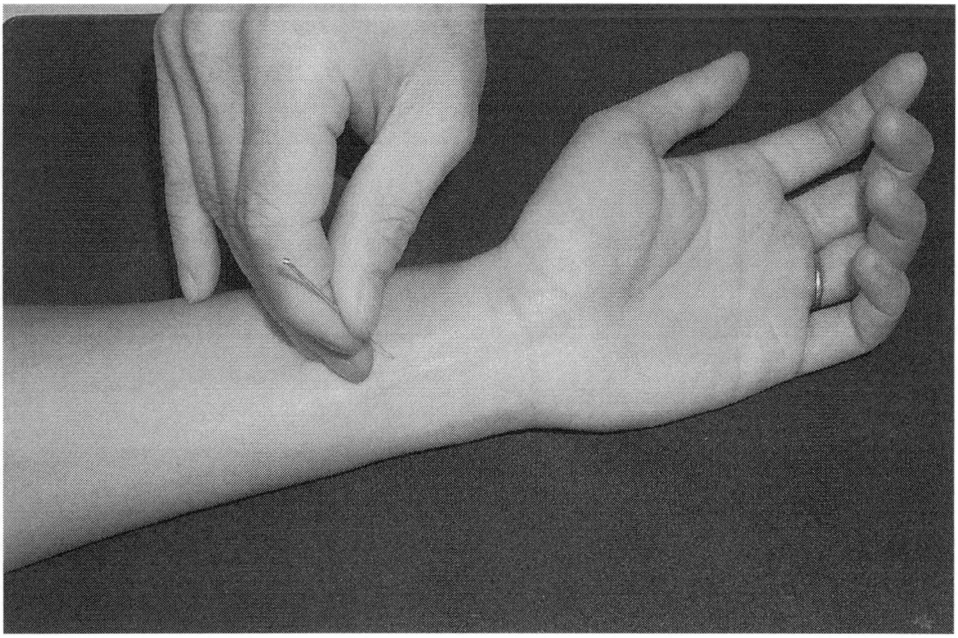

Figure 10.1 Location of the pericardium meridian point 6 acupoint.

the function of the stomach to reduce the adverse flow of *qi*, PC6 acupoint stimulation may prevent nausea and vomiting[6]. However, from a Western evidence-based medicine perspective, the mechanism by which PC6 stimulation helps manage PONV is unclear.

Prevention

In the recent update of a Cochrane systematic review[7] on the effectiveness of PC6 acupoint stimulation for the prevention of PONV, 10 types of PC6 acupoint stimulation were examined in 59 trials published between 1986 and 2015 involving 7,667 participants. The invasive types of PC6 acupoint stimulation included the following techniques that penetrated the skin: needle acupuncture (five trials), acupuncture needle infiltration of PC6 acupoint with dextrose (four trials) or droperidol (one trial), semipermanent needles (one trial) and electrical stimulation of needles (six trials). The noninvasive types of PC6 acupoint stimulation that did not penetrate the skin included the following techniques: transcutaneous electrical nerve or acupoint stimulation (five trials), laser stimulation (two trials), acustimulation device (six trials), acupressure wristbands (25 trials), capsicum plaster (two trials) and conventional peripheral nerve stimulation (three trials). PC6 stimulation was compared with six different antiemetic drugs: metoclopramide (five trials), cyclizine (one trial), prochlorperazine (two trials), droperidol (five trials), ondansetron (nine trials) and dexamethasone plus ondansetron (one trial).

Of the 59 trials, only two were considered as at low risk of bias, 32 at moderate risk of bias and 25 at high risk of bias. Thus, the results as shown in Table 10.1 should be interpreted with a degree of caution. There were wide variations in the type of surgery patients underwent, the PC6 acupoint therapy technique (type, timing and duration), comparison (sham or antiemetic) and the follow-up time for assessing PONV (from postanesthesia care unit (PACU) to 72 h). However, the risks of POV were similar between subgroups.

Most trials compared PC6 acupoint stimulation versus sham and showed that PC6 acupoint stimulation was effective for preventing PONV and reduced the need for rescue antiemetics (Table 10.1). Although the overall evidence was low due to underlying high risk of bias in a small proportion of trials and a moderate level of heterogeneity, we would expect 54 (95% confidence interval (CI), 48–62) and 48 (95% CI, 41–57) fewer nausea and vomiting episodes per 100 high-risk patients, respectively, when the underlying control risk is set at 80 per 100. In the trials directly comparing PC6 acupoint stimulation before and after induction of anesthesia against sham[9,10], the risk reduction in PONV was similar in magnitude regardless of the timing of PC6 acupoint stimulation.

In contrast, there was a moderate level of evidence to support PC6 acupoint stimulation being comparable to an antiemetic to prevent PONV (Table 10.1). There is also emerging evidence, albeit low quality, to suggest that the combined effect of P6 acupoint stimulation and antiemetic was more effective than an antiemetic alone in reducing the risk of vomiting and the need for a rescue antiemetic. The risk reduction associated with the combined effect of the PC6 acupoint stimulation and an antiemetic was consistent with the multimodal concept of using a combination of antiemetic therapy to provide a "synergistic" effect. Overall, the side effects associated with PC6 acupoint stimulation were minor and self-limiting.

Treatment

Few trials have been conducted to examine the use of PC6 acupoint stimulation for the management of established PONV. One trial showed that, for established postoperative nausea associated with the use of morphine patient-controlled analgesia, a greater reduction was observed in the severity of nausea on a 100-mm visual analog scale with bilateral PC6 acupuncture for 2 min compared with sham acupuncture (mean difference 29; 95% CI, 16–43) [11]. Rescue metoclopramide was more likely to be required in the sham acupressure group (100%) than in the PC6 acupressure group (47%; $P = 0.001$). Another trial showed that, in addition to intravenous (IV) metoclopramide 10 mg or droperidol 0.625 mg prophylaxis after induction of anesthesia, the combination of a wristband acustimulation device and ondansetron for the treatment of established emetic symptoms was more effective than the acustimulation device group, but was similar in the effectiveness to the ondansetron group (complete response rate without need for rescue therapy 73%, 40% and 57%, respectively) [12]. The results of these two trials suggest that PC6 acupoint stimulation may be a promising nonpharmacologic technique for the treatment of established PONV in those patients who may have had contraindications to taking an antiemetic.

Whilst many different techniques of PC6 acupoint stimulation have been examined in approximately 7,800 patients, there is currently a lack of widespread uptake of the technique. This may be due to a lack of evidence in the optimal timing, duration and method of PC6 acupoint stimulation[13]. In addition, invasive PC6 acupoint stimulation requires trained professionals to administer the technique that often takes up to 30 min; in contrast, the pharmacologic effect of an antiemetic is immediate. New research methods, such as network meta-analysis, may offer fresh insights into the comparative effectiveness of PC6 acupoint stimulation techniques against sham or antiemetics to answer the question of which types of PC6 acupoint stimulation technique are most effective to prevent PONV.

Table 10.1 Results of meta-analyses of PC6 acupoint stimulation trials for preventing PONV

Outcome	Studies	Patients	RR (95% CI)	Quality of evidence
Acupoint PC6 stimulation versus sham				
Nausea				Low[a]
All groups	40	4,742	0.68 (0.60–0.77)	
Invasive	7	896	0.56 (0.39–0.80)	
Noninvasive	33	3,846	0.71 (0.62–0.81)	
Vomiting				Low[a]
All groups	45	5,147	0.60 (0.51–0.71)	
Children	6	542	0.67 (0.46–0.97)	
Adults	37	4,465	0.61 (0.51–0.72)	
Mixed age groups	2	410	0.24 (0.07–0.79)	
Invasive	7[b]	896	0.51 (0.34–0.76)	
Noninvasive	37[b]	4,151	0.60 (0.50–0.73)	
Need for rescue antiemetic	39	4,622	0.64 (0.55–0.73)	Low[a]
Acupoint PC6 stimulation versus antiemetic				
Nausea				Moderate[c]
All groups	14	1,332	0.91 (0.75–1.10)	
Invasive	5	559	0.69 (0.41–1.14)	
Noninvasive	9	773	0.95 (0.78–1.16)	
Vomiting				Moderate[c]
All groups	19	1,708	0.93 (0.74–1.17)	
Invasive	8	734	0.99 (0.70–1.41)	
Noninvasive	12	974	0.90 (0.67–1.21)	
Need for rescue antiemetic	9	895	0.87 (0.65–1.16)	Moderate[c]
Combined PC6 stimulation and antiemetic versus antiemetic				
Nausea	8	642	0.79 (0.55–1.13)	Very low[d]
Vomiting	9	687	0.56 (0.35–0.91)	Very low[d]
Need for rescue antiemetic	5	419	0.61 (0.44–0.86)	Low[e]

CI, confidence interval; PC6, pericardium meridian point 6 acupoint; RR, relative risk.

[a] Evidence graded low due to a large proportion of underlying trials with moderate-to-high risk of bias and moderate degree of heterogeneity.

[b] Shenkman et al.[8] not included in subgroup analysis as the intervention involved the use of both acupuncture and acupressure wristband.

[c] Evidence graded moderate due to a large proportion of underlying trials with moderate-to-high risk of bias.

[d] Evidence graded very low due to a large proportion of underlying trials with moderate-to-high risk of bias, imprecision and moderate degree of heterogeneity.

[e] Evidence graded low due to trials with imprecision and moderate-to-high risk of bias.

Ginger

Prevention

Ginger *(Zingiber officinale)* is a common herb used in TCM. The pharmacologically active component of ginger, 6-gingerol, has antiserotonin and anticholinergic actions in the gastrointestinal tract[14]. As with all herbs, it is difficult to standardize the active extracts, which may partly explain the mixed results from clinical trials. A pharmacokinetic analysis showed that the half-lives of ginger metabolites were 1–3 h in human plasma and did not accumulate

Table 10.2 Results of meta-analyses of oral ginger capsules for preventing PONV

Outcome	Studies	Patients	RR (95% CI)	Quality of evidence
		Ginger versus placebo		
Nausea				Low[a]
All groups	7	778	0.87 (0.74–1.03)	
Dose ≥1g	6	549	0.82 (0.65–1.02)	
Dose <1g	2	229	1.05 (0.79–1.39)	
Vomiting				Moderate[b]
All groups	9	878	0.77 (0.56–1.05)	
Dose ≥1g	8	649	0.64 (0.49–0.84)	
Dose <1g	2	229	1.42 (0.91–2.22)	
Need for rescue antiemetic	6	550	0.61 (0.30–1.23)	Low[a]
		Ginger versus antiemetic		
Nausea	2	136	0.93 (0.62–1.39)	Moderate[c]
Vomiting	3	176	0.96 (0.56–1.67)	Moderate[c]
Need for rescue antiemetic	3	176	0.51 (0.23–1.15)	Moderate[c]
		Combined ginger and antiemetic versus antiemetic		
Nausea	2	176	1.10 (0.60–2.01)	Moderate[c]
Vomiting	2	176	1.66 (0.69–4.00)	Moderate[c]
Need for rescue antiemetic	2	220	0.75 (0.45–1.26)	Moderate[c]

CI, confidence interval; RR, relative risk.

[a] Evidence graded low due to a large proportion of underlying trials with moderate-to-high risk of bias and moderate degree of heterogeneity that cannot be explained by different dosages.

[b] Evidence graded moderate due to a large proportion of underlying trials with moderate-to-high risk of bias.

[c] Evidence graded moderate due to imprecision of the estimate.

after multiple daily dosing of 2 g over 1 month[15]. It appears that ginger supplements do not have clinically important anticoagulant effects[16].

This section reviews the RCTs of ginger powder in capsules on the prevention of PONV and updates the published trials included in a 2006 systematic review[17]. There were 11 oral ginger trials[14,18–27] published between 1990 and 2014 involving 1,228 participants. In all trials, the oral ginger, placebo and antiemetics (metoclopramide, dexamethasone and droperidol) were given 1 h before induction of anesthesia. The dose of ginger powder ranged from 0.3 g[21] to 2 g[27], with one trial[19] comparing 0.5 g and 1 g against a placebo. Trials were mainly conducted in women undergoing gynecologic surgery[14,18–21,24,25,27]. Follow-up time for PONV ranged from 2 to 24 h. Of the 11 trials, only two were considered as at low risk of bias[19,21], seven at moderate risk of bias and two at high risk of bias[18,23].

The results of meta-analyses of ginger comparisons are shown in Table 10.2. In comparing ginger with placebo, there was no subgroup difference on nausea by dose ($P = 0.17$). However, there was a subgroup difference on vomiting by dose ($P < 0.01$), with a significant risk reduction in trials with doses 1 g or above compared to placebo ($P = 0.001$). A sensitivity analysis based on low-to-moderate risk of bias trials with ginger doses 1 g or above showed that ginger was more effective than placebo in reducing the risk of vomiting (relative risk (RR) 0.66; 95% CI, 0.49–0.88). The effects of ginger or combined ginger with an antiemetic were similar to the antiemetic control group (Table 10.2). The reported side effects (abdominal discomfort and heartburn) associated with ginger were infrequent[18,19,25].

Treatment

No RCTs of oral ginger powder for treating established PONV are available.

Aromotherapy

Aromotherapy can be defined as the inhalation of vapors of essential oils or any substances for the purposes of a therapeutic benefit[28]. Most common vapors used to prevent or treat postoperative nausea are isopropyl alcohol, peppermint oil and ginger oil. The mechanism by which aromatherapy alleviates nausea is unclear. A disadvantage of aromatherapy is the risk of degradation of essential oils by oxidation or evaporation[28].

Prevention

In an RCT of 80 women undergoing laparoscopic and gynecologic surgery, half were allocated to inhale three deep nasal inhalations of 70% isopropyl alcohol before oxygenation and the other half were given no treatment[29]. Both groups were given ondansetron 4 mg IV before the end of surgery. The risk of postoperative nausea was similar between the isopropyl alcohol inhalation group and control group (47% versus 32%, respectively; $P = 0.16$). Although the outcome assessors were blinded to the treatment allocation, the patients and attending anesthesiologists were not blinded.

Treatment

This section updates a systematic review of RCTs on aromatherapy for the treatment of PONV[28], with the primary outcome of the need for rescue antiemetic. Trials published as conference abstracts were excluded. We found seven trials[30–36] published between 1999 and 2014 involving 613 patients with PONV symptoms. One trial[35] was conducted in children undergoing general anesthesia for outpatient surgery. Patients were asked to deeply inhale the scent of isopropyl alcohol[30–33,35,36], peppermint[30,34], ginger[32], blended oils[32] or placebo[30,32,34,35] three times at 5-min intervals for up to a maximum of three times, or were given an antiemetic as standard treatment[31,33,36]. Of the seven trials, three were at high risk of bias[32,34,36].

In trials comparing aromatherapy with placebo, the high degree of heterogeneity was likely due to the type of essential oils used as there was a significant subgroup difference detected ($P = 0.03$) (Figure 10.2). Figure 10.2 suggests that aromotherapy using ginger or blended oils was more effective in reducing the need for rescue antiemetic than placebo aromatherapy, but these results are based upon one low-quality trial[32]. Whilst isopropyl alcohol is readily available in the PACU (in the form of injection site "prep-pads"), there was no reduction in the proportion of patients needing rescue antiemetic compared to placebo aromatherapy (RR 0.85; 95% CI, 0.69–1.05). Thus, the overall evidence to support the use of aromatherapy over placebo is rated "very low" due to the imprecision of results (total sample size of 415) and the inclusion of a large proportion of high risk of bias trials.

Compared to standard care of treating PONV with an antiemetic, the risk of requiring rescue antiemetic in the isopropyl alcohol group was similar in the pooled results from three trials (RR 0.67; 95% CI, 0.31–1.45). The overall quality of evidence is rated "low" due to imprecision of results and inclusion of moderate-to-high risk of bias trials.

Study or Subgroup	Experimental Events	Experimental Total	Placebo Events	Placebo Total	Weight	Risk Ratio IV, Random, 95% CI
2.1.1 Isopropyl alcohol						
Anderson 2004	5	11	3	6	3.8%	0.91 [0.32, 2.54]
Hunt 2013	56	78	20	25	27.0%	0.90 [0.71, 1.14]
Wang 1999	11	20	15	19	14.0%	0.70 [0.44, 1.10]
Subtotal (95% CI)		**109**		**50**	**44.8%**	**0.85 [0.69, 1.05]**
Total events	72		38			
Heterogeneity: Tau² = 0.00; Chi² = 0.93, df = 2 (P = 0.63); I² = 0%						
Test for overall effect: Z = 1.50 (P = 0.13)						
2.1.2 Peppermint						
Anderson 2004	6	10	3	6	4.5%	1.20 [0.47, 3.09]
Sites 2014	11	26	6	16	6.3%	1.13 [0.52, 2.45]
Subtotal (95% CI)		**36**		**22**	**10.8%**	**1.16 [0.63, 2.11]**
Total events	17		9			
Heterogeneity: Tau² = 0.00; Chi² = 0.01, df = 1 (P = 0.92); I² = 0%						
Test for overall effect: Z = 0.47 (P = 0.63)						
2.1.3 Ginger						
Hunt 2013	42	76	20	24	24.7%	0.66 [0.51, 0.87]
Subtotal (95% CI)		**76**		**24**	**24.7%**	**0.66 [0.51, 0.87]**
Total events	42		20			
Heterogeneity: Not applicable						
Test for overall effect: Z = 2.98 (P = 0.003)						
2.1.4 Blended oils						
Hunt 2013	30	74	19	24	19.8%	0.51 [0.36, 0.72]
Subtotal (95% CI)		**74**		**24**	**19.8%**	**0.51 [0.36, 0.72]**
Total events	30		19			
Heterogeneity: Not applicable						
Test for overall effect: Z = 3.81 (P = 0.0001)						
Total (95% CI)		**295**		**120**	**100.0%**	**0.74 [0.60, 0.91]**
Total events	161		86			
Heterogeneity: Tau² = 0.03; Chi² = 9.87, df = 6 (P = 0.13); I² = 39%						
Test for overall effect: Z = 2.79 (P = 0.005)						
Test for subgroup differences: Chi² = 8.92, df = 3 (P = 0.03), I² = 66.4%						

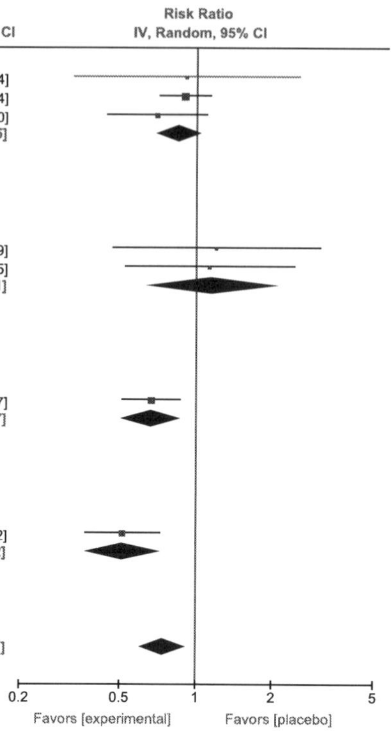

Figure 10.2 Results of total and subgroup meta-analyses on the need for rescue antiemetic in trials comparing aromatherapy and placebo inhalation. CI, confidence interval; IV, inverse-variance.

Summary

Nonpharmacologic therapies are attractive alternatives to antiemetics, with benefits including low cost, noninvasive nature of administration and infrequent side effects. The results of this chapter suggests that compared to placebo, there is low evidence to support the use of PC6 acupoint stimulation for the prevention of PONV and moderate evidence to support the use of oral ginger capsules at a dose of 1 g or more to prevent POV in high-risk patients who have contraindications to the use of standard antiemetics. There is insufficient evidence to support the widespread use of aromatherapy for treatment of PONV at this point in time.

References

1. Gan TJ, Diemunsch P, Habib AS, et al. Consensus guidelines for the management of postoperative nausea and vomiting. *Anesth Analg* 2014; 118: 85–113.
2. Higgins JPT Green S. Cochrane Handbook for Systematic Reviews of Interventions, version 5.1.0 (updated March 2011). The Cochrane Collaboration, 2011. www.cochrane-handbook.org (accessed January 16, 2015).
3. Guyatt G, Oxman AD, Akl EA, et al. GRADE guidelines: 1. Introduction – GRADE evidence profiles and summary of findings tables. *J Clin Epidemiol* 2011; 64: 383–94.

4. Balshem H, Helfand M, Schunemann HJ, et al. GRADE guidelines: 3. Rating the quality of evidence. *J Clin Epidemiol* 2011; 64: 401–06.
5. Yang LC, Jawan B, Chen CN, et al. Comparison of P6 acupoint injection with 50% glucose in water and intravenous droperidol for prevention of vomiting after gynecological laparoscopy. *Acta Anaesthesiol Scand* 1993; 37: 192–4.
6. Lv JQ, Feng RZ, Li N. P6 acupoint stimulation for prevention of postoperative nausea and vomiting in patients undergoing craniotomy: study protocol for a randomized controlled trial. *Trials* 2013; 14: 153.
7. Lee A, Chan SK, Fan LT. Stimulation of the wrist acupuncture point PC6 for preventing postoperative nausea and vomiting. *Cochrane Database Syst Rev* 2015; 11: CD003281.
8. Shenkman Z, Holzman RS, Kim C, et al. Acupressure-acupuncture anti-emetic prophylaxis in children undergoing tonsillectomy. *Anesthesiology* 1999; 90: 1311–6.
9. Frey UH, Scharmann P, Lohlein C, et al. P6 acustimulation effectively decreases postoperative nausea and vomiting in high-risk patients. *Br J Anaesth* 2009; 102: 620–5.
10. Frey UH, Funk M, Lohlein C, et al. Effect of P6 acustimulation on postoperative nausea and vomiting in patients undergoing a laparoscopic cholecystectomy. *Acta Anaesthesiol Scand* 2009; 53: 1341–7.
11. McConaghy P, Bland D, Swales H. Acupuncture in the management of postoperative nausea and vomiting in patients receiving morphine via a patient-controlled analgesia system. *Acup Med* 1996; 14: 2–5.
12. Coloma M, White PF, Ogunnaike BO, et al. Comparison of acustimulation and ondansetron for the treatment of established postoperative nausea and vomiting. *Anesthesiology* 2002; 97: 1387–92.
13. Streitberger K, Kranke P. Evidence for the efficacy of acupressure for preventing post-operative nausea and vomiting: an ongoing debate. *Eur J Anaesthesiol* 2011; 28: 396–8.
14. Nanthakomon T, Pongrojpaw D. The efficacy of ginger in prevention of postoperative nausea and vomiting after major gynecologic surgery. *J Med Assoc Thai* 2006; 89(Suppl 4): S130–6.
15. Yu Y, Zick S, Li X, et al. Examination of the pharmacokinetics of active ingredients of ginger in humans. *AAPS J* 2011; 13: 417–26.
16. Stanger MJ, Thompson LA, Young AJ, et al. Anticoagulant activity of select dietary supplements. *Nutr Rev* 2012; 70: 107–17.
17. Chaiyakunapruk N, Kitikannakorn N, Nathisuwan S, et al. The efficacy of ginger for the prevention of postoperative nausea and vomiting: a meta-analysis. *Am J Obstet Gynecol* 2006; 194: 95–9.
18. Apariman S, Ratchanon S, Wiriyasirivej B. Effectiveness of ginger for prevention of nausea and vomiting after gynecological laparoscopy. *J Med Assoc Thai* 2006; 89: 2003–9.
19. Arfeen Z, Owen H, Plummer JL, et al. A double-blind randomized controlled trial of ginger for the prevention of postoperative nausea and vomiting. *Anaesth Intensive Care* 1995; 23: 449–52.
20. Bone ME, Wilkinson DJ, Young JR, et al. Ginger root – a new anti-emetic. The effect of ginger root on postoperative nausea and vomiting after major gynaecological surgery. *Anaesthesia* 1990; 45: 669–71.
21. Eberhart LH, Mayer R, Betz O, et al. Ginger does not prevent postoperative nausea and vomiting after laparoscopic surgery. *Anesth Analg* 2003; 96: 995–8.
22. Mandal P, Das A, Majumdar S, et al. The efficacy of ginger added to ondansetron for preventing postoperative nausea and vomiting in ambulatory surgery. *Pharmacognosy Res* 2014; 6: 52–7.

23. Montazeri AS, Hamidzadeh A, Raei M, et al. Evaluation of oral ginger efficacy against postoperative nausea and vomiting: a randomized, double- blinded clinical trial. *Iran Red Crescent Med J* 2013; 15: e12268.

24. Phillips S, Ruggier R, Hutchinson SE. *Zingiber officinale* (ginger) – an anti-emetic for day case surgery. *Anaesthesia* 1993; 48: 715–7.

25. Pongrojpaw D, Chiamchanya C. The efficacy of ginger in prevention of post-operative nausea and vomiting after outpatient gynecological laparoscopy. *J Med Assoc Thai* 2003; 86: 244–50.

26. Tavlan A, Tuncer S, Erol A, et al. Prevention of postoperative nausea and vomiting after thyroidectomy: combined anti-emetic treatment with dexamethasone and ginger versus dexamethasone alone. *Clin Drug Investig* 2006; 26: 209–14.

27. Visalyaputra S, Petchpaisit N, Somcharoen K, et al. The efficacy of ginger root in the prevention of postoperative nausea and vomiting after outpatient gynaecological laparoscopy. *Anaesthesia* 1998; 53: 506–10.

28. Hines S, Steels E, Chang A, et al. Aromatherapy for treatment of postoperative nausea and vomiting. *Cochrane Database Syst Rev* 2012; 4: CD007598.

29. Radford KD, Fuller TN, Bushey B, et al. Prophylactic isopropyl alcohol inhalation and intravenous ondansetron versus ondansetron alone in the prevention of postoperative nausea and vomiting in high-risk patients. *AANA J* 2011; 79(4 Suppl): S69–74.

30. Anderson LA, Gross JB. Aromatherapy with peppermint, isopropyl alcohol, or placebo is equally effective in relieving postoperative nausea. *J Perianesth Nurs* 2004; 19: 29–35.

31. Cotton JW, Rowell LR, Hood RR, et al. A comparative analysis of isopropyl alcohol and ondansetron in the treatment of postoperative nausea and vomiting from the hospital setting to the home. *AANA J* 2007; 75: 21–6.

32. Hunt R, Dienemann J, Norton HJ, et al. Aromatherapy as treatment for postoperative nausea: a randomized trial. *Anesth Analg* 2013; 117: 597–604.

33. Pellegrini J, DeLoge J, Bennett J, et al. Comparison of inhalation of isopropyl alcohol vs promethazine in the treatment of postoperative nausea and vomiting (PONV) in patients identified as at high risk for developing PONV. *AANA J* 2009; 77: 293–9.

34. Sites DS, Johnson NT, Miller JA, et al. Controlled breathing with or without peppermint aromatherapy for postoperative nausea and/or vomiting symptom relief: a randomized controlled trial. *J Perianesth Nurs* 2014; 291: 12–9.

35. Wang SM, Hofstadter MB, Kain ZN. An alternative method to alleviate postoperative nausea and vomiting in children. *J Clin Anesth* 1999; 11: 231–4.

36. Winston AW, Rinehart RS, Riley GP, et al. Comparison of inhaled isopropyl alcohol and intravenous ondansetron for treatment of postoperative nausea. *AANA J* 2003; 71: 127–32.

Chapter 11

Combination antiemetics

Jessica Carter, Amy Mauritz and Ashraf S. Habib

None of the currently available antiemetics are entirely effective for the prophylaxis against postoperative nausea and vomiting (PONV). The best number needed-to-treat (NNT) for the most effective antiemetics investigated in meta-analyses is about four, meaning that four patients have to receive antiemetic prophylaxis for one patient to benefit from such intervention. The limited efficacy of single-agent antiemetic prophylaxis, particularly in high-risk patients, has led to increased interest in combination antiemetic therapy. The concept of combination antiemetic prophylaxis originated in 1988 for the management of chemotherapy-induced nausea and vomiting (CINV)[1]. Investigating combination antiemetic therapy for PONV prophylaxis followed the encouraging results in CINV.

The use of combination antiemetic therapy has sound physiologic basis. The vomiting center is located in the lateral reticular formation of the medulla and is triggered by activating stimuli from several areas within the central nervous system (CNS), including the chemoreceptor trigger zone in the area postrema, the vestibular apparatus, the vagus nerve, the solitary tract nucleus, the forebrain and other higher cortical centers[2]. These various sites contain receptors for serotonin, histamine, dopamine, acetylcholine, neurokinin (NK), opioids and many other endogenous neurotransmitters[3]. Antagonists at those receptors form the mainstay of most of the currently available antiemetics. Since the etiology of PONV is multifactorial, improved antiemetic prophylaxis might be achieved by using a combination of antiemetic drugs that work at different receptor sites. This chapter will focus on the following aspects relating to combination antiemetic therapy.

- Combination of two antiemetics for PONV prophylaxis.
- Combination of more than two antiemetics and the multimodal approach for PONV prophylaxis.
- Comparison between different antiemetic combinations.
- Side effects of combination antiemetic therapy.
- Efficacy of combination therapy for postdischarge nausea and vomiting (PDNV).
- Combination therapy for the treatment of established PONV.

Combination of two antiemetics for PONV prophylaxis

Numerous combinations of two antiemetics have been investigated. A comprehensive list of all the combinations studied is beyond the scope of this chapter. In general, a combination

Postoperative Nausea and Vomiting: A Practical Guide, eds. Tong Joo Gan and Ashraf S. Habib. Published by Cambridge University Press.

of two effective antiemetic interventions has been associated with improved PONV prophylaxis compared to either intervention alone. The combination of first-generation serotonin antagonists with dexamethasone or droperidol has been the most frequently studied combination. The following combination of two antiemetics will be reviewed:

- combination of 5-HT_3 receptor antagonists with dexamethasone
- combination of 5-HT_3 receptor antagonists with droperidol
- combination of dexamethasone and droperidol
- combination of ondansetron and scopolamine
- combinations involving metoclopramide
- combinations involving NK type 1 (NK_1)-receptor antagonists
- other combinations.

5-HT_3 receptor antagonists + dexamethasone

The combination of dexamethasone with a 5-HT_3 receptor antagonist is one of the most commonly used combinations in current practice. It has been previously suggested that there might be synergy between 5-HT_3 receptor antagonists and dexamethasone stemming from the corticosteroid's ability to slow the turnover of serotonin in the CNS[4]. However, a large multicenter study suggested that the interaction between ondansetron and dexamethasone is additive and not synergestic[5].

Combination of dexamethasone with first-generation 5-HT_3 receptor antagonists

Ondansetron was the first 5-HT_3 receptor antagonist reported in the medical literature in 1988 for the management of CINV and in 1991 for PONV[6,7], and has been the most extensively studied agent. One of the first randomized controlled trials (RCTs) of the combination of ondansetron and dexamethasone was published in 1996 by Lopez-Olaondo et al., who performed a double-blind RCT of women undergoing elective gynecologic surgery[8]. They reported that dexamethasone 8 mg combined with ondansetron 4 mg was more effective at preventing PONV than either agent alone or placebo; the incidence of PONV at 48 h was 80% with placebo, 48% with ondansetron, 40% with dexamethasone and 16% in the combination therapy group.

Subsequently, numerous studies investigated this combination and confirmed its superiority to single agent prophylaxis[9]. In a large European multicenter study of factorial design involving patients with at least 40% risk for PONV, according to the Apfel simplified risk score, Apfel et al. reported that the combination of ondansetron 4 mg with dexamethasone 4 mg was more effective than each agent alone (37% PONV with monotherapy versus 28% with combination therapy)[5]. Comparable results have been obtained with the combination of dexamethasone with granisetron[10], tropisetron[11,12] and dolasetron[13,14]. A number of meta-analyses have also confirmed the superiority of the combination of dexamethasone with first-generation 5-HT_3 receptor antagonists compared to prophylaxis with a single agent[15–17].

Combination of dexamethasone with second-generation 5-HT_3 receptor antagonists

Palonosetron, a second-generation 5-HT_3 receptor antagonist, first appeared in the literature for the prevention of delayed CINV in 2003 and for PONV prevention in 2008[18,19].

Since palonosetron is a newer agent, data on combination therapies including palonosetron are still sparse. Bala et al. assessed PONV prophylaxis with palonosetron 0.075 mg/dexamethasone 8 mg combination therapy compared to palonosetron alone in patients undergoing laparoscopic cholecystectomy[20]. In the first 24 postoperative hours, the combination therapy group had significantly lower PONV episodes compared to monotherapy (26.3% versus 76.2%, $P = 0.004$). Other studies, however, did not confirm the superiority of this combination. In a high-risk population with two or more PONV risk factors undergoing gynecologic, ear or thyroid surgery, Park et al. found no difference in PONV severity scores between the palonosetron 0.075 mg versus palonosetron 0.075 mg plus dexamethasone 8 mg groups[21]. Similarly, Blitz et al. included patients with three or more PONV risk factors undergoing laparoscopic surgery and showed no difference in PONV incidence between the palonosetron and palonosetron plus dexamethasone groups[22]. More studies are needed to assess whether there is added benefit of combining dexamethasone with palonosetron compared to prophylaxis with palonosetron alone.

5-HT$_3$ receptor antagonists + droperidol

The combination of ondansetron and droperidol was one of the most commonly investigated combinations. The greater antinausea efficacy of droperidol combined with the good efficacy of ondansetron against vomiting provides a good rationale for this combination. Further, droperidol seems to have a protective effect against headache, a common side effect of ondansetron[23]. In 2000, Eberhart et al. performed a meta-analysis of eight studies including 881 patients and reported that seven of the eight studies reported increased antiemetic efficacy of the combination, but the results were not statistically significant[15]. When those studies were pooled in a meta-analysis, the differences were still not statistically significant (NNT = 12 for PONV with the combination versus droperidol alone and NNT = 14 for PONV with the combination versus 5-HT$_3$ receptor antagonists alone). Habib et al. reported comparable results in a subsequent meta-analysis[16]. In a large European multicenter study of factorial design, however, Apfel et al. reported that the combination of droperidol 1.25 mg and ondansetron 4 mg was significantly more effective than each agent alone[5]. Following the US Food and Drug Administration (FDA) black box warning on droperidol, the use of this agent has decreased and some studies began to investigate the use of haloperidol for PONV prophylaxis. Data on combination therapy involving haloperidol are limited, but one study reported that the combination of haloperidol 2 mg with ondansetron 4 mg was associated with a higher complete response (79%) compared with haloperidol (61%) or ondansetron (62%) alone[24].

Dexamethasone + droperidol

The combination of dexamethasone with droperidol has been less frequently investigated. In a large European multicenter study, the combination of dexamethasone 4 mg with droperidol 1.25 mg was found to be more effective than each agent alone[5]. Following the FDA black box warning on droperidol, some studies investigated the combination of dexamethasone with haloperidol. Chu et al. found that the 24 h incidence of PONV was significantly reduced with the combination of haloperidol 2 mg with dexamethasone 5 mg (19%) compared with each agent alone or droperidol 1.25 alone (36–38%) or placebo (65%)[25].

Ondansetron + transdermal scopolamine

In a large multicenter study involving 620 females undergoing outpatient laparoscopic or breast surgery, Gan et al. reported that the combination of transdermal scopolamine (TDS) patch 1.5 mg applied 2 h before surgery and ondansetron 4 mg administered at induction of anesthesia was associated with a higher 24-h complete response (no vomiting/retching or need for rescue) (48%) compared with ondansetron alone (39%)[26]. Interestingly, the incidence of side effects was also lower in the combination group. Other studies have also confirmed the superior antiemetic efficacy of this combination compared with ondansetron alone[27,28].

Combinations involving metoclopramide

Studies evaluating the combination of metoclopramide 10 mg with other antiemetics have, in general, showed limited benefit compared to single-agent prophylaxis with the antiemetics[9]. For instance, the combination of metoclopramide 10 mg with droperidol[29] or dexamethasone[30] was no better than the other antiemetic alone. In a recent meta-analysis[31], there were limited studies investigating combinations involving metoclopramide 10 mg, and those studies have shown no benefit of combinations involving metoclopramide, except for early (1–6 h) nausea, which was reduced with the combination compared to placebo with a NNT of 10, but were not compared to single-agent prophylaxis. Higher doses of metoclopramide might, however, have a more consistent antiemetic effect. A large German multicenter study involving 3,140 patients confirmed that metoclopramide 10 mg combined with dexamethasone 8 mg did not result in improved PONV prophylaxis compared with dexamethasone alone. Higher doses of metoclopramide of 25 and 50 mg combined with dexamethasone were associated with lower PONV rates (17% and 15%, respectively) compared with dexamethasone alone (21%)[32].

Combinations involving NK_1-receptor antagonists

There are relatively few data on combination therapy involving the NK_1 receptor antagonists. A summary of studies investigating combinations with NK_1 receptor antagonists is presented in Table 11.1. In females undergoing abdominal hysterectomy, the combination of ondansetron 4 mg plus the NK_1 receptor antagonist (CP-122, 721) was significantly better than each agent alone in prolonging the time to the first administration of rescue antiemetic and in reducing the incidence of vomiting (4% combination group versus 24% ondansetron group and 6% CP-122, 721 group)[33]. The combination of casopitant with ondansetron was also more effective than ondansetron alone in achieving a higher complete response rate[34,35]. Aprepitant, the only FDA-approved NK_1-receptor antagonist, was studied in combination with ondansetron compared to ondansetron alone in three studies[36–38], with all showing lower incidence of vomiting with the combination compared to ondansetron alone. Interestingly, only one study used the FDA-approved PONV aprepitant prophylaxis dose of 40 mg[38], while the other two used higher doses[36,37]. Similarly, the combination of aprepitant 80 mg with ramosetron 0.3 mg was more effective than ramosetron alone in reducing the incidence of nausea and vomiting as well as the severity of nausea[39]. Finally, the combination of aprepitant 80 mg with dexamethasone 8 mg was more effective than dexamethasone alone in reducing the incidence of vomiting and the severity of nausea[40]. Interestingly, none of those studies compared the combination to a

Table 11.1 Studies of combination antiemetic therapy involving the use of NK_1-receptor antagonists

Study	Type of surgery	Groups (*n*)	Nausea (%)	Vomiting (%)	Complete response (%)	Results of statistical analysis
Gesztesi et al. [33]	Hysterectomy	O 4 mg (52) CP122, 7211 200 mg (52) O 4 mg + CP122, 721 200 mg (53)	98 96 98	24 6 4		Nausea: NS Vomiting: CP122, 721 = O + CP122, 721 > O
Altorjay et al. [34]	Breast, shoulder, gynecologic, or thyroid surgeries, cholecystectomy, hysterectomy	O 4 mg IV (237) O 4 mg IV + C 50 mg PO (235)		25.1 10.3	58.7 68.7	Vomiting and CR: O + C > O
Singla et al. [35]	Laparoscopic or open gynecologic surgery, laparoscopic cholecystectomy	O 4 mg IV (129) O 4 mg IV + C 50 mg PO (135) O 4 mg IV + C 100 mg PO (130) O 4 mg IV + C 150 mg PO (128) C 150 mg PO (126)	67.1 70 63.6 66.4 72.5	28.6 9.3 4.3 7.1 7	40 59.3 62.1 60.7 50	Nausea: NS Vomiting and CR: all O + C groups > O
Lim et al. [36]	Rhinolaryngologic	O 4 mg IV (26) O 4 mg IV + A 80 mg PO (28) O 4 mg IV + A 125 mg PO (24)			70.8 82.1 96.1	PONV: O + A 125 mg > O
Sinha et al. [37]	Laparoscopic bariatric surgery	O 4 mg IV (60) O 4 mg IV + A 80 mg PO (64)		15 3.1	36.7 42.2	Vomiting: O + A > O CR: NS
Vallejo et al. [38]	Ambulatory plastic surgery	O 4 mg IV (75) O 4 mg IV + A 40 mg PO (75)		29.7 9.3	26.7 34.7	Vomiting: O + A > O CR: NS
Lee[39]	Gynecologic surgery	R 0.3 mg IV (42) R 0.3 mg IV + A 80 mg PO (42)	80.9 50	42.8 4.7	47.6 19.1	Nausea, vomiting and PONV: R + A > R
Kawano et al. [40]	Knee surgery	Dex 8 mg IV (30) Dex 8 mg IV + A 80 mg PO (30)		27 3		Vomiting: Dex + A > Dex
Green et al. [41]	Any surgery	A 40 mg PO (57) A 40 mg PO + TDS 1.5 mg (58)	35 45	3.5 8.6	63 57	Nausea, vomiting and CR: NS

A, aprepitant; C, casopitant; CR, complete response; Dex, dexamethasone; IV, intravenous; NS, no statistically significant differences; O, ondansetron; PO, oral; R, ramosetron; TDS, transdermal scopolam ne; >, statistically significant difference. Data are 24-h data unless studies reported data at other time points not including 24 h.

group receiving aprepitant only prophylaxis; therefore, it is not clear if those combinations are superior to single-agent prophylaxis with aprepitant. The only study comparing combination therapy to monotherapy with aprepitant was in patients with at least two of the four Apfel risk factors who received prophylaxis with aprepitant 40 mg alone or combined with TDS[40]. Interestingly, the addition of TDS did not confer any improved antiemetic efficacy compared to aprepitant alone.

Other combinations

Lee et al. evaluated the combination of TDS with intravenous dexamethasone in patients receiving patient-controlled epidural analgesia after major orthopedic surgery, and reported that the combination was more effective in preventing PONV than dexamethasone alone or dexamethasone plus ramosetron[42]. The combination of cyclizine 50 mg and ondansetron 4 mg was more effective than ondansetron alone in preventing PONV in women undergoing ambulatory gynecologic surgery[43]. Khalil et al. compared the combination of ondansetron 2 mg and promethazine 12.5 mg with ondansetron 4 mg, promethazine 25 mg or placebo in 87 patients scheduled for middle ear surgery[44]. During the 24-h postoperative period, the incidence of PONV was lower in the combination (29%) and promethazine (39%) groups compared with the placebo group (74%). Whilst the incidence of PONV in the ondansetron group (48%) was higher than the combination group, the difference was not statistically significant since the study was not powered to detect differences between the combination group and single agent group, which is also the case in many other published studies comparing combination therapy versus the two active agents and placebo. Gan et al. compared the combination of promethazine 6.25 mg with granisetron 0.1 mg versus each agent alone in women undergoing outpatient laparoscopy[45]. Prophylaxis with oral promethazine 12.5 mg, granisetron 1 mg or both was started in the respective groups 12 h after the end of surgery and continued every 12 h until postoperative day 3. Patients in the combination group had a higher total response rate (no PONV and no rescue) at 6, 24, 48 and 72 h after surgery compared with those who received promethazine alone (at 24 h combination 69.6%, promethazine 36.2%, granisetron 53.3%; $P = 0.0079$). The maximum nausea scores were also lower in the combination group compared to both single-agent groups.

Combination of more than two antiemetics and the multimodal approach for PONV prophylaxis

The concept of the multimodal approach involves the use of strategies to minimize the baseline risk of PONV in addition to using combination antiemetic therapy. Scuderi et al. investigated a multimodal approach to the management of PONV in female patients undergoing outpatient laparoscopy[46]. Their multimodal algorithm consisted of total intravenous anesthesia (TIVA) with propofol and remifentanil, no nitrous oxide, no neuromuscular blockade, aggressive intravenous hydration, triple prophylactic antiemetics (ondansetron 1 mg, droperidol 0.625 mg and dexamethasone 10 mg) and ketorolac 30 mg. Control groups included inhaled anesthetic, nitrous oxide, fentanyl and muscle relaxation with neostigmine reversal with or without 4 mg ondansetron prophylaxis. Complete response rate (no PONV and no rescue) in the postanesthesia care unit occurred in 98% of patients in the multimodal group compared with 76% in the ondansetron group and 59% in the placebo group

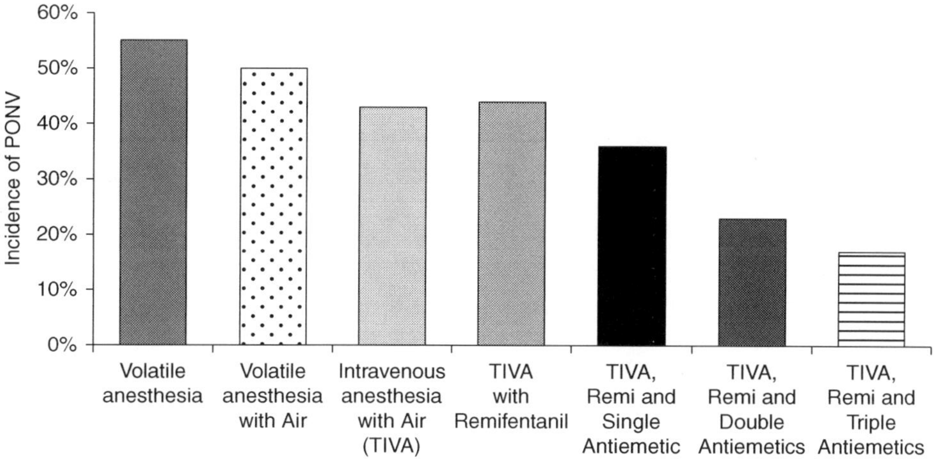

Figure 11.1 Incidence of postoperative nausea and vomiting (PONV) with various combinations of anesthetic – omission of nitrous oxide (air), use of total intravenous anesthesia (TIVA) with propofol and use of remifentanil (remi) – and antiemetic interventions (single, double or triple antiemetics of the following: ondansetron 4 mg, droperidol 1.25 mg and dexamethasone 4 mg).

($P < 0.0001$). Readiness to discharge was also sooner in the multimodal group ($P < 0.001$). Habib et al. also found that a multimodal approach incorporating TIVA with propofol combined with ondansetron 4 mg and droperidol 0.625 mg, together with ketorolac and local anesthetic infiltration, was more effective than the combination of the two antiemetics alone or TIVA alone in achieving a complete response (no PONV and no rescue) at 24 h following laparoscopic cholecystectomy (80%, 63% and 43%, respectively)[47]. The contribution of each component to the antiemetic effect, however, was not assessed in those studies. In a multicenter study of factorial design involving 5,161 patients with at least two of the four Apfel risk factors, a multimodal approach was assessed involving three antiemetic interventions (ondansetron 4 mg, droperidol 1.25 mg and dexamethasone 4 mg) and three anesthetic interventions (TIVA with propofol, omission of nitrous oxide and use of remifentanil for intraoperative analgesia); the antiemetic efficacy of various combinations of those interventions was evaluated[5]. The incidence of PONV was 17% in patients who received all six interventions compared to 59% in those who did not receive any of those interventions. The progressive reduction in the risk of PONV with each added intervention is shown in Figure 11.1[5]. Each antiemetic reduced the incidence of PONV by 26%, TIVA with propofol reduced it by 19% and omission of nitrous oxide reduced it by 12%. The use of remifentanil intraoperatively instead of fentanyl did not confer any additional benefit. The interaction between those interventions was additive and not synergistic.

Comparison between different antiemetic combinations

There are relatively few studies comparing the efficacy of different antiemetic combinations. This is partly due to the fact that a large sample size is needed to demonstrate differences between different antiemetic combinations. In a meta-analysis involving 3,447 patients, Habib et al. reported no difference in antiemetic efficacy between the combination of 5-HT_3

receptor antagonists with droperidol and their combination with dexamethasone[16]. Similarly, Apfel et al. reported no difference in antiemetic efficacy between three combinations: ondansetron 4 mg with dexamethasone 4 mg, ondansetron 4 mg with droperidol 1.25 mg and dexamethasone 4 mg with droperidol 1.25 mg[5]. Gan et al. reported that low-dose granisetron 0.1 mg plus dexamethasone 8 mg was as effective as ondansetron 4 mg plus dexamethasone 8 mg IV in women undergoing abdominal hysterectomy[48].

Side effects of combination antiemetic therapy

Studies have reported no increased risk of side effects when using combination antiemetic therapy compared with single-agent prophylaxis. A meta-analysis involving 3440 patients reported no increase in side effects with the combination of 5-HT_3 receptor antagonists with dexamethasone or droperidol compared to monotherapy, except for an increased risk of headache with the combination of 5-HT_3 receptor antagonists with dexamethasone compared to dexamethasone alone (odds ratio (OR), 1.75; 95% confidence interval (CI), 1.01–3.03)[49]. The combination of 5-HT_3 receptor antagonists with droperidol was associated with fewer headaches than 5-HT_3 receptor antagonists alone (OR, 0.35; 95% CI, 0.18–0.69). Whilst 5-HT_3 antagonists and droperidol have been associated with prolongation of the QT interval, there is no significant increase in QT-interval prolongation when these medications are used in combination compared to each agent alone[50,51].

Efficacy of combination therapy for PDNV

In 2003, Gupta et al. performed a meta-analysis assessing the efficacy of monotherapy and combination therapy for the prophylaxis against PDNV. They reported that, compared with placebo, ondansetron reduced the risk of PDNV with an NNT of 14, while the NNT for the combination of ondansetron with another antiemetic was 5[52]. Pan et al. compared single-agent prophylaxis with ondansetron 4 mg versus the combination of ondansetron 4 mg and dexamethasone 8 mg with postdischarge 8 mg ondansetron oral disintegrating tablet administered on the morning of postoperative days 1 and 2[53]. The combination group had a lower incidence of postdischarge nausea (57% versus 20%), and postdischarge vomiting (20% versus 3%) compared with the ondansetron monotherapy group. Quality of recovery scores were also higher in the combination group. Studies on combination antiemetic therapy involving longer-acting antiemetics in the context of PDNV are lacking.

Combination therapy for the treatment of established PONV

Whilst most studies evaluate the efficacy of different antiemetics for PONV prophylaxis, there are few data on the efficacy of these drugs for the treatment of established PONV, particularly with regards to the use of combination therapy. Rusch et al. evaluated the recurrence of PONV over 24 h in 228 patients with established PONV who received rescue with a single agent (dolasetron or haloperidol) alone or with added dexamethasone 8 mg[54]. The addition of dexamethasone significantly reduced PONV recurrence from 51 to 33% (P = 0.005). Ormel et al. evaluated 80 gynecologic day surgery patients with established PONV who were randomized to treatment with triple therapy consisting of ondansetron, droperidol and dexamethasone versus ondansetron and droperidol[55]. There was a significant reduction in PONV in the first 6 h with triple therapy (81.4%) compared with dual therapy regimen (65%, P = 0.04).

Summary

Combination therapy is more effective than single-agent prophylaxis, with no increase in side effects associated with its use. Patients at moderate-to-high risk for PONV benefit most from combination antiemetic prophylaxis and the multimodal approach. Studies of combinations involving newer, longer-acting antiemetics and focusing on PDNV are needed.

References

1. Parikh PM, Charak BS, Banavali SD, et al. A prospective, randomized double-blind trial comparing metoclopramide alone with metoclopramide plus dexamethasone in preventing emesis induced by high-dose cisplatin. *Cancer* 1988; 62: 2263–6.
2. Watcha MF, White PF. Postoperative nausea and vomiting. Its etiology, treatment, and prevention. *Anesthesiology* 1992; 77: 162–84.
3. Miller AD, Leslie RA. The area postrema and vomiting. *Front Neuroendocrinol* 1994; 15: 301–20.
4. Fredrikson M, Hursti T, Furst CJ, et al. Nausea in cancer chemotherapy is inversely related to urinary cortisol excretion. *Br J Cancer* 1992; 65: 779–80.
5. Apfel CC, Korttila K, Abdalla M, et al. A factorial trial of six interventions for the prevention of postoperative nausea and vomiting. *N Engl J Med* 2004; 350: 2441–51.
6. Leeser J, Lip H. Prevention of postoperative nausea and vomiting using ondansetron, a new, selective, 5-HT3 receptor antagonist. *Anesth Analg* 1991; 72: 751–5.
7. Kris MG, Gralla RJ, Clark RA, et al. Dose-ranging evaluation of the serotonin antagonist GR-C507/75 (GR38032F) when used as an antiemetic in patients receiving anticancer chemotherapy. *J Clin Oncol* 1988; 6: 659–62.
8. Lopez-Olaondo L, Carrascosa F, Pueyo FJ, et al. Combination of ondansetron and dexamethasone in the prophylaxis of postoperative nausea and vomiting. *Br J Anaesth* 1996; 76: 835–40.
9. Habib AS, Gan TJ. Combination antiemetics: what is the evidence? *Int Anesthesiol Clin Fall* 2003; 41: 119–144.
10. Biswas BN, Rudra A. Comparison of granisetron and granisetron plus dexamethasone for the prevention of postoperative nausea and vomiting after laparoscopic cholecystectomy. *Acta Anaesthesiol Scand* 2003; 47: 79–83.
11. Eberhart LH, Buning EK, Folz B, et al. Anti-emetic prophylaxis with oral tropisetron and/or dexamethasone. *Eur J Clin Invest* 2006; 36: 580–7.
12. Zhou H, Xu H, Zhang J, et al. Combination of dexamethasone and tropisetron before thyroidectomy to alleviate postoperative nausea, vomiting, and pain: randomized controlled trial. *World J Surg* 2012; 36: 1217–24.
13. Coloma M, White PF, Markowitz SD, et al. Dexamethasone in combination with dolasetron for prophylaxis in the ambulatory setting: effect on outcome after laparoscopic cholecystectomy. *Anesthesiology* 2002; 96: 1346–50.
14. Piper SN, Triem JG, Rohm KD, et al. [Prevention of post-operative nausea and vomiting. Randomised comparison of dolasetron versus dolasetron plus dexamethasone]. *Anaesthesist* 2003; 52: 120–6.
15. Eberhart LH, Morin AM, Georgieff M. [Dexamethasone for prophylaxis of postoperative nausea and vomiting. A meta-analysis of randomized controlled studies]. *Anaesthesist* 2000; 49: 713–20.
16. Habib AS, El-Moalem HE, Gan TJ. The efficacy of the 5-HT(3) receptor antagonists combined with droperidol for PONV prophylaxis is similar to their combination with dexamethasone. A meta-analysis of randomized controlled trials. *Can J Anesth* 2004; 51: 311–9.

17. Shen YD, Chen CY, Wu CH, et al. Dexamethasone, ondansetron, and their combination and postoperative nausea and vomiting in children undergoing strabismus surgery: a meta-analysis of randomized controlled trials. *Paediatr Anaesth* 2014; 24: 490–8.

18. Gralla R, Lichinitser M, Van Der Vegt S, et al. Palonosetron improves prevention of chemotherapy-induced nausea and vomiting following moderately emetogenic chemotherapy: results of a double-blind randomized phase III trial comparing single doses of palonosetron with ondansetron. *Ann Oncol* 2003; 14: 1570–7.

19. Kovac AL, Eberhart L, Kotarski J, et al. A randomized, double-blind study to evaluate the efficacy and safety of three different doses of palonosetron versus placebo in preventing postoperative nausea and vomiting over a 72-hour period. *Anesth Analg* 2008; 107: 439–44.

20. Bala I, Bharti N, Murugesan S, et al. Comparison of palonosetron with palonosetron–dexamethasone combination for prevention of postoperative nausea and vomiting in patients undergoing laparoscopic cholecystectomy. *Minerva Anestesiol* 2014; 80: 779–84.

21. Park JW, Jun JW, Lim YH, et al. The comparative study to evaluate the effect of palonosetron monotherapy versus palonosetron with dexamethasone combination therapy for prevention of postoperative nausea and vomiting. *Korean J Anesthesiol* 2012; 63: 334–9.

22. Blitz JD, Haile M, Kline R, et al. A randomized double blind study to evaluate efficacy of palonosetron with dexamethasone versus palonosetron alone for prevention of postoperative and postdischarge nausea and vomiting in subjects undergoing laparoscopic surgeries with high emetogenic risk. *Am J Ther* 2012; 19: 324–9.

23. Kazemi-Kjellberg F, Henzi I, Tramer MR. Treatment of established postoperative nausea and vomiting: a quantitative systematic review. *BMC Anesthesiol* 2001; 1: 2.

24. Feng PH, Chu KS, Lu IC, et al. Haloperidol plus ondansetron prevents postoperative nausea and vomiting in patients undergoing laparoscopic cholecystectomy. *Acta Anaesthesiol Taiwan* 2009; 47: 3–9.

25. Chu CC, Shieh JP, Tzeng JI, et al. The prophylactic effect of haloperidol plus dexamethasone on postoperative nausea and vomiting in patients undergoing laparoscopically assisted vaginal hysterectomy. *Anesth Analg* 2008; 106: 1402–6.

26. Gan TJ, Sinha AC, Kovac AL, et al. A randomized, double-blind, multicenter trial comparing transdermal scopolamine plus ondansetron to ondansetron alone for the prevention of postoperative nausea and vomiting in the outpatient setting. *Anesth Analg* 2009; 108: 1498–504.

27. Sah N, Ramesh V, Kaul B, et al. Transdermal scopolamine patch in addition to ondansetron for postoperative nausea and vomiting prophylaxis in patients undergoing ambulatory cosmetic surgery. *J Clin Anesth* 2009; 21: 249–52.

28. Jones S, Strobl R, Crosby D, et al. The effect of transdermal scopolamine on the incidence and severity of postoperative nausea and vomiting in a group of high-risk patients given prophylactic intravenous ondansetron. *Aana j* 2006; 74: 127–32.

29. Nesek-Adam V, Grizelj-Stojcic E, Mrsic V, et al. Prophylactic antiemetics for laparoscopic cholecystectomy: droperidol, metoclopramide, and droperidol plus metoclopramide. *J Laparoendosc Adv Surg Tech A* 2004; 14: 212–8.

30. Nesek-Adam V, Grizelj-Stojcic E, Rasic Z, et al. Comparison of dexamethasone, metoclopramide, and their combination in the prevention of postoperative nausea and vomiting after laparoscopic cholecystectomy. *Surg Endosc* 2007; 21: 607–12.

31. De Oliveira GS Jr, Castro-Alves LJ, Chang R, et al. Systemic metoclopramide to prevent postoperative nausea and vomiting: a meta-analysis without Fujii's studies. *Br J Anaesth* 2012; 109: 688–97.

32. Wallenborn J, Gelbrich G, Bulst D, et al. Prevention of postoperative nausea and vomiting by metoclopramide combined with dexamethasone: randomised double blind multicentre trial. *BMJ* 2006; 333: 324.

33. Gesztesi Z, Scuderi PE, White PF, et al. Substance P (neurokinin-1) antagonist prevents postoperative vomiting after abdominal hysterectomy procedures. *Anesthesiology* 2000; 93: 931–7.

34. Altorjay A, Melson T, Chinachoit T, et al. Casopitant and ondansetron for postoperative nausea and vomiting prevention in women at high risk for emesis: a phase 3 study. *Arch Surg* 2011; 146: 201–6.

35. Singla NK, Singla SK, Chung F, et al. Phase II study to evaluate the safety and efficacy of the oral neurokinin-1 receptor antagonist casopitant (GW679769) administered with ondansetron for the prevention of postoperative and postdischarge nausea and vomiting in high-risk patients. *Anesthesiology* 2010; 113: 74–82.

36. Lim CS, Ko YK, Kim YH, et al. Efficacy of the oral neurokinin-1 receptor antagonist aprepitant administered with ondansetron for the prevention of postoperative nausea and vomiting. *Korean J Anesthesiol* 2013; 64: 212–7.

37. Sinha AC, Singh PM, Williams NW, et al. Aprepitant's prophylactic efficacy in decreasing postoperative nausea and vomiting in morbidly obese patients undergoing bariatric surgery. *Obes Surg* 2014; 24: 225–31.

38. Vallejo MC, Phelps AL, Ibinson JW, et al. Aprepitant plus ondansetron compared with ondansetron alone in reducing postoperative nausea and vomiting in ambulatory patients undergoing plastic surgery. *Plast Reconstr Surg* 2012; 129: 519–26.

39. Lee SJ, Lee SM, Kim SI, et al. The effect of aprepitant for the prevention of postoperative nausea and vomiting in patients undergoing gynecologic surgery with intravenous patient controlled analgesia using fentanyl: aprepitant plus ramosetron vs ramosetron alone. *Korean J Anesthesiol* 2012; 63: 221–6.

40. Kawano H, Matsumoto T, Hamaguchi E, et al. Antiemetic efficacy of combined aprepitant and dexamethasone in patients at high-risk of postoperative nausea and vomiting from epidural fentanyl analgesia. *Minerva Anestesiol* 2014

41. Green MS, Green P, Malayaman SN, et al. Randomized, double-blind comparison of oral aprepitant alone compared with aprepitant and transdermal scopolamine for prevention of postoperative nausea and vomiting. *Br J Anaesth* 2012; 109: 716–22.

42. Lee HK, Lee JH, Chon SS, et al. The effect of transdermal scopolamine plus intravenous dexamethasone for the prevention of postoperative nausea and vomiting in patients with epidural PCA after major orthopedic surgery. *Korean J Anesthesiol* 2010; 58: 50–5.

43. Ahmed AB, Hobbs GJ, Curran JP. Randomized, placebo-controlled trial of combination antiemetic prophylaxis for day-case gynaecological laparoscopic surgery. *Br J Anaesth* 2000; 85: 678–82.

44. Khalil S, Philbrook L, Rabb M, et al. Ondansetron/promethazine combination or promethazine alone reduces nausea and vomiting after middle ear surgery. *J Clin Anesth* 1999; 11: 596–600.

45. Gan TJ, Candiotti KA, Klein SM, et al. Double-blind comparison of granisetron, promethazine, or a combination of both for the prevention of postoperative nausea and vomiting in females undergoing outpatient laparoscopies. *Can J Anaesth* 2009; 56: 829–36.

46. Scuderi PE, James RL, Harris L, et al. Multimodal antiemetic management prevents early postoperative vomiting after outpatient laparoscopy. *Anesth Analg* 2000; 91: 1408–14.

47. Habib AS, White WD, Eubanks S, et al. A randomized comparison of a multimodal management strategy versus combination antiemetics for the prevention of postoperative nausea and vomiting. *Anesth Analg* 2004; 99: 77–81.

48. Gan TJ, Coop A, Philip BK. A randomized, double-blind study of granisetron plus dexamethasone versus ondansetron plus dexamethasone to prevent postoperative nausea and vomiting in patients undergoing abdominal hysterectomy. *Anesth Analg* 2005; 101: 1323–9.

49. Leslie JB, Gan TJ. Meta-analysis of the safety of 5-HT3 antagonists with dexamethasone or droperidol for prevention of PONV. *Ann Pharmacother* 2006; 40: 856–72.

50. Charbit B, Alvarez JC, Dasque E, et al. Droperidol and ondansetron-induced QT interval prolongation: a clinical drug interaction study. *Anesthesiology* 2008; 109: 206–12.

51. Chan MT, Choi KC, Gin T, et al. The additive interactions between ondansetron and droperidol for preventing postoperative nausea and vomiting. *Anesth Analg* 2006; 103: 1155–62.

52. Gupta A, Wu CL, Elkassabany N, et al. Does the routine prophylactic use of antiemetics affect the incidence of postdischarge nausea and vomiting following ambulatory surgery?: A systematic review of randomized controlled trials. *Anesthesiology* 2003; 99: 488–95.

53. Pan PH, Lee SC, Harris LC. Antiemetic prophylaxis for postdischarge nausea and vomiting and impact on functional quality of living during recovery in patients with high emetic risks: a prospective, randomized, double-blind comparison of two prophylactic antiemetic regimens. *Anesth Analg* 2008; 107: 429–38.

54. Rusch D, Arndt C, Martin H, et al. The addition of dexamethasone to dolasetron or haloperidol for treatment of established postoperative nausea and vomiting. *Anaesthesia* 2007; 62: 810–7.

55. Ormel G, Romundstad L, Lambert-Jensen P, et al. Dexamethasone has additive effect when combined with ondansetron and droperidol for treatment of established PONV. *Acta Anaesthesiol Scand* 2011; 55: 1196–205.

Chapter 12

Management of postoperative nausea and vomiting in pediatric patients

Imelda Tjia, Michelle Dalton and Mehernoor F. Watcha

Although postoperative nausea and vomiting (PONV) has been called the big "little problem" in anesthesia, it remains a major cause of patient dissatisfaction and increased perioperative costs from delayed discharge and unplanned hospital admission[1–3]. Postoperative vomiting (POV) occurs in 30% of adults, nausea in 50% and postdischarge nausea and vomiting in 37%, with rates as high as 80% for various subsets of adults[2,4]. In pediatric patients, the incidence of PONV in children may be underestimated as many younger pediatric patients cannot report the sensation of nausea[2,5]. In pediatric studies, the rate of POV is therefore used as an endpoint and the incidence of POV is higher in children than adults.

PONV rates are increasingly considered to be quality-of-care markers as life-threatening anesthetic related events are now rare[1]. This focus on PONV led to the establishment of expert consensus guidelines for the management of PONV by the Society for Ambulatory Anesthesia, with endorsement of the 2014 revised guidelines by many professional anesthesiology associations around the world[2]. The guidelines recommended: the identification of at-risk patients; the reduction of risk factors; the administration of prophylaxis commensurate with the degree of risk in the individual, including children; rescue treatment for patients in whom prophylaxis either failed or was not given; ensuring that recommendations for prevention and treatment of PONV were actually implemented; and facilitation of such implementation by a multimodal approach[2]. This chapter will be based on these guidelines and will focus on POV in children.

Physiology of nausea and vomiting

The physiology of vomiting in adults was described by Borison and Wang[6] and is discussed in more detail elsewhere. In summary, vomiting is controlled by two areas of the brain – the chemoreceptor trigger zone (CTZ) located in the area postrema in the floor of the fourth ventricle, and the emetic center in the lateral reticular formation of the brainstem. These areas coordinate interactions between smooth and striated muscles of the gut to produce vomiting.

Although vomiting occurs at every age, including the neonatal period, there are very few data available on the age-related development of the emetic center and CTZ. Anesthetic agents have a neuroapoptotic effect on the developing brain in animals[7]. However, it is unclear if exposure to anesthetics leads to neuroapoptosis in the emetic center and the CTZ of humans, and if this has any short- or long-term clinical significance.

Postoperative Nausea and Vomiting: A Practical Guide, eds. Tong Joo Gan and Ashraf S. Habib. Published by Cambridge University Press.

PONV risk factors in children

Whilst many factors are associated with increased PONV, the consensus guidelines recommended focusing on the ones shown to be independent risk factors in large cohort studies after accounting for confounding factors. There is a dose-dependent effect of volatile agents and postoperative opioids on PONV[4,8]. Increased PONV with abdominal surgery in adults may represent the effect of confounding issues, such as duration of surgery or increased opioid use rather than being an independent risk factor[9].

The factors used in pediatric risk stratification scores differ from those in adult subjects[10]. Eberhart et al. identified four factors in children: duration of surgery >30 min; age >3 years; prior POV in the patient, parent or sibling; and strabismus surgery. If 0, 1, 2, 3 or 4 of these factors were present, the patient's risk for POV was approximately 9%, 10%, 30%, 55% and 70%, respectively[10]. This score was validated in another institution where children not undergoing strabismus surgery and not receiving antiemetic prophylaxis had a POV incidence of 3.4%, 11.6%, 28.2% and 42.3% in the presence of 0, 1, 2 or 3 factors, respectively[11]. Bourdaud et al. studied 2,392 children undergoing general anesthesia and created a new, simplified 6-point score based on age, predisposition to POV, duration of anesthesia >45 min, type of surgery and use of multiple doses of opioids (Table 12.1)[12]. The relationship between age and risk of POV was not linear but highest for ages between 6 and 13 years, with twice the risk compared to children between 3 and 6 years or above 13 years, while children <3 years had the lowest risk. A predisposition to POV was defined as prior history of POV, motion sickness or family history of POV. The study also identified tonsillectomy and tympanoplasty in addition to strabismus surgery as independent risk factors. The authors considered patients with a risk score of 0–1 as being at low risk, 2–3 as moderate and 4–6 as high risk for POV. This new pediatric vomiting in the postoperative period (VPOP) score[12] had a greater area under the receiver-operating characteristics curve compared to the score by Eberhart et al.[10]. If these findings are confirmed in other studies, the VPOP score could be used to guide therapy for POV in children.

Factors that have been disproved or of limited clinical relevance in adults have been discussed in other chapters. In children, preoperative anxiety was not found to be associated with increased POV[13], and routine gastric suctioning and intraoperative therapeutic suggestion did not reduce POV[5,13–15]. Whilst airway and pulmonary complications are higher in children coming from households with smokers, the effect of second-hand smoking on POV in children is unknown[2,5,16,17]. The preoperative visit may be an opportunity to introduce the child's caretakers to smoking cessation programs.

Reducing baseline risks of POV

Strategies recommended to reduce baseline risk and incidence of POV include[2,5]:

- the avoidance of general anesthesia by the use of regional anesthesia
- preferential use of propofol infusions
- avoidance of nitrous oxide
- avoidance of volatile anesthetics
- minimization of perioperative opioids
- adequate hydration.

Table 12.1 Clinical risk score for VPOP[a,b]

	Point score		
Factor	**0**	**1**	**2**[c]
Age	Below 3 years of age	3–6 years or >13 years of age	Between 6 and 13 years of age
Predisposition to POV (previous POV, motion sickness or family history of POV)	No predisposition	Predisposition present	NA
Duration of anesthesia >45 min	No	Yes	NA
High-risk surgery (tonsillectomy, tympanoplasty strabismus)	*Not* high PONV risk procedures	High PONV risk (tonsillectomy, tympanoplasty strabismus)	NA
Multiple doses of opioids	No	Yes	NA

NA, not applicable; PONV, postoperative nausea and vomiting; POV, postoperative vomiting; VPOP, vomiting in the postoperative period.

[a] Adapted with permission[12].

[b] Low risk: total score of 0–1; moderate risk: total score of 2–3; high risk: total score of 4–6.

[c] The factors of predisposition to POV, duration of anesthesia >45 mins, high-risk surgery and multiple doses of opioids are scored as 0 or 1 only. Age is scored as 0, 1 or 2 according to criteria listed above.

Regional anesthesia is associated with less PONV than general anesthesia in both children and adults[2]. In the pediatric patient population, regional anesthesia is usually performed after induction of general anesthesia to reduce stress associated with inserting needles. A major benefit of a combined general and regional anesthetic technique is the reduction in perioperative opioid requirements, and consequently, reduced postoperative emesis. Children randomized to a wrist block during hand surgery had less emesis than those receiving perioperative opioids[18]. Similarly, children receiving a peribulbar block, subtenon block or topical lidocaine during strabismus repair had less emesis than a control group[19,20].

When general anesthesia is required, use of propofol for induction and maintenance of anesthesia lowers the incidence of early PONV occurring within the first 6 h[21]. Children receiving intraoperative propofol in subhypnotic doses (bolus of 1 mg/kg followed by an infusion at 20 μg/kg/min), combined with dexamethasone or tropisetron during tonsillectomy procedures, had less emesis than those receiving dexamethasone or tropisetron alone[22,23]. However, single induction doses of propofol have no effect on POV[2].

The combination of propofol and air/oxygen (total intravenous anesthesia) has additive effects, reducing PONV risk by approximately 25% in adults[24,25]. Nitrous oxide has little impact when the baseline risk for PONV is low, but avoidance of nitrous oxide is associated with decreased POV in high-risk subjects[5,26].

Baseline risk for PONV can also be reduced by minimizing perioperative opioids by supplemental nonopioid analgesics or regional nerve blocks. Perioperative nonsteroidal anti-inflammatory drugs (NSAIDs), cyclooxygenase-2 inhibitors, alpha-2 agonists, such as clonidine and dexmedetomidine, and ketamine may have a morphine-sparing effect with decreased opioid-related PONV[27–32]. A systematic review of 12 trials with 928 children showed less emesis in a group receiving NSAIDs (odds ratio, 0.49; 95% confidence interval (CI), 0.29–0.83)[28].

Adequate hydration is another simple strategy to reduce emesis. High-dose intravenous fluids at 30 mL/kg are associated with less emesis than the standard 10 mL/kg therapy in children[33,34]. However, routine gastric decompression and limiting oral intake after surgery are ineffective in reducing pediatric POV[35,36]. Other strategies initially thought to be effective were later shown to have minimal or no effect, including supplemental oxygen and minimization of neostigmine[2].

Prophylactic antiemetic therapy in children at increased risk for POV

In children, the POV rate can be twice as high as in adults, which suggests a greater need for POV prophylaxis in this population. Many drugs are effective for POV prophylaxis in children including 5-HT_3 antagonists, steroids, antihistamines, anticholinergic drugs and dopamine antagonists, such as butyrophenones, phenothiazines and benzamides (Table 12.2).

Ondansetron and other 5-HT_3 antagonists

There is good evidence from meta-analyses and large studies to suggest that 5-HT_3 antagonists and dexamethasone are the most effective antiemetics in the prophylaxis of pediatric POV[37–39]. Ondansetron was more effective than metoclopramide in 557 children undergoing adenotonsillectomy[37]. In a systematic review of children undergoing this procedure, the 5-HT_3 antagonists and dexamethasone were found to be the most effective prophylactic antiemetics, with insufficient evidence for the efficacy of dimenhydrinate, droperidol or perphenazine in children[38]. Perphenazine was effective compared to placebo in children, but a 5-HT_3 antagonist (ondansetron or granisetron) was more effective[40]. In a Bayesian meta-analysis of six single-drug therapies and five combinations of antiemetics in children, Engelman et al. noted that the most pessimistic expectations of single-drug prophylaxis with the 5-HT_3 receptor antagonists or dexamethasone would result in a 50–60% relative risk (RR) reduction, and that the expected RR reduction of the combination is 80%[39]. In this study, the risk reduction with droperidol was 40%.

Ondansetron is effective in children as young as 1 month[41] and the pharmacokinetics have been established in children between 1 and 48 months[42]. Clearance decreased by 31%, 53% and 76% for the typical 6-, 3- and 1-month-old, respectively, compared to published data in older children aged 3–12 years, and was attributed to immaturity of cytochrome P450 enzymes. Ondansetron 0.1 mg/kg in children <6 months produced exposure similar to a 0.15 mg/kg dose in older children, suggesting a need for close monitoring when used in children <4 months old[42].

There is greater experience with ondansetron, the first available antiserotonin drug compared to other 5-HT_3 antagonists, such as granisetron, dolasetron or tropisetron, but little evidence to suggest improved efficacy with any one of these drugs. Dolasetron is no longer available in the USA because of risks of cardiac arrhythmias. Tropisetron is not available in the USA but has been used in Europe. There are also no published pediatric data to make recommendations on the use of palonosetron in pediatric POV. A randomized controlled trial without a placebo arm showed no differences in the 48-h rates of POV in children receiving 0.5, 1.0 or 1.5 mg/kg palonosetron[43]. The low cost of generic ondansetron and similar efficacy makes it difficult to show any advantage in using the other first-generation antiserotonin drugs.

Table 12.2 Antiemetic doses for POV prophylaxis in children[2]

Drug	Dose	Maximum
Dexamethasone	150 μg/kg	5 mg
Dimenhydrinate	0.5 mg/kg	25 mg
Droperidol[a]	10–15 μg/kg	1.25 mg
5-HT_3 antagonists:		
Ondansetron	50–100 μg/kg	4 mg
Tropisetron	0.1 mg/kg	2 mg
Granisetron	40 μg/kg	0.6 mg
Dolasetron	350 μg/kg	12.5 mg

[a] FDA black box warning calls for 12-lead electrocardiogram to rule out prolonged QT syndrome before administering droperidol and continuous electrocardiogram monitoring for at least 2–3 h after administering droperidol.

Data to base a recommendation on the timing of administration of these drugs in children are sparse. No differences were found in POV in children who received tropisetron immediately after induction or at the end of surgery during short tonsillectomy procedures[44].

Dexamethasone

Corticosteroids have been shown to be very effective in the prevention of POV in children, with administration at induction recommended rather than toward the end of anesthesia[39]. The mechanism of action of steroids in POV prophylaxis may be related to depletion of the serotonin precursor tryptophan, prevention of release of gut serotonin and 5-HT_3 receptor sensitization to other antagonists[45]. Most studies have been with dexamethasone 0.5 mg/kg, but methylprednisolone 2.5 mg /kg is noninferior[46]. However, the dose–effect relationship of dexamethasone in POV prophylaxis is unclear. Kim et al. did not find differences in POV rates or secondary outcomes in children receiving 0.0625, 0.125, 0.25, 0.5 or 1 mg/kg (maximum dose 24 mg) during adenotonsillectomy procedures[47]. Another study of the same patient population showed a dose-dependent reduction in POV, with the best response in children receiving 0.5 mg/kg compared to 0.05 and 0.15 mg/kg doses[48]. An updated Cochrane review of steroids for tonsillectomy patients stated that "the question of appropriate dosing remains unanswered and final recommendations must await randomized dose-control trials"[49].

Older drugs

A number of older drugs are also effective in POV management. These include antihistamines (dimenhydrinate), dopamine antagonists such as butyrophenones (e.g., droperidol and haloperidol), phenothiazines (promethazine, prochlorperazine and perphenazine), benzamides (metoclopramide) and cholinergic antagonists (scopolamine). There are few dose-ranging data and limited evidence for the efficacy of these drugs. In addition, the 5-HT_3 antagonists are more effective and associated with a lower side-effect profile[38,39]. Concerns about the effect of droperidol on cardiac rhythms have led to a black box warning that may not be entirely justified as similar effects on cardiac rhythm are seen with other antiemetics[50]. Side effects for metoclopramide and phenothiazines also include extrapyramidal symptoms (Table 12.3). With the availability of lower-priced generic ondansetron,

Table 12.3 Older drugs to be used as a second-line option[a]

Drug	Dose (mg/kg)	Maximum single dose (mg)	Side effects
Diphenhydramine	1.0	25	Sedation, dry mouth, blurred vision, urinary retention
Metoclopramide	0.25[b]	10	Extrapyramidal reactions more common in children. Not recommended below 1 year of age
Phenothiazines:			Sedation, hypotension (particularly in hypovolemic patients), extrapyramidal syndromes can occur with phenothiazines
Perphenazine	0.07	2.0	
Prochlorperazine[c]	0.1–0.2	2.5	
Promethazine[d]	0.25–0.5	25	Promethazine is contraindicated in children below 2 years. It is also an IV irritant with a risk for severe tissue injury
Scopolamine (IM, IV, SC)[e]	0.006	0.3	Drowsiness, dry mouth, visual disturbances, dizziness

IM, intramuscular; IV, intravenous; SC, subcutaneous.

[a] Dose: ranging and efficacy studies are sparse for these older drugs. These drugs may be used for rescue therapy after failure of 5-HT_3 antagonists and are usually not used for routine prophylaxis.

[b] Although higher doses may be more effective, there is a higher incidence of side effects.

[c] Prochlorperazine is not recommended for children under the age of 2 years or less than 10 kg body weight.

[d] Promethazine has two black box warnings by the FDA: (1) not to be used below 2 years because of the potential risks of fatal respiratory depression, and (2) severe tissue injury and gangrene with perivascular extravasation or unintentional intra-arterial injection. The preferred route of administration is deep IM injection and SC injection is contraindicated[51].

[e] Scopolamine patches should not be divided. The patch should not be used in children below 12 years of age.

the use of the older drugs is now limited to second-line options as rescue therapy when other drugs have failed or when 5-HT_3 antagonists are contraindicated.

Nonpharmacologic therapy

Two meta-analyses show acupuncture and acustimulation are effective in reducing POV in children, with no differences between the two methods[52,53]. Pooled data from 12 studies show all modalities reduce vomiting (RR, 0.69; 95% CI, 0.59–0.8).

Combination therapy

Prophylaxis with drugs acting at different receptor sites may be more effective even if this is an additive and not a synergistic effect[24]. Whilst low-risk patients may not require prophylactic antiemetics, those with a moderate-to-high risk of POV and children with a potential for medical sequelae from emesis (e.g., wound dehiscence, wired jaws) should receive prophylactic combination therapy with two or three antiemetics from different classes[2]. The prophylactic use of a combination of dexamethasone and ondansetron is strongly recommended in most pediatric patients at highest risk for POV unless there are contraindications (Table 12.4)[2]. This is similar to the recommendation by the Association of Paediatric Anaesthetists of Great Britain and Ireland[5].

Table 12.4 Antiemetic combination therapy in children[2]

Drug (1)	Dose		Drug (2)	Dose
Ondansetron	0.05 mg/kg	+	Dexamethasone	0.015 mg/kg
Ondansetron	0.1 mg/kg	+	Droperidol	0.015 mg/kg
Tropisetron	0.1 mg/kg	+	Dexamethasone	0.5 mg/kg

Side effects of drugs

Cardiovascular complications with ondansetron and droperidol

Cardiovascular complications have been reported after ondansetron therapy in children. An 11-year-old child with an undiagnosed long QT syndrome developed ventricular tachycardia after receiving ondansetron and dimenhydrinate[54]. Fatal ventricular tachycardia occurred in a child after receiving ondansetron in the emergency department, and severe bradycardia has been reported during incision and drainage of an abscess[55,56]. The effects of droperidol and ondansetron on myocardial repolarization have been studied when given alone or in combination to healthy children[50]. There were clinically insignificant changes with lengthening of the QT intervals by 10–17 ms and of the interval between the peak and end of the T-wave (Tp-e) intervals by 0–7 ms without any differences between the groups. This may have clinical relevance in children with prolonged QT syndrome.

Steroids

Tumor lysis syndrome has been reported in children with leukemia who received intraoperative dexamethasone[57,58]. One patient with an undiagnosed acute lymphoblastic leukemia developed hyperkalemia and a fatal cardiac arrest during a tonsillectomy procedure[57].

A study of steroids in children undergoing tonsillectomies was terminated early because of increased bleeding in patients receiving dexamethasone[48]. There has been considerable discussion about this unexpected finding as it was a secondary outcome and was not adjusted for other risk factors[59]. Other studies, including a meta-analysis and retrospective reviews, have failed to show increased postoperative bleeding between patients receiving dexamethasone and controls, but one meta-analysis suggested increased risk of re-operation with dexamethasone[60]. The American Academy of Otolaryngology–Head and Neck Surgery continues to make a strong recommendation for the use of a single dose of dexamethasone in children undergoing tonsillectomy[61].

Scopolamine

The incidence of complications with scopolamine patches may be higher in children than adults. It is difficult to control the dose received when a patch is divided as the distribution of the drug in the patch may not be uniform. In addition, continued absorption from the skin site may occur even after the patch is removed. These concerns have lead many anesthesiologists to avoid the use of scopolamine patches in younger children.

Rescue therapy for those who have received no prophylaxis or when prophylaxis has failed

Some low-risk patients who have received no prophylaxis and higher-risk patients who received prophylactic therapy may still experience POV. When factors such as blood draining down the throat or bowel obstruction have been eliminated as causes for emesis, rescue therapy should be initiated, preferably with a 5-HT_3 antagonist if no prophylaxis was used. Rescue therapy should not be with a drug from the same class of antiemetics administered for prophylaxis[62]. If rescue therapy is needed more than 6 h after the previous dose, medication given for prophylaxis may be repeated (except dexamethasone or transdermal scopolamine)[2]. Although these recommendations are based on adult data, it is reasonable to extend this approach to children in the absence of contradictory evidence from pediatric studies.

Research agenda

Despite the large volume of literature on this topic, considerable gaps in knowledge remain in the pediatric patient population. A research agenda should focus on providing evidence to support clinical practices. An important unanswered question is a recommendation for rescue therapy after failed prophylaxis with a combination of steroids and ondansetron[2]. Studies are also required to determine the role of neurokinin type 1-receptor antagonists for both prophylaxis and rescue therapy in children as pediatric POV data on this class of drugs are unavailable.

A major problem is the inability to assess the subjective symptoms of nausea in the younger child. The visual analog scale for nausea is a validated tool for adults, but may not be valid in children <9 years who may not be able to grade the severity of subjective symptoms with reliability. Because pictorial scales appear to have better reliability and validity in young children, the pictorial Baxter Animated Retching Faces (BARF) scale was developed using a series of cartoon faces with expressions of increasing nausea (Figure 12.1)[63]. The BARF scale demonstrated convergent and discriminant validity, with the ability to detect change after antiemetic treatment. Studies need to be done to show if treatment of nausea can be based on this scale.

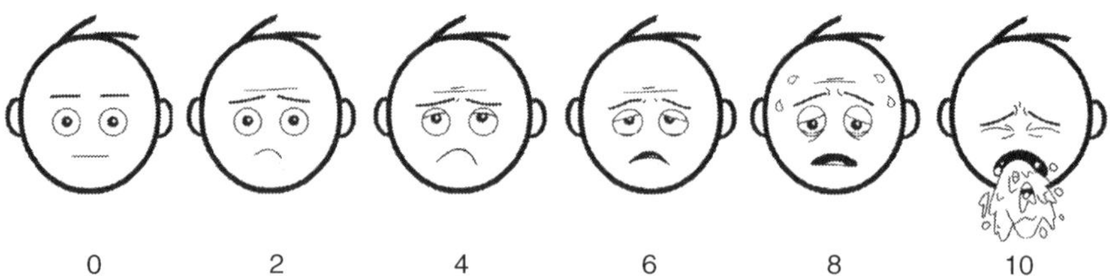

Figure 12.1 Baxter Animated Retching Faces (BARF) scale for nausea
Script for the BARF scale: "Have you thrown up or felt like you were going to throw up before? How did your tummy feel then? We call that feeling of being sick to the stomach "nausea". These faces show children who feel no nausea at all, who feel a little bit nauseated, who feel even more nauseated, and these are children who have the most nausea it is possible to feel". (Point to each face at the appropriate time.) "Which face is more like you feel right now?" Reproduced with permission[63].

Summary

POV occurs more frequently in children than adults. This chapter has discussed the risk factors and recommended the use of a combination of a 5-HT_3 antagonist and a steroid (usually ondansetron and dexamethasone) for prophylaxis in most high-risk patients, unless there is a contraindication. Older drugs should be reserved for rescue therapy when steroids and ondansetron have failed. A research agenda is proposed.

Acknowledgment

Contents are partly based on contributions by M.F. Watcha, MD to the article by Gan et al.[2].

References

1. Benn J, Arnold G, Wei I, et al. Using quality indicators in anaesthesia: feeding back data to improve care. *Br J Anaesth.* 2012; 109(1):80–91.
2. Gan TJ, Diemunsch P, Habib AS, et al. Consensus Guidelines for the Management of Postoperative Nausea and Vomiting. *Anesth Analg* 2014; 118(1):85–113.
3. Kapur PA. The big "little problem". *Anesth Analg* 1991; 73(3):243–5.
4. Apfel CC Philip PB, Cakmakkaya OS, et al. Who is at risk for postdischarge nausea and vomiting after ambulatory surgery? *Anesthesiology* 2012; 86:475–86.
5. Carr AS, Courtman S, Holtby H, et al. Guidelines on the Prevention of Post-operative Vomiting in children: Association of Paediatric Anaesthetists of Great Britain & Ireland, 2009. http://www.apagbi.org.uk/sites/default/files/APA_Guidelines_on_the_Prevention_of_Postoperative_Vomiting_in_Children.pdf (accessed September 17, 2014).
6. Borison HL, Wang SC. Physiology and pharmacology of vomiting. *Pharmacol Rev* 1953; 5:193–230.
7. Creeley CE, Olney JW. The young: neuroapoptosis induced by anesthetics and what to do about it. *Anesth Analg* 2010; 110(2):442–8.
8. Apfel CC, Kranke P, Katz MH, et al. Volatile anaesthetics may be the main cause of early but not delayed postoperative vomiting: a randomized controlled trial of factorial design. *Br J Anaesth* 2002; 88:659–68.
9. Apfel CC, Kranke P, Eberhart LH. Comparison of surgical site and patient's history with a simplified risk score for the prediction of postoperative nausea and vomiting. *Anaesthesia* 2004; 59:1078–82.
10. Eberhart LH, Geldner G, Kranke P, et al. The development and validation of a risk score to predict the probability of postoperative vomiting in pediatric patients. *Anesth Analg* 2004; 99(6):1630–7.
11. Kranke P, Eberhart LH, Toker H, et al. A prospective evaluation of the POVOC score for the prediction of postoperative vomiting in children. *Anesth Analg* 2007 105(6):1592–7.
12. Bourdaud N, Devys J-M, Bientz J, et al. Development and validation of a risk score to predict the probability of postoperative vomiting in pediatric patients: the VPOP score. *Pediatric Anesth* 2014; 24(9):945–52.
13. Wang SM, Kain ZN. Preoperative anxiety and postoperative nausea and vomiting in children: is there an association? *Anesth Analg* 2000; 90(3):571–5.
14. Fortier MA, Weinberg M, Vitulano LA, et al. Effects of therapeutic suggestion in children undergoing general anesthesia: a randomized controlled trial. *Paediatr Anaesth* 2010; 20(1):90–9.

15. Jones JE, Tabaee A, Glasgold R, et al. Eficacy of gastric aspiration in reducing posttonsillectomy vomiting. *Arch Otolaryngol Head Neck Surg* 2001; 127(8):980–4.
16. Aydogan MS, Ozturk E, Erdogan MA, et al. The effects of secondhand smoke on postoperative pain and fentanyl consumption. *J Anesth* 2013; 27(4):569–74.
17. Drongowski RA, Lee D, Reynolds PI, et al. Increased respiratory symptoms following surgery in children exposed to environmental tobacco smoke. *Pediatr Anesth* 2003; 13(4):304–10.
18. De Windt AC, Asehnoune K, Roquilly A, et al. An opioid-free anaesthetic using nerve blocks enhances rapid recovery after minor hand surgery in children. *Eur J Anaesthesiol* 2010; 27(6):521–5.
19. Gupta N, Kumar R, Kumar S, et al. A prospective randomised double blind study to evaluate the effect of peribulbar block or topical application of local anaesthesia combined with general anaesthesia on intra-operative and postoperative complications during paediatric strabismus surgery. *Anaesthesia* 2007; 62(11):1110–3.
20. Steib A, Karcenty A, Calache E, et al. Effects of subtenon anesthesia combined with general anesthesia on perioperative analgesic requirements in pediatric strabismus surgery. *Reg Anesth Pain Med* 2005; 30(5):478–83.
21. Visser K, Hassink EA, Bonsel GJ, et al. Randomized controlled trial of total intravenous anesthesia with propofol versus inhalation anesthesia with isoflurane-nitrous oxide – postoperative nausea and vomiting and economic analysis. *Anesthesiology* 2001; 95(3):616–26.
22. Erdem AF, Yoruk O, Alici HA, et al. Subhypnotic propofol infusion plus dexamethasone is more effective than dexamethasone alone for the prevention of vomiting in children after tonsillectomy. *Paediatr Anaesth* 2008; 18(9):878–83.
23. Erdem AF, Yoruk O, Silbir F, et al. Tropisetron plus subhypnotic propofol infusion is more effective than tropisetron alone for the prevention of vomiting in children after tonsillectomy. *Anaesth Intensive Care* 2009; 37(1):54–9.
24. Apfel CC, Korttila K, Abdalla M, et al. A factorial trial of six interventions for the prevention of postoperative nausea and vomiting. *N Eng J Med* 2004; 350(24):2441–51.
25. Tramer M, Moore A, McQuay H. Meta-analytic comparison of prophylactic antiemetic efficacy for postoperative nausea and vomiting: propofol anaesthesia vs omitting nitrous oxide vs total i.v. anaesthesia with propofol. *Br J Anaesth* 1997; 78(3):256–9.
26. Tramer M, Moore A, McQuay H. Omitting nitrous oxide in general anaesthesia: meta-analysis of intraoperative awareness and postoperative emesis in randomized controlled trials. *Br J Anaesth* 1996; 76(2):186–93.
27. Blaudszun G, Lysakowski C, Elia N, et al. Effect of perioperative systemic α2 agonists on postoperative morphine consumption and pain intensity: systematic review and meta-analysis of randomized controlled trials. *Anesthesiology* 2012; 116:1312–22.
28. Lewis SR, Nicholson A, Cardwell ME, et al. Nonsteroidal anti-inflammatory drugs and perioperative bleeding in paediatric tonsillectomy. *Cochrane Database Syst Rev* 2013; (7):CD003591.
29. Elia N, Lysakowski C, Tramer MR. Does multimodal analgesia with acetaminophen, nonsteroidal antiinflammatory drugs, or selective cyclooxygenase-2 inhibitors and patient-controlled analgesia morphine offer advantages over morphine alone? Meta-analyses of randomized trials. *Anesthesiology* 2005; 103:1296–304.
30. Elia N, Tramer M. Ketamine and postoperative pain – a quantitative systematic review of randomized trials. *Pain* 2005; 113:61–70.
31. Gan TJ, Joshi G, Zhao SZ, et al. Presurgical intravenous parecoxib sodium and follow-up oral valdecoxib for pain management after laparoscopic

cholecystectomy surgery reduces opioid requirements and opioid related adverse effects. *Acta Anaesthesiol Scand* 2004; 48:1194–207.

32. Gurbet A, Basagan-Mogol E, Turker G, et al. Intraoperative infusion of dexmedetomidine reduces perioperative analgesic requirements. *Can J Anaesth* 2006; 53:646–52.

33. Elgueta MF, Echevarría GC, De la Fuente N, et al. Effect of intravenous fluid therapy on postoperative vomiting in children undergoing tonsillectomy. *Br J Anaesth* 2013; 110(4):607–14.

34. Goodarzi M, Matar MM, Shafa M, et al. A prospective randomized blinded study of the effect of intravenous fluid therapy on postoperative nausea and vomiting in children undergoing strabismus surgery. *Paediatr Anaesth* 2006; 16(1):49–53.

35. Chukudebelu O, Leonard DS, Healy A, et al. The effect of gastric decompression on postoperative nausea and emesis in pediatric tonsillectomy patients. *Int J Pediatr Otorhinolaryngol* 2010; 74(6):674–6.

36. Radke OC, Biedler A, Kolodzie K, et al. The effect of postoperative fasting on vomiting in children and their assessment of pain. *Paediatr Anaesth* 2009; 19(5):494–9.

37. Bolton CM, Myles PS, Carlin JB, et al. Randomized, double-blind study comparing the efficacy of moderate-dose metoclopramide and ondansetron for the prophylactic control of postoperative vomiting in children after tonsillectomy. *Br J Anaesth* 2007; 99(3):699–703.

38. Bolton CM, Myles PS, Nolan T, et al. Prophylaxis of postoperative vomiting in children undergoing tonsillectomy: a systematic review and meta-analysis. *Br J Anaesth* 2006; 97(5):593–604.

39. Engelman E, Salengros J-C, Barvais L. How much does pharmacologic prophylaxis reduce postoperative vomiting in children? Calculation of prophylaxis effectiveness and expected incidence of vomiting under treatment using Bayesian meta-analysis. *Anesthesiology* 2008; 109(6):1023–35.

40. Schnabel A, Eberhart LH, Muellenbach R, et al. Efficacy of perphenazine to prevent postoperative nausea and vomiting: a quantitative systematic review. *Eur J Anaesthesiol* 2010; 27(12):1044–51.

41. Khalil SN, Roth AG, Cohen IT, et al. A double-blind comparison of intravenous ondansetron and placebo for preventing postoperative emesis in 1- to 24-month-old pediatric patients after surgery under general anesthesia. *Anesth Analg* 2005; 101(2):356–61.

42. Mondick JT, Johnson BM, Haberer LJ, et al. Population pharmacokinetics of intravenous ondansetron in oncology and surgical patients aged 1–48 months. *Eur J Clin Pharmacol* 2010; 66(1):77–86.

43. Bicer C, Aksu R, Ulgey A, et al. Different doses of palonosetron for the prevention of postoperative nausea and vomiting in children undergoing strabismus surgery. *Drugs R D* 2011; 11(1):29–36.

44. Gross D, Reuss S, Dillier CM, et al. Early vs late intraoperative administration of tropisetron for the prevention of nausea and vomiting in children undergoing tonsillectomy and/or adenoidectomy. *Paediatr Anaesth* 2006; 16(4):444–50.

45. Henzi I, Walder B, Tramer MR. Dexamethasone for the prevention of postoperative nausea and vomiting: a quantitative systematic review. *Anesth Analg* 2000; 90(1):186–94.

46. Aouad MT, Nasr VG, Yazbeck-Karam VG, et al. A comparison between dexamethasone and methylprednisolone for vomiting prophylaxis after tonsillectomy in inpatient children: a randomized trial. *Anesth Analg* 2012; 115(4):913–20.

47. Kim MS, Cote CJ, Cristoloveanu C, et al. There is no dose-escalation response to dexamethasone (0.0625–1.0 mg/kg) in pediatric tonsillectomy or adenotonsillectomy patients for preventing vomiting, reducing pain, shortening time to first liquid intake, or the incidence of voice change. *Anesth Analg* 2007; 104(5):1052–8.

48. Czarnetzki C, Elia N, Lysakowski C, et al. Dexamethasone and risk of nausea and vomiting and postoperative bleeding after tonsillectomy in children: a randomized trial. *JAMA* 2008; 300(22):2621–30.

49. Steward DL, Grisel J, Meinzen-Derr J. Steroids for improving recovery following tonsillectomy in children. *Cochrane Database Syst Rev* 2011 (8):CD003997.

50. Mehta D, Sanatani S, Whyte SD. The effects of droperidol and ondansetron on dispersion of myocardial repolarization in children. *Paediatr Anaesth* 2010; 20(10):905–12.

51. US Food and Drug Administration. Information for Healthcare Professionals: Intravenous promethazine and severe tissue injury, including gangrene. http://www.fda.gov/Drugs/DrugSafety/PostmarketDrugSafetyInformationforPatientsandProviders/DrugSafetyInformationforHeathcareProfessionals/ucm182169.htm (accessed March 15, 2015).

52. Dune LS, Shiao S-YPK. Metaanalysis of acustimulation effects on postoperative nausea and vomiting in children. *Explore (NY)*. 2006; 2(4):314–20.

53. Jindal V, Ge A, Mansky PJ. Safety and efficacy of acupuncture in children: a review of the evidence. *J Pediatr Hematol Oncol* 2008; 30(6):431–42.

54. McKechnie K, Froese A. Ventricular tachycardia after ondansetron administration in a child with undiagnosed long QT syndrome. *Can J Anaesth* 2010; 57(5):453–7.

55. Afonso N, Dang A, Namshikar V, et al. Intravenous ondansetron causing severe bradycardia: two cases. *Ann Cardiac Anaesth* 2009; 12(2):172–3.

56. Chandrakala R, Vijayashankara CN, Kumar KK, et al. Ondansetron induced fatal ventricular tachycardia. *Indian J Pharmacol* 2008; 40(4):186–7.

57. McDonnell C, Barlow R, Campisi P, et al. Fatal peri-operative acute tumour lysis syndrome precipitated by dexamethasone. *Anaesthesia* 2008; 63(6):652–5.

58. Osthaus WA, Linderkamp C, Bunte C, et al. Tumor lysis associated with dexamethasone use in a child with leukemia. *Paediatr Anaesth* 2008; 18(3):268–70.

59. Gunter JB, Willging JP, Myer CM 3rd. Dexamethasone and postoperative bleeding after tonsillectomy in children. *JAMA* 2009; 301(17):1764–5; author reply 1765–6.

60. Plante J, Turgeon AF, Zarychanski R, et al. Effect of systemic steroids on post-tonsillectomy bleeding and reinterventions: systematic review and meta-analysis of randomised controlled trials. *BMJ* 2012; 345:e5389.

61. Baugh RF, Archer SM, Mitchell RB, et al. Clinical practice guideline: tonsillectomy in children. *Otolaryngol Head Neck Surg* 2011; 144(1 Suppl):S1–30.

62. Kovac AL, O'Connor TA, Pearman MH, et al. Efficacy of repeat intravenous dosing of ondansetron in controlling postoperative nausea and vomiting: a randomized, double-blind, placebo-controlled multicenter trial. *J Clin Anesth* 1999; 11(6):453–9.

63. Baxter AL, Watcha MF, Baxter WV, et al. Development and validation of a pictorial nausea rating scale for children. *Pediatrics* 2011; 127(6):e1542–9. [Erratum appears in *Pediatrics* 2011; 128(5):1004].

Chapter 13

Management of postoperative nausea and vomiting in inpatients and ambulatory patients

Brian Donnenfeld and Beverly K. Philip

Postoperative nausea and vomiting background

Postoperative nausea and vomiting (PONV) is one of the most troublesome postoperative complications, with an incidence of between 20% and 30%[1], and up to 80% in high-risk individuals[2]. PONV results in significant patient discomfort, and can lead to prolonged recovery room stay, unplanned admission and the need for pharmacologic treatment, all of which increase overall healthcare costs[3]. PONV is one of the leading causes of unanticipated hospital admission after ambulatory surgery[4], and can lead to suture dehiscence, aspiration, increases in intraocular and intracranial pressure, esophageal rupture, pneumothorax and hematoma formation[5,6]. A solid understanding of the etiology, biochemical pathways, risk factors and the available treatment modalities is essential in order to provide excellent anesthesia care to both the ambulatory and inpatient surgical population.

PONV is a multifactorial process, involving several well-described pathways and receptor types, including, but not limited to: serotonergic, dopaminergic, muscarinic, cholinergic, histaminergic, neurokinin (NK) and opioid. A multimodal approach to the problem, utilizing a validated risk assessment model, combined with risk-reducing anesthetic techniques and prophylaxis/treatment with medications of different pharmacologic classes, provides the clinician with the proper tools to manage the at-risk patient.

Risk reduction

Risk factors for PONV have been well described, and can be categorized into anesthetic risk factors, patient-specific risk factors and surgical risk factors. Modifiable anesthetic risk factors include exposure to volatile anesthetics and nitrous oxide, as well as postoperative opioid use[7]. A volatile-free technique, utilizing propofol for anesthetic maintenance, has been demonstrated to reduce baseline risk by 19%[8]. Omitting nitrous oxide in favor of nitrogen as a carrier gas yields a risk reduction of 12%[8]. The risk-reducing effects of total intravenous anesthesia (TIVA) has a similar risk reduction as the commonly used agents, ondansetron, dexamethasone and droperidol[8] (Table 13.1). Avoidance of general anesthesia with the use of peripheral nerve blocks also significantly decreases the risk of PONV[9]. When compared with monitored anesthesia care and regional anesthesia, general anesthesia is associated with an 11-fold increase in the risk of PONV[10].

The effects of neostigmine on PONV are controversial. One meta-analysis demonstrated an increased risk of PONV with neostigmine doses ≥2.5 mg[11]. A more recent

Postoperative Nausea and Vomiting: A Practical Guide, eds. Tong Joo Gan and Ashraf S. Habib. Published by Cambridge University Press.

Table 13.1 Risk of PONV according to patients' randomly assigned interventions[a]

Intervention	Received intervention: Yes	No	Percent RR (95% CI)	*P* value[b]
	Number with PONV/total number (%)[c]			
Ondansetron (versus no ondansetron)	735/2,576 (28.5)	996/2,585 (38.5)	−26.0 (−31.5 to −19.9)	<0.001
Dexamethasone (versus no dexamethasone)	739/2,596 (28.5)	992/2,565 (38.7)	−26.4 (−31.9 to −20.4)	<0.001
Droperidol (versus no droperidol)	742/2,573 (28.8)	989/2,588 (38.2)	−24.5 (-30.2 to −18.4)	<0.001
Propofol (versus inhalational anesthetic)	1,066/3,427 (31.1)	665/1,734 (38.4)	−18.9 (−25.0 to −12.3)	<0.001
Nitrogen as carrier gas (versus nitrous oxide)	668/2,146(31.1)	755/2,131 (35.4)	−12.1 (−19.3 to −4.3)	0.003
Remifentanil (versus fentanyl)	827/2,386 (34.7)	792/2,403 (33.0)	5.2 (−2.9 to 13.8)	0.21

CI, confidence interval; PONV, postoperative nausea and vomiting; RR, relative risk.
[a] Reproduced with permission[8].
[b] *P* values were calculated using the chi-square test.
[c] The numbers shown are the numbers of patients who had postoperative nausea, vomiting or both divided by the total numbers of patients randomly assigned to the specified intervention for whom complete outcome data could be analyzed. The data are based on all 5,161 randomly assigned patients who completed the study, with the exceptions of the data for carrier gas (4,277 patients) and for remifentanil versus fentanyl (4,789 patients).

meta-analysis demonstrated insufficient evidence to recommend either a dose reduction or omission of neostigmine as an effective strategy to reduce baseline risk of PONV[12].

Opioids have become the cornerstone of pain management, yet they are associated with numerous side effects, including sedation, respiratory depression, pruritus, constipation, urinary retention and PONV[13]. The incidence of PONV is increased in a dose-dependent manner by the total amount of opioid administered[14]. A zero-effect dose has not been identified. Avoidance or minimization of opioid use via a multimodal analgesic approach utilizing nonsteroidal anti-inflammatory drugs (NSAIDs) [15], cyclooxygenase-2 inhibitors[16] and beta-blockers [17,18] have been shown to reduce PONV risk, as well as alpha-2 agonists[19], gabapentinoids[20,21] and ketamine[22] to a lesser extent. The opioid-sparing effects of NSAIDs is associated with a 30% reduction in PONV[15] compared with a side-effect profile that includes gastrointestinal (GI) mucosal injury, renal toxicity and bleeding.

Pharmacologic therapies

PONV prophylaxis

In order to maximize benefit and minimize both cost and the risk of adverse effects, it is necessary to identify medium-to-high risk patients using a risk stratification tool before instituting a prophylactic regimen. Apfel et al. have created a simple, validated scoring system for PONV risk assessment in adult inpatients, using four independent risk factors: female gender, history of PONV or motion sickness, nonsmoker and postoperative opioid use[1]. In their scoring system, each risk factor is associated with a 20% increase in the risk of developing PONV, with a baseline risk of 10%. Application of this scoring system in decision-making regarding instituting PONV prophylaxis has been shown to be effective in reducing institutional rates of PONV[8,23]. Cost of prophylaxis should also be considered recognizing that newer classes of antiemetic agents, such as the neurokinin type 1 (NK_1)-receptor antagonists, are more expensive than older agents like dexamethasone and droperidol. PONV prophylaxis for the low-risk patient should be carefully balanced against both cost and side-effect profile. Other factors to consider are surgical/medical implications of vomiting, including increases in intracranial pressure, and increases in intra-abdominal pressure after hernia repair and esophageal surgery[2].

5-HT_3 receptor antagonists

The 5-HT_3 receptor antagonists (ondansetron, dolasetron, granisetron, tropisetron, palonosetron and ramosetron) are highly effective for PONV prophylaxis and treatment. Because of their safety profile and efficacy, they have become the mainstay of PONV management. As a class, the 5-HT_3 receptor antagonists have more antivomiting than antinausea effects[2]. The 5-HT_3 RAs are most effective when administered at the end of surgery (ondansetron has a half-life of 4 h), with the exception of the second-generation 5-HT_3 antagonist palonosetron, which has a half-life of 40 h and is typically given after induction[2,24].

Ondansetron, the most commonly used antiemetic from this class, reduces PONV risk by approximately 25%[7]. Optimal dosing is 4 mg intravenous (IV), with a number needed-to-treat (NNT) of approximately 6 for the prevention of postoperative vomiting (POV), and an NNT of approximately 7 for the prevention of postoperative nausea[2,25]. While ondansetron has efficacy for both the prevention and treatment of PONV, there is no benefit to repeat dosing in patients whom ondansetron prophylaxis has failed[26], supporting the concept of using a different pharmacologic class of antiemetics for rescue treatment. As a group, the 5-HT_3 antagonists are very well tolerated. Side effects include QTc prolongation, headaches, constipation and transient elevations in liver enzymes.

Corticosteroids

Dexamethasone is highly effective in preventing PONV up to 24 h postoperatively, with an NNT of 4[27], and has similar efficacy to both ondansetron and droperidol[8]. The recommended dose for PONV prophylaxis is 4–5 mg, and optimal timing of administration is preinduction or immediately postinduction[2,28]; however, the high incidence of perineal pain on injection limits its use at preinduction[29]. Peak effect is reached between 45 min and 1 h. Higher doses, 0.1 mg/kg, have been demonstrated to reduce postoperative pain and opioid consumption[29], as well as to reduce time to discharge readiness and to improve postdischarge recovery at 24 h in ambulatory gynecologic surgery and laparoscopic cholecystectomy[30,31].

Dexamethasone is thought to exert its antiemetic effects via several mechanisms: prostaglandin antagonism, decreased serotonin release in the GI tract and depletion of tryptophan, a serotonin precursor, in neural tissue[27]. As a class, corticosteroids have a host of adverse effects including cortisol suppression, GI bleeding and perforation, avascular necrosis of the femoral head, hyperglycemia, immune suppression and impaired wound healing[32]. There is a paucity of data to support any adverse effects of single-dose dexamethasone, except for mild hyperglycemia following administration[29,33]. Even at high doses administered during cardiac surgery, 1 mg/kg dexamethasone has not been shown to impair wound healing[34]. The hyperglycemic effects of dexamethasone 8 mg given during major noncardiac surgery was shown to be limited, and less in diabetics than nondiabetics[35].

Anticholinergics

Scopolamine is a belladonna alkaloid, which possesses centrally acting anticholinergic effects, producing sedation and antiemetic effects[36]. Transdermal scopolamine (TDS) is a patch that delivers 1.5 mg of scopolamine over 72 h and possesses the same antiemetic efficacy as ondansetron and droperidol[37], with an NNT of 6[38]. Unlike the butyrophenones (droperidol and haloperidol) and the 5-HT_3 antagonists, TDS does not increase the QTc interval. Optimal timing of administration is either the night before surgery or preoperatively, with no difference in its efficacy for PONV prophylaxis[39]. Onset of effect is between 2 and 4 h[39]. Because of its long duration of action, up to 72 h, TDS might confer an advantage for the prevention of postdischarge nausea and vomiting (PDNV). However, the results of a large meta-analysis of TDS demonstrated no statistically significant benefit during the late postoperative period (24–48 h after surgery), which might be related to the limited number of studies looking at PDNV specifically[39], and to the low overall incidence of nausea and vomiting later after surgery.

Side effects of TDS include sedation, agitation, confusion, urinary retention, visual disturbances and dry mouth, the latter two being the most common adverse reactions, with numbers needed-to-harm of 5.6 and 12.5, respectively[38]. However, a recent meta-analysis of TDS demonstrated no difference in the anticholinergic side effects in the postoperative period, compared to placebo, other than visual disturbances between 24 and 48 h[39]. As elderly patients might be more susceptible to the anticholinergic effects such as confusion and agitation, caution should be exercised when considering TDS in the elderly patient[39].

Butyrophenones

Droperidol

Droperidol is a butyrophenone, first approved by the US Food and Drug Administration (FDA) in 1970 for use as an antiemetic[40]. Droperidol has similar efficacy for PONV prophylaxis as ondansetron and dexamethasone[8]. The dosing range for PONV prophylaxis is 0.625 mg to 1.25 mg IV, with an NNT of 5 for the prevention of PONV[41]. Unlike the 5-HT_3 antagonists, droperidol has more pronounced antinausea effects than antivomiting effects[25,41,42]. Optimal timing of administration is at the end of surgery.

Side effects of droperidol include extrapyramidal symptoms, sedation, dizziness, and QTc prolongation. In 2001, the FDA mandated that a black box warning be placed on the package insert of droperidol, warning of the risk of serious ventricular arrhythmias including torsades de pointes and sudden death, and requiring electrocardiogram monitoring after its administration. The majority of the deaths involving droperidol were at doses ranging from 25 to 250 mg[40], well above doses used for PONV prophylaxis and treatment. Several large studies comparing the safety and efficacy of droperidol and ondansetron have shown them to be equally efficacious for PONV prophylaxis, with similar safety profiles[8,41,42].

When compared to the 5-HT_3 antagonist ondansetron, droperidol was associated with similar clinically relevant QTc prolongations[43].

Haloperidol

Haloperidol is a butyrophenone with a high affinity for the dopamine D_2 receptor[44]. Haloperidol is highly effective at preventing PONV at doses between 0.5 and 2 mg IV or IM, well below the doses used for its antipsychotic properties[44]. Haloperidol has similar antiemetic efficacy to droperidol, and ondansetron, with an NNT of 4–6[44,45]. The timing of administration does not influence its antiemetic efficacy[46]. It can be given either postinduction or 30 min before the end of surgery, possibly related to its longer elimination half-life of 12–35 h[46]. As is the case with droperidol, its antinausea effects are more pronounced than its antivomiting effects[44]. Haloperidol is also effective for the treatment of established PONV; a 2-mg intramuscular (IM) dose was effective for the treatment of nausea[44].

The side-effect profile of haloperidol is similar to droperidol, with adverse effects that include extrapyramidal symptoms, sedation and a dose-dependent increase in the QTc interval. Extrapyramidal symptoms are rare at antiemetic doses. A meta-analysis of 806 patients receiving haloperidol for the prevention of PONV, at doses between 0.25 and 5 mg IV, revealed a single case of mild extrapyramidal symptoms[44]. Unlike droperidol, haloperidol does not possess an FDA black box warning on its package insert, making it a suitable replacement for droperidol, in terms of cost, efficacy and safety profile. Clinically, its effects on the QTc are identical to droperidol. Of the almost 1,400 patients receiving haloperidol in one meta-analysis, there were no reported cases of arrhythmias, torsades or sudden cardiac death[44].

Phenothiazine derivatives

Promethazine

Promethazine, an aliphatic phenothiazine derivative, has pharmacologic activity at several receptors involved in PONV, including dopamine, histamine and muscarinic acetylcholine[47]. Optimal dosing for PONV is 6.25–25 mg IV, IM or orally (PO) given at induction[48], or as a rescue agent if PONV prophylaxis fails. Promethazine can cause sedation, lethargy, dry mouth, urinary retention and extrapyramidal effects. When compared with ondansetron, placebo and combination therapy for PONV prophylaxis in middle ear surgery, promethazine was shown to reduce the incidence of nausea, but not vomiting during the first 24 h postoperatively, at a dose of 25 mg IV[47]. A dose of 12.5 mg IV was used for combination therapy with ondansetron and was shown to be effective for preventing both nausea and vomiting during the first 24 h[47]. A dose of 6.25 mg IV appears to be sufficient for PONV efficacy, with no increase in sedation compared with ondansetron 4 mg[49]. Promethazine appears to also have opioid-sparing effects, which might contribute to its antiemetic effects[50]. A small study involving abdominal hysterectomy patients demonstrated a 30% reduction in opioid consumption and reduction in PONV immediately postoperatively, and decreased need for rescue antiemetics on the first postoperative day[50]. The timing of administration, either pre- or postoperatively, did not significantly alter its efficacy. Currently, there is an FDA black box warning on the package insert advising against arterial administration or subcutaneous administration because of the risk of severe tissue injury and/or gangrene .

Prochlorperazine

Prochlorperazine, a heterocyclic phenothiazine derivative, shares a similar mechanism of action with promethazine, exerting its antiemetic effects via antidopaminergic, antihistaminergic and anticholinergic activity, with a similar side-effect profile. Dosing is 5–10 mg IV, IM or PO[48]. Promethazine and prochlorperazine are equally effective for PONV prevention, with promethazine causing more postoperative sedation and being associated with a higher risk of extrapyramidal side effects[51]. A small trial comparing 10 mg IM prochlorperazine to 4 mg IV ondansetron for the prevention of PONV for knee/hip arthroplasty demonstrated superior control of PONV in the prochlorperazine group[52].

NK_1-receptor antagonists

Substance P is a regulatory peptide that is released from enterochromaffin cells and binds to NK_1 receptors located in the GI tract and in the nucleus tractus solitarius and area postrema[53,54]. NK_1 receptor antagonists (aprepitant, casopitant and rolapitant) were first used to prevent chemotherapy-induced nausea and vomiting (CINV). Aprepitant has been shown to be at least equal to ondansetron for the prevention of nausea and the need for rescue antiemetics; however, aprepitant was shown to be superior to ondansetron for the prevention of vomiting in the first 24–48 h[53,55]. Patients taking ondansetron were twice as likely to experience vomiting during the first 24 h when compared with those taking aprepitant[55]. Adverse effects, including headache and QTc prolongation, did not differ between the groups[53]. The most common side effects of aprepitant are pyrexia, constipation, headache and bradycardia[55]. Aprepitant has a half-life of approximately 9–12 h[53]. Advantages of NK_1-receptor antagonists for the prevention of PONV compared with other classes of antiemetics include absence of sedation or QTc prolongation, superiority for the prevention of POV compared to all other antiemetics, and a long half-life, which might make them an ideal candidate to prevent PDNV[54]. Limitations include cost and inhibition of CYP3A4, which metabolizes common anesthetic drugs including fentanyl and midazolam, as well as coumadin[53,54].

Metoclopramide

Metoclopramide is a dopamine D_2 antagonist that possesses both central and peripheral serotonergic antagonism. Centrally, it is a 5-HT_3 antagonist, contributing to its antiemetic efficacy. Peripherally, metoclopramide is a 5-HT_4 antagonist, with prokinetic effects[56]. It has been widely used for the prevention of PONV. Historical dosing of metoclopramide for PONV has been 10 mg IV, compared to 2 mg/kg for prevention of CINV[57]. A large meta-analysis of over 3,000 patients receiving metoclopramide for PONV demonstrated a lack of effectiveness for preventing PONV at a 10 mg dose compared with placebo[56]. Ideal dosing for prevention of PONV appears to be at least 20 mg; however, literature supporting a dose–response relationship is lacking. In one study of ondansetron versus metoclopramide 0.4 mg/kg, metoclopramide was shown to be equally efficacious for the prevention of PONV[58]. Adverse effects include extrapyramidal side effects, sedation, drowsiness, dizziness, vertigo and headache; these effects are rare at the low doses used for PONV prophylaxis.

Ephedrine

Ephedrine, a sympathomimetic, has long been used for the prevention and treatment of PONV, particularly in patients with orthostatic hypotension. It has been postulated that a sympathomimetic agent would counteract postoperative vagal tone and its associated cholinergic activity at the vomiting center in the nucleus tractus solitarius[59]. Two studies of intramuscular ephedrine at a dose of 0.5 mg/kg, given at the end of surgery, showed ephedrine to have equal efficacy for the prevention of PONV as droperidol, with superiority over placebo[59,60]. When compared with droperidol and placebo, patients who received ephedrine had lower sedation scores, with a trend towards shorter time to discharge[59]. No significant differences in mean arterial pressure between the three groups were noted. When compared with placebo, the antiemetic effects of IM ephedrine were short-lived, extending to the first 3 h postoperatively, with no benefit over placebo between 3 and 24 h, and a trend towards less sedation was noticed, without any significant hemodynamic differences between the two groups[60]. Low cost, efficacy and decreased postoperative sedation make it an attractive agent, particulary in the ambulatory surgical patient. Potential for increased wakefulness and shorter recovery time might be an added benefit.

Antihistamines

Dimenhydrinate

Dimenhydrinate, an antihistamine derived from diphenhydramine, is an older antiemetic, used commonly for motion sickness. It is inexpensive and has a safety record that spans almost 70 years. The main side effect is drowsiness. In a meta-analysis of almost 1,400 patients receiving dimenhydrinate for prevention of PONV, dimenhydrinate was shown to be effective for preventing PONV in high-risk patients (baseline risk of 60%) with an NNT of 5, similar to the 5-HT_3 antagonists dexamethasone and droperidol[61]. The recommended dose is 1 mg/kg[62]. Whilst clearly not a first-line agent for the prevention of treatment of PONV, dimenhydrinate is inexpensive, has a long safety record with few side effects and has efficacy in high-risk patients.

Propofol

Propofol is one of the most commonly used sedative hypnotics for the induction of general anesthesia and maintenance of sedation. The antiemetic effects of propofol are widely accepted. Apfel et al. demonstrated an almost 25% risk reduction when using propofol as part of TIVA for the maintenance of general anesthesia, compared with maintenance of general anesthesia with one of the volatile agents[8]. Propofol has also been shown to have antiemetic properties in subhypnotic doses, requiring a plasma concentration of approximately 340 ng/mL[63,64]. When compared with placebo, 10 mg of IV propofol was effective in treating established PONV, with an absolute risk reduction of 46% and a 30-min relapse rate of 28% with no accompanying increase in sedation scores[64]. Efficacy of propofol compared with intralipid emulsion has been shown, demonstrating a unique antiemetic effect of propofol rather than its lipid emulsion[65]. When used as an induction agent only or administered at the end of surgery, propofol appears to lack antiemetic efficacy after the first hour postoperatively, likely related to lower postoperative plasma concentrations[66]. Subhypnotic doses of propofol appear to have similar efficacy compared to ondansetron[67].

The mechanism of action for the antiemetic effect of propofol is unclear. Possible mechanisms of action include a direct depressant effect on the chemoreceptor trigger zone and vagal nuclei[66] or by causing a decrease in serotonin concentrations in the area postrema[68].

Benzodiazepines

Midazolam is the most commonly used preoperative medication in the ambulatory setting, likely due to its rapid onset, short half-life, good safety profile and its efficacy in preoperative anxiolysis[69]. In addition to providing anxiolysis with dose-related anterograde amnesia, midazolam is effective at reducing PONV and improving patient satisfaction. When compared with placebo, 0.04 mg/kg of IV midazolam significantly reduced PONV from 50% to 25% with an NNT of 4, reduced POV from 21% to 8% and was associated with an increase in patient satisfaction, without an increase in postanesthesia care unit length of stay[70].

The antiemetic effects of midazolam appear to extend past its use preoperatively. When compared with 4 mg of IV ondansetron, 2 mg of IV midazolam given 30 min before the end of surgery had similar efficacy for the prevention of PONV as ondansetron, without an increase in time to awakening or time to reach an Aldrete score of 10[71]. Midazolam also has efficacy when used postoperatively for the treatment of established PONV. When compared with ondansetron 4 mg IV and propofol 15 mg IV, midazolam effectively treated established PONV; a 2-mg dose had greater efficacy for PONV treatment than a 1-mg dose, with slightly higher sedation scores[67].

The exact mechanism by which benzodiazepines exert their antiemetic effects is unclear. They are effective for anticipatory nausea, likely inhibiting cortical afferent signals to the vomiting center; however, this would not account for their action in the treatment of established PONV. Possible mechanisms include glycine-mimetic inhibitory effects, enhanced adenosinergic effects and inhibition of dopamine release[67].

Nonpharmacologic therapies

Pericardium P6 point acupucture/acupressure

The P6 point, also known as the pericardium point, is located between the tendons of the palmaris longus and flexor carpi radialis muscles, 4 cm proximal to the wrist crease[72]. A recent Cochrane meta-analysis of 40 trials involving 4,858 participants demonstrated that when compared with sham treatment, P6 acupoint stimulation significantly reduced nausea, vomiting and the need for rescue antiemetics[72]. Both the mechanism of action and the optimal timing of acupressure are unclear, although one study suggests maximal efficacy when used postoperatively[73]. Many devices exist to stimulate the P6 point, including acupuncture needles, disposable acupressure devices and transcutaneous nerve stimulators. One study demonstrated a 25% reduction in PONV over 24 h when monitoring neuromuscular blockade at the P6 acupuncture point (median nerve), compared with monitoring over the ulnar nerve[74]. The effects were primarily in reduction of nausea, rather than vomiting, which matched the risk reduction of the commonly used medications for PONV prophylaxis.

IV hydration

Intravascular volume depletion in the fasting patient has been thought to play a role in PONV. As crystalloid solutions are well tolerated, inexpensive and relatively void of side effects, they might be an ideal agent for the prevention of PONV. Several studies have demonstrated that preoperative fluid replacement with a crystalloid solution is an effective strategy for reducing the risk of PONV when given from doses of 2 mL/kg for every hour of fasting up to 20 mL/kg[75,76]. Benefits were seen in other patient outcomes, including thirst, drowsiness, dizziness, speed of recovery after surgery[75], as well as decreased postoperative pain scores[76]. Further, the benefits of a preoperative large-volume crystalloid resuscitation extended up to 72 h postoperatively[76].

Another study, using an esophageal Doppler probe for goal-directed therapy aimed at maintaining stroke volume during major surgery, found a quicker return of bowel function, shorter length of stay and decreased risk of PONV[77], possibly indicating hypovolemia, bowel hypoperfusion and bowel dysfunction as a cause of PONV.

Postdischarge nausea and vomiting

Definition and risk assessment

Postdischarge nausea and vomiting (PDNV), roughly defined as nausea and/or vomiting up to 48 h postdischarge, occurs in 35–50% of patients[78]. Lack of access to highly effective treatment options, including those requiring IV access, make this a significant problem for the ambulatory surgical patient[79]. A simplified scoring system to predict PONV risk, the "Apfel score," has been validated for PONV risk assessment in the inpatient setting[1]. Apfel et al. have developed and validated a second scoring system to assess the risk of PDNV, including five independent risk factors: age <50 years, female gender, prior history of PONV, immediate postoperative nausea and postoperative opioid administration[79]. Presence of zero, one, two, three, four and five risk factors were associated with a PDNV incidence of 7%, 20%, 28%, 53%, 60% and 89%, respectively (Figure 13.1)[79]. Since many of our highly effective antiemetic agents have relatively short half-lives, different strategies must be used to prevent PDNV, utilizing a combination of oral and IV medications with longer half-lives.

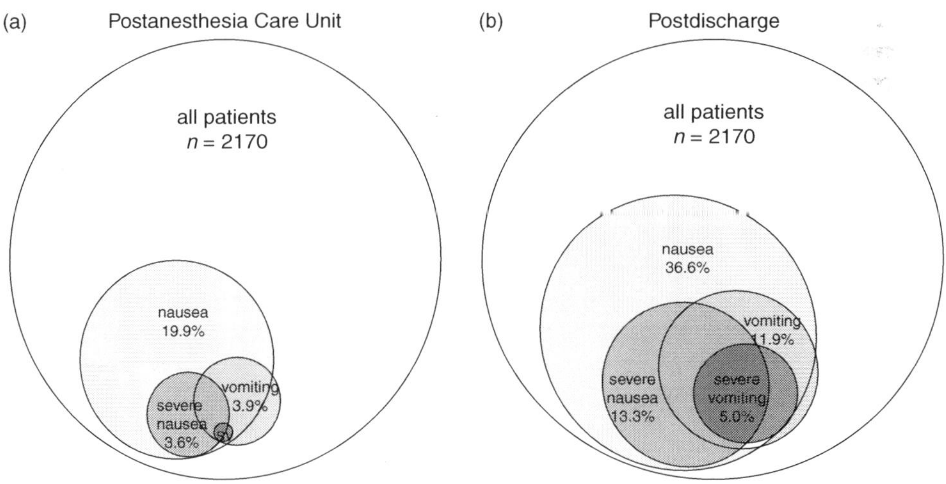

Figure 13.1 Percentage of patients who experienced nausea and/or vomiting (a) in the postanesthesia care unit and (b) postdischarge. The incidence of severe vomiting in the postanesthesia care unit was 0.2%. Reproduced with permission.

Strategies for reducing the risk of PDNV

Successful strategies for reducing the risk of PDNV take into account both the pharmacokinetics of the antiemetic agent as well as the principle of multimodal prophylaxis, utilizing agents of different pharmacologic classes. Ondansetron, the most commonly used 5-HT_3 antagonist, has little efficacy in preventing PDNV because of its short half-life of approximately 3 h[79]. Palonosetron, a second-generation 5-HT_3 antagonist with a half-life of 40 h, has been shown to reduce the risk of PONV for up to 72 h compared with placebo[80], with no effect on the QTc interval[81]. The use of propofol as part of TIVA compared with volatile anesthetics, reduces immediate postoperative nausea/vomiting; however, that benefit is likely lost in the late postoperative period, due to the short half-life of propofol[82]. When compared with the 5-HT_3 antagonists, dexamethasone appears to significantly reduce PDNV[79]. Dexamethasone has a biological half-life of 36–72 h[27], giving it a potential advantage for the prevention of PDNV.

The NK_1 receptor antagonist, aprepitant, has a relatively long half-life of between 9 and 12 h compared to ondansetron. When compared with ondansetron, aprepitant has been shown to be superior for the prevention of vomiting and reducing nausea severity over the first 48 h, likely related to a combination of superior antivomiting efficacy, as well as its significantly longer half-life[53,55]. The combination of greater antivomiting efficacy and longer half-life make aprepitant an ideal prophylactic agent for use in preventing PDNV. Rolapitant, an NK_1 receptor antagonist with an extremely long half-life of 180 h and a lack of enzyme inhibition, has been shown to be equally efficacious as ondansetron for the prevention of PONV during the first 24 h, with a decreased risk of emesis at 72 and 120 h postoperatively[83].

Although the benefits of TDS for the prevention of PDNV, between 24 and 48 h postoperatively, have not been demonstrated in a large meta-analysis[39], its long duration of action, up to 72 h, would appear to make it an ideal agent for the prevention of PDNV. More studies are needed to better evaluate the efficacy of TDS for the prevention of PDNV. However, adverse effects of TDS, specifically visual disturbances, might limit its use during this time period[39].

Strategies for managing established PONV

The successful management of established PONV must take into account both the pharmacokinetics and the pharmacodynamics of our antiemetic agents. Several of our highly effective agents for PONV prevention have poor utility for the treatment of established PONV. Dexamethasone exerts in pharmacologic activity for the prevention of PONV via its anti-inflammatory effects and prostaglandin inhibition, making it a poor choice for PONV treatment. Transdermal scopolamine is an equally poor choice because of its relatively long onset time, 2–4 h. When PONV prophylaxis fails, consideration should be given to using medications from other pharmacologic classes for treatment[2,84,85]. The 5-HT_3 antagonists have been well studied for the treatment of established PONV and are very effective for the treatment of POV, less so for the treatment of postoperative nausea[86]. There does not appear to be dose responsiveness of ondansetron for the treatment of established PONV, a dose of 1 mg IV should be considered to minimize the risk of adverse effects, specifically headache[86]. If prophylaxis with a 5-HT_3 antagonist fails, there is little evidence to support re-administering a second dose[85]. In patients who have failed prophylaxis with either ondansetron or droperidol, promethazine (6.25–25 mg IV) and dimenhydrinate (25–50 mg

IV) have been shown to be significantly more effective for treatment than either of the two prophylactic agents[84].

Although its use for the treatment of established PONV has not been rigorously studied, IM ephedrine might be an ideal medication for a specific subset of patients undergoing ambulatory surgery. Its unique mechanism of action compared to first-line prophylactic agents, efficacy for the prevention of PONV and its tendency towards less sedation and shorter recovery times might make it a useful adjunct for PONV treatment[60].

References

1. Apfel CC, Laara E, Koivuranta M, et al. A simplified risk score for predicting postoperative nausea and vomiting. *Anesthesiology* 1999; 91:693–700.
2. Gan TJ, Diemunsch P, Habib AS, et al. Consensus Guidelines for the Management of Postoperative Nausea and Vomiting. *Anasth Analg* 2014; 118:85–113.
3. Fortier J, Chung F, Su J. Unanticipated admission after ambulatory surgery – a prospective study. *Can J Anaesth* 1998; 45:612–9.
4. Gold BS, Kitz DS, Lecky JH, et al. Unanticipated admission to the hospital following ambulatory surgery. *JAMA* 1989; 262:3008–10.
5. Brenner WG, Kumar CM. Delayed surgical emphysema, pneumomediastinum and bilateral pneumothoraces after postoperative vomiting. *Br J Anaesth* 1993; 71: 296–7.
6. Eberhart LHJ, Morin AM, Kranke P, et al. Prevention and control of post-operative nausea and vomiting in post-craniotomy patients. *Best Pract Res Clin Anaesthesiol* 2008; 22(1): 575–593.
7. Apfel CC, Heidrich FM, Jukar-Rao S, et al. Evidence-based analysis of risk factors for postoperative nausea and vomiting. *Br J Anaesth* 2012; 109:742–53
8. Apfel CC, Kortilla K, Abdalla M, et al. IMPACT Investigators. A factorial trial of six interventions for the prevention of postoperative nausea and vomiting. *N Engl J Med* 2004; 350:2441–51.
9. Liu SS, Strodtbeck WM, Richman JM, et al. A comparison of regional versus general anesthesia for ambulatory anesthesia: a meta-analysis of randomized controlled trials. *Anesth Analg* 2005; 101:1634–42.
10. Sinclair DR, Chung F, Mezei G. Can postoperative nausea and vomiting be predicted. *Anesthesiology* 1999; 91:109–18.
11. Tramer MR, Fuchs-Buder T. Omitting antagonism of neuromuscular block: effect on postoperative nausea and vomiting and risk of residual paralysis: a systematic review. *Br J Anaesth* 1999; 82:379–86.
12. Cheng CR, Sessler DI, Apfel CC. Does neostigmine administration produce a clinically important increase in postoperative nausea and vomiting? *Anesth Analg* 2005; 101:1349–55.
13. Wheeler M, Oderda GM, Ashburn MA, et al. Adverse events associated with postoperative opioid analgesia: a systematic review. *J Pain* 2002; 3:159–80.
14. Roberts GW, Bekker TB, Carlsen HH, et al. Postoperative nausea and vomiting are strongly influenced by postoperative opioid use in a dose-related manner. *Anesth Analg* 2005; 101:1343–8.
15. Marret E, Kurdi O, Zufferey P, et al. Effects of nonsteroidal antiinflammatory drugs on patient-controlled analgesia morphine side effects: meta-analysis of randomized controlled trials. *Anesthesiology* 2005; 102:1249–60.
16. Gan TJ, Joshi GP, Zhao SZ, et al. Presurgical intravenous parecoxib sodium and follow-up oral valdecoxib for pain management after laparoscopic cholecystectomy surgery reduces opioid requirements and opioid-related adverse effects. *Acta Anaesthesiol Scand* 2004; 48:1194–207.

17. Lee SJ, Lee JN. The effect of perioperative esmolol infusion on the post-operative nausea, vomiting and pain after laparoscopic appendectomy. *Korean J Anesthesiol* 2010; 59:179–84.

18. Collard V, Mistraletti G, Taqi A, et al. Intraoperative esmolol infusion in the absence of opioids spares postoperative fentanyl in patients undergoing ambulatory Laparoscopic cholecystectomy. *Anesth Analg* 2007; 105:1255–62.

19. Gurbet A, Basagan-Mogol E, Turker G, et al. Intraoperative infusion of dexemedetomodine reduces perioperative analgesic requirements. *Can J Anaesth* 2006; 53:646–52.

20. Tiippana EM, Hamunen K, Kontinen VK, et al. Do surgical patients benefit from perioperative gabapenin/pregabalin? A systematic review of efficacy and safety. *Anesth Anal* 2007; 104:1545–57.

21. Hurley RW, Cohen SP, Williams KA, et al. The analgesic effect of perioperative gabapentin on postoperative pain: a meta-analysis. *Reg Anesth Pain Med* 2006; 31:237–47.

22. Bell RF, Dahl JB, Moore RA, et al. Peri-operative ketamine for acute post-operative pain: a quantitative and qualitative systematic review (Cochrane review). *Acta Anesthesiol Scand* 2005; 49:1405–28.

23. Pierre S, Corno G, Benais H, et al. A risk score-dependent antiemetic approach effectively reduces postoperative nausea and vomiting – a continuous quality improvement initiative. *Can J Anaesth* 2004; 51:320–5

24. Kovac AL, Eberhart L, Kotarski J, et al. A randomized, double-blind study to evaluate the efficacy and safety of three different doses of palonosetron versus placebo in preventing postoperative nausea and vomiting over a 72-hour period. *Anesth Analg* 2008; 107:439–44.

25. Tramer MR, Reynolds JM, Moore RA, et al. Efficacy, dose–response and safety of ondansetron in prevention of postoperative nausea and vomiting. *Anesthesiology* 1997; 87:1277–89.

26. Kovac AL, O'Connor TA, Pearman MH, et al. Efficacy of repeat intravenous dosing of ondansetron in controlling postoperative nausea and vomiting: a randomized, double-blind, placebo-controlled multicenter trial. *J Clin Anesth* 1999; 11:453–9.

27. Henzi I, Walder B, Tramer MR. Dexamethasone for the prevention of postoperative nausea and vomiting. A quantitative systematic review. *Anesth Analg* 2000; 90:186–94.

28. Wang JJ, Ho ST, Tzeng JI, et al. The effect of timing of dexamethasone administration on its efficacy as a prophylactic antiemetic for postoperative nausea and vomiting. *Anesth Analg* 2000; 91:136–39.

29. De Oliveira GS, Almeida MD, Benzon HT, et al. Perioperative single dose systemic dexamethasone for postoperative pain. *Anesthesiology* 2011; 115:575–88.

30. De Oliveira GS, Ahmad S, Fitzgerald PC, et al. Dose ranging study on the effect of preoperative dexamethasone on postoperative quality of recovery and opioid consumption after ambulatory gynaecologic surgery. *Br J Anaesth* 2011; 107:362–71.

31. Murphy GS, Szokol JW, Greenberg MD, et al. Preoperative dexamethasone enhances quality of recovery after laparoscopic cholecytectomy. *Anesthesiology* 2011; 114:882–90.

32. Khan SA, McDonagh DL, Gan TJ. Wound complications with dexamethasone for postoperative nausea and vomiting prophylaxis: a moot point? *Anesth Analg* 2013; 116:966–7.

33. Cowie BS, Allen KJ, Said SA, et al. Anti-emetic doses of dexamethasone suppress cortisol response in laparoscopic cholecystectomy. *Anaesth Intensive Care* 2010; 38:667–70.

34. Dieleman JM, Nierich AP, Rosseel et al. Dexamethasone for Cardiac Surgery (DECS) Study Group. Intraoperative high-dose dexamethasone for cardiac surgery: a randomized controlled trial. *JAMA* 2012; 308:1761–7.

35. Abdelmalak B, Bonilla AM, Yang D, et al. The hyperglycemic response to major noncardiac surgery and the added effect of steroid administration in patients with and without diabetes. *Anesth Analg* 2013; 116:1116–22.

36. Pergolizzi JV, Philip BK, Taylor RJ. Perspectives on transdermal scopolamine for the treatment of postoperative nausea and vomiting. *J Clin Anesth* 2012; 24:334–45.

37. White PF, Tang J, Song D, et al. Transdermal scopolamine: an alternative to ondansetron and droperidol for the prevention of postoperative and postdischarge emetic symptoms. *Anesth Analg* 2007; 104:92–96.

38. Kranke P, Morin AM, Roewer N, et al. The efficacy and safety of transdermal scopolamine for the prevention of postoperative nausea and vomiting: a quantitative systematic review. *Anesth Analg* 2002; 95:133–43.

39. Apfel, CC, Zhang K, George E, et al. Transdermal scopolamine for the prevention of postoperative nausea and vomiting: a systematic review and meta-analysis. *Clin Ther* 2010; 32:1987–2002.

40. White, P. Droperidol: a cost-effective antiemetic for over thirty years. *Anesth Analg* 2002; 95:789–90.

41. Henzi I, Sonderegger J, Tramer M. Efficacy, dose–response, and adverse effects of droperidol for prevention of postoperative nausea and vomiting. *Can J Anaesth* 2000; 47:537–551.

42. Fortney J, Gan TJ, Graczyk S, et al. A comparison of the efficacy, safety, and patient satisfaction of ondansetron versus droperidol as antiemetics for elective outpatient surgical procedures. *Anesth Analg* 1998; 86:731–8.

43. Charbit B, Albaladejo P, Funck-Brentano C, et al. Prolongation of QT_c interval after postoperative nausea and vomiting treatment by droperidol or ondansetron. *Anesthesiology* 2005; 102:1094–100.

44. Buttner M, Walder B, von Elm E, et al. Is low-dose haloperidol a useful antiemetic? A meta-analysis of published and unpublished randomized trials. *Anesthesiology* 2004; 101:1454–63.

45. Lee Y, Wang PK, Lai HY, et al. Haloperidol is as effective as ondansetron for preventing postoperative nausea and vomiting. *Can J Anaesth* 2007; 54:349–54.

46. Yang YL, Lai HY, Wang JJ, et al. The timing of haloperidol administration does not affect is prophylactic antiemetic efficacy. *Can J Anaesth* 2008; 55:270–5.

47. Khalil S, Philbrook L, Rabb M, et al. Ondansetron/promethazine combination or promethazine alone reduces nausea and vomiting after middle ear surgery. *J Clin Anesth* 1999; 11:596–600.

48. Gan TJ, Meyer TA, Apfel CC, et al. Society for Ambulatory Anesthesia Guidelines for the Management of Postoperative Nausea and Vomiting. *Anesth Analg* 2007; 105:1615–24.

49. Moser JD, Caldwell JB, Rhule FJ. No more than necessary: safety and efficacy of low-dose promethazine. *Ann Pharmacother* 2006; 40:45–8.

50. Chia YY, Lo Y, Liu K, et al. The effect of promethazine on postoperative pain: a comparison of preoperative, postoperative, and placebo administration in patients following total abdominal hysterectomy. *Acta Anaesthesiol Scand* 2004; 48:625–30.

51. Kovac AL. Prevention and treatment of postoperative nausea and vomiting. *Drugs* 2000; 59: 213–43.

52. Chen JJ, Frame DG, White TJ. Efficacy of ondansetron and prochlorperazine for the prevention of postoperative nausea and vomiting after total hip replacement or total knee replacement produres. *Arch Intern Med* 1998; 158:2124–29.

53. Gan TJ, Apfel CC, Kovac A, et al. Aprepitant-PONV Study Group. A randomized, double-blind comparison of the NK1 antagonist, aprepitant, versus ondansetron for the prevention of postoperative nausea and vomiting. *Anesth Analg* 2007; 104:1082–9.

54. Apfel CC, Malhotra A, Leslie JB. The role of neurokinin-1 receptor antagonists for the management of postoperative nausea

and vomiting. *Curr Opin Anesth* 2008; 21:427–32.

55. Diemunsch P, Gan TJ, Philip BK, et al. Aprepitant-PONV Protocol 091 International Study Group. Single-dose aprepitant vs ondansetron for the prevention of postoperative nausea and vomiting: a randomized, double-blind Phase III trial in patients undergoing open abdominal surgery. *Br J Anaesth* 2007; 99:202–11.
56. Henzi I, Walder B, Tramer MR. Metoclopramide in the prevention of postoperative nausea and vomiting: a quantitative systematic review of randomized, placebo-controlled studies. *Br J Anaesth* 1999; 83:761–7.
57. Gralla RJ, Itri LM, Pisko SE, et al. Antiemetic efficacy of high-dose metoclopramide: randomized trials with placebo and prochlorperazine in patients with chemotherapy-induced nausea and vomiting. *N Engl J Med* 1981; 305:905–9.
58. Monagle J, Barnes R, Goodchild C, et al. Ondansetron is not superior to moderate dose metoclopramide in the prevention of post-operative nausea and vomiting after gynaecologic surgery. *Eur J Anaesth* 1997; 14:604–9.
59. Rothenberg DM, Parnass SM, Litwack K, et al. Efficacy of ephedrine in the prevention of postoperative nausea and vomiting. *Anesth Analg* 1991; 72:58–61.
60. Hageman E, Halvorson A, Holgersen O, et al. Intramuscular ephedrine reduces emesis during the first three hours after abdominal hysterectomy. *Acta Anaesthesiol Scand* 2000; 44:107–11.
61. Kranke P, Morin AM, Roewer N, et al. Dimenhydrinate for prophylaxis of postoperative nausea and vomiting: a meta-analysis of randomized controlled trials. *Acta Anaesthesiol Scand* 2002; 46:238–44.
62. Eberhart LHJ, Seeling W, Bopp TI, et al. Dimenhydrinate for prevention of post-operative nausea and vomiting in female in-patients. *Eur J Anaesthesiol* 1999; 16:284–9.
63. Gan TJ, Glass PSA, Howell ST, et al. Determination of plasma concentration of propofol associated with 50% reduction in postoperative nausea. *Anesthesiology* 1997; 87:779–84.
64. Borgeat A, Wilder-Smith OHG, Saiah M, et al. Subhypnotic doses of propofol possess direct antiemetic properties. *Anesth Analg* 1992; 74:539–41.
65. Ostman PL, Faure E, Glosten B, et al. Is the antiemetic effect of the emulsion formulation of propofol due to the lipid emulsion? *Anesth Analg* 1990; 71:536–40.
66. Gan TJ, Ginsberg B, Grant P, et al. Double-blind, randomized comparison of ondansetron and intraoperative propfol to prevent postoperative nausea and vomiting. *Anesthesiology* 1996; 85:1036–42.
67. Unlugenc H, Guler T, Gunes Y, et al. Comparative study of the antiemetic efficacy of ondansetron, propofol and midazolam in the early postoperative period. *Eur J Anaesthesiol* 2004; 21:60–5.
68. Diab A, Gelb AW, Cechetto DF. Effects of the anesthetic propofol on 5-HT and FOS in the rat brain [Abstract]. *Neuroscience* 1994; 20:1169.
69. Kain ZN, Mayes LC, Bell C, et al. Premedication in the United States: a status report. *Anesth Analg* 1997; 84:427–32.
70. Bauer KP, Dom PM, Ramirez AM, et al. Preoperative intravenous midazolam: benefits beyond anxiolysis. *J Clin Anesth* 2004; 16:177–83.
71. Lee Y, Wang JJ, Yang YL, et al. Midazolam vs ondansetron for preventing postoperative nausea and vomiting: a randomised controlled trial. *Anaesthesia* 2007; 62:18–22.
72. Lee A, Fan LT. Stimulation of the wrist acupuncture point P6 for preventing postoperative nausea and vomiting. *Cochrane Database Syst Rev* 2009; (2):CD003281.
73. White PF, Hamza MA, Recart A, et al. Optimal timing of acustimulation for antiemetic prophylaxis as an adjunct to ondansetron in patients undergoing plastic surgery. *Anesth Analg* 2005; 100:367–72

74. Arnberger M, Stadelmann K, Alischer P, et al. Monitoring of neuromuscular blockade at the P6 acupuncture point reduces the incidence of postoperative nausea and vomiting. *Anesthesiology* 2007; 107:903–908

75. Yogendran S, Asokumar B, Cheng DCH, et al. A prospective randomized double-blinded study of the effect of intravenous fluid therapy on adverse outcomes on outpatient surgery. *Anesth Analg* 1995; 80:682–6.

76. Maharaj CH, Kallam SR, Malik A, et al. Preoperative intravenous fluid therapy decreases postoperative nausea and pain in high risk patients. *Anesth Analg* 2005; 100:675–82.

77. Gan TJ, Soppitt A, Maroof M, et al. Goal-directed intraoperative fluid administration reduces length of hospital stay after major surgery. *Anesthesiology* 2002; 97:820–26.

78. Gupta A, Wu CL, Elkassabany N, et al. Does the routine prophylactic use of antiemetics affect the incidence of postdischarge nausea and vomiting following ambulatory surgery? *Anesthesiology* 2003; 99:488–95.

79. Apfel C, Philip B, Cakmakkaya OS, et al. Who is at risk for postdischarge nausea and vomiting after ambulatory surgery? *Anesthesiology* 2012; 117: 475–86.

80. Kovac AL, Eberhart L, Kotarski J, et al. Palonosetron 04-07 Study Group. A randomized, double-blind study to evaluate the efficacy and safety of three different doses of palonosetron versus placebo in preventing postoperative nausea and vomiting over a 72-hour period. *Anesth Analg* 2008; 107:439–44.

81. George E, Hornuss C, Apfel CC. Neurokinin-1 and novel seratonin antagonists for postoperative and postdischarge nausea and vomiting. *Curr Opin Anesth* 2010; 23:714–21.

82. Apfel CC, Kranke P, Katz MH, et al. Volatile anaesthetics may be the main cause of early but not delayed postoperative vomiting: a randomized controlled trial of factorial design. *Br J Anesth* 2002; 88:659–68.

83. Gan TJ, Gu J, Singla N, et al. Rolapitant Investigation Group. Rolapitant for the prevention of postoperative nausea and vomiting: a prospective, double-blinded, placebo-controlled randomized trial. *Anesth Analg* 2011; 112:804–12.

84. Habib A, Gan TJ. The effectiveness of rescue antiemetics after failure of prophylaxis with ondansetron or droperidol: a preliminary report. *J Clin Anesth* 2005; 17:62–5.

85. Kovac A, O'Connor TA, Pearman MH, et al. Efficacy of repeat intravenous dosing of ondansetron in controlling postoperative nausea and vomiting: a randomized, double-blind, placebo-controlled multicenter trial. *J Clin Anesth* 1999; 11:453–9.

86. Kazemi-Kjellberg F, Henzi I, Tramer MR. Treatment of established postoperative nausea and vomiting: a quantitative systematic review. *BMC Anesthesiol* 2001; 1:2. http://www.biomedcentral .com/1471–2253/1/2.

Chapter 14

Postoperative nausea and vomiting management: cost-effectiveness and patient outcome

Paul S. Myles

Postoperative nausea and vomiting (PONV) and postdischarge nausea and vomiting (PDNV) are distressing to patients and staff, delay recovery after surgery and are costly[1–15]. There is abundant knowledge regarding the prevention and treatment of PONV, and some information regarding cost-effectiveness, but the weakest link in the chain is implementation of evidence-based strategies. Some have proposed that near-universal multimodal PONV prophylaxis may represent a simpler and more reliable approach to reducing the incidence of PONV[16]. The low cost of most of the currently available antiemetics and their low incidence of side effects suggest that a liberal antiemetic prophylaxis regimen could be a rational option to eliminate or substantially reduce the big "little problem"[17]. Such opinions, however, require our deliberation and critique, and it is fortunate that there is a growing body of literature to guide such decision-making.

Decisions about drug choices and administration should consider the cost and benefits of relevant drugs, as well as the option of not using drug therapy. Information is available on how to consider drug cost-effectiveness[18], and such studies should be conducted according to established guidelines[18–22]. Until recently, most costing studies of PONV therapies have been incomplete and not conducted in accordance with these recommendations[20,23].

It might be useful to consider what, exactly, are the costs or consequences of PONV and PDNV. It many cases the avoidance or early treatment of PONV leads to a beneficial effect on patient comfort and quality of recovery after surgery. Most patients and clinicians want to avoid any PONV – the resultant consequences of discomfort and emotional distress are probably sufficient reasons to avoid PONV. Most patients, however, would not suffer PONV irrespective of treatment, and of those who are given antiemetic prophylaxis, only about one-third will benefit from this practice. There are of course economic costs of PONV: requirements for treatment, delayed discharge from the postanaesthesia care unit (PACU), unplanned readmission, and for patients discharged home there may be limitations on return to work or increased need for domiciliary assistance. Some patients' prior experience of PONV fuels an ongoing aversion to further surgery and anesthesia.

Postoperative Nausea and Vomiting: A Practical Guide, eds. Tong Joo Gan and Ashraf S. Habib. Published by Cambridge University Press.

Methodology of cost-effectiveness studies

There are several different ways health costing studies can be considered and quantified. Approaches to analyses typically include the following:

- **Cost-of-illness** The direct economic impact of an illness or adverse event, including treatment costs. For PONV this would include drug acquisition costs, extra time in the PACU and loss of earnings.
- **Cost-minimization** To determine the least costly alternative treatment assumed to produce equivalent outcomes. This would include the option of no prophylaxis or treatment.
- **Cost-effectiveness** A ratio of monetary costs with outcomes quantified in non-monetary units – that is, the impact of reduced PONV on overall health status.
- **Cost–utility** A ratio of monetary costs with outcomes quantified in terms of their utility to the patient. This type of analysis typically uses quality-adjusted life years (QALYs).
- **Cost–benefit** A ratio of costs and benefits, both quantified in monetary units.

The perspective of a cost analysis refers to who is bearing the costs. This may be the patient, the hospital, a third-party payer or society overall. It is generally recommended that all costs and outcomes should be considered from a societal perspective, because the patient or anesthesiologist may not appreciate what is truly cost-effective, and they or the hospital are not usually responsible for all cost outlays.

In cost-effectiveness analysis, it is conventional to distinguish between the direct costs and the indirect costs associated with the treatment, perhaps including intangibles, which may be difficult to quantify, but are often consequences of treatment or opting for no treatment. Direct costs might include drug and disposables costs, staff time to deal with PONV, cleaning and linen, and any other patient expenses associated with PONV. Indirect costs include family burdens and productivity losses; intangibles might include patient distress and other adverse effects.

In 1994, it was estimated that each episode of emesis delays discharge from PACU by approximately 20 min[24]. These costs are likely to be a lot higher in contemporary settings.

The incremental cost-effectiveness ratio (ICER) is the ratio of the change in costs to incremental benefits of a therapeutic intervention or treatment, calculated as[22]:

$$ICER = (C1 - C2) / (E1 - E2)$$

where:

C1 and E1 are the cost and effect in the treatment group, and
C2 and E2 are the cost and effect in the control group.

Costs are described in monetary units and benefit/effect on health status is usually measured in terms of QALYs gained or lost. That is, the numerator measures treatment costs and the denominator places a monetary cost on the health consequences. Increased *length* of life, and/or *quality* of life, will increase QALYs. One QALY is equal to 1 year of life lived in perfect health. A medical complication leading to a 25% reduction in quality of life but with no effect on longevity will result in a 0.75 QALY. QALYs can be used to rank any number of competing treatment options or to compare two treatment options.

Most national drug approval or funding agencies expect cost-effectiveness to be expressed as a cost per QALY gained or lost. That is, in terms of society's willingness to pay for an additional unit of health gain.

In the UK, the National Institute for Health and Clinical Excellence (NICE) uses QALYs as the "common currency" to enable comparisons across therapeutic areas. The ICER is expressed as the cost per QALY gained and can be compared with those of other interventions or with a national threshold value of what is considered to represent cost-effectiveness. NICE has a range of acceptable cost-effectiveness of around £25,000 (US$55,000) per QALY[10].

Another approach that has been used in the PONV literature is the *willingness to pay* method. For example, several studies have found that patients are willing to pay approximately $100 to avoid experiencing PONV[25,26], and another study found parents are willing to spend approximately $80 to prevent postoperative vomiting (POV) in their children[27]. The threshold for the willingness to pay method is about $50–100,000 in the USA[28]. A willingness to pay rate of $100 per case avoided makes PONV prophylaxis cost-effective in clinical settings with a baseline incidence of PONV of 40%.

The QALY approach can be modified to suit a perioperative, particularly ambulatory surgery setting, such as if a proposed prophylactic treatment costs $11.00 and on average increases a person's quality of recovery score 2 points on a 0–10 point scale, say from 6 to 8, for the next 24-h period and they otherwise recover fully at home (i.e., they will eventually recover full health), we can calculate a QALY as:

- QALY without PONV prophylaxis is: 6/10 × 1 (day) + 364 (remaining days in the year, ignoring the leap year), so 364.6 QALYs
- QALY with PONV prophylaxis is 364.8
- The gain in QALYs with PONV prophylaxis is 0.2/365 (=0.0.0005479)
- The ICER will then be $11/0.0005479 = $20,077 per QALY. This is a cost-effective treatment and can be recommended.

Estimates of cost-effectiveness can vary markedly because of different assumptions relating to the cost of treatment and impact on "outcomes," particularly measures of resultant health status. Costing studies should include some sensitivity analysis, to explore the effect of changes in the underlying assumptions of the costs and benefits. For example, if the drug acquisition and disposables cost were twice as much or the benefit of reduced PONV on overall health status was less.

The practicality of developing evidence on drug cost-effectiveness has been addressed in other specialties[29], and can be explored in perioperative practice. It is not too difficult to obtain cost data on types of treatments available, dosages, and sundry equipment and staffing. It is therefore possible to estimate incremental cost-effectiveness to facilitate informed decision-making by both payers and physicians. This can improve quality of care and enhance the efficient allocation of resources.

Patient-centered outcome measures and PONV

In the USA, the Patient Protection and Affordable Care Act was devised with the aim of improving quality of healthcare, outcomes and cost-efficiency. The Patient-Centered Outcomes Research Institute (PCORI) was established to encourage and support more comparative effectiveness research[30]. These changes place much greater emphasis on outcomes research, knowledge translation, and the need to incorporate patient preferences in clinical decision-making. Patient outcomes are also related to the level of communication with and trust in the doctor[31,32].

Patient-reported outcomes are events directly reported by patients or their surrogates about experiences with care, including symptoms, functional status or quality of life[33]. In the perioperative setting, this would include quality of recovery[34–37]. These are necessary and important outcome measures used by drug registration agencies, as well as to provide clinicians and the patients they treat with clinically useful information. This is in contrast to studies focusing on surrogate outcome measures[38,39]; many are of questionable significance and often have no convincing relationship with patient outcome.

Whilst some have argued that PONV is not necessarily an adverse patient outcome[40]; there is little doubt that many PONV episodes are clinically important[41,42]. It is, however, necessary to include some measure(s) of patient outcome over and above the incidence of PONV in perioperative research. This may include quantifying the clinical importance of PONV[41], or including one or more measures of patient quality of recovery or satisfaction with care[40].

Several quality of recovery (QoR) scores are available[32,43–47], but the most stringently studied has been the QoR-40[48]. For example, several groups have identified interventions that not only reduce PONV but also the resultant effect on QoR[49,50]. Quantitative measures of quality of recovery provide a numerical value for health status, and so can be used to calculate QALYs and ICER.

Myles and Wengritzky[41] developed a simple-to-use measure of the intensity and clinical impact of PONV. They found that around one in five patients with PONV had features that could classify them as having clinically important PONV; that is, where the PONV episode had a demonstrable effect on measures of health status. Patients with clinically important PONV had a much poorer quality of recovery ($P < 0.0005$), needed more antiemetic administrations for treatment ($P < 0.0005$), and were more likely to have consequences and complications of PONV ($P < 0.01$) when compared with those with lesser degrees of PONV.

PONV cost-evaluation studies

Whilst prophylactic antiemetic therapy reduces the incidence of PONV, it is unclear whether there is net benefit (less patient discomfort, delayed recovery, less staff resources) or harm (drug administration costs, side effects). Most patients do not benefit when given prophylactic antiemetic therapy, but all are exposed to potential harms.

Carlisle and Stevenson[51] performed a systematic review and meta-analysis of randomized controlled trials, which compared PONV prophylaxis with placebo. They identified 737 trials involving 103,237 patients and found that eight drugs were efficacious in preventing PONV when compared with placebo: dexamethasone, droperidol, metoclopramide, ondansetron, tropisetron, dolasetron, granisetron and cyclizine. The relative risks (RR) were between 0.60 and 0.80, depending upon the drug and outcome, indicating a 20–40% reduction in risk. Most of the original studies did not report side effects, but there was evidence of excess sedation with droperidol (RR 1.32) and headache with ondansetron (RR 1.16). The authors concluded that for each 100 patients given one of the above drugs, of whom 30 would report PONV without prophylaxis, 10 people would benefit from treatment and 90 people would not.

Failure to treat and overtreatment are two ends of a poor cost-effectiveness spectrum. Risk scores can identify patients at increased risk of PONV, and may therefore aid cost-effectiveness. An electronic decision-support clinical information system can assist[52]. Quality metrics to improve the cost-effective management of PONV have been proposed[53].

Pierre et al.[54] triaged surgical patients into three groups: (i) those at low risk of PONV that did not receive any antiemetic prophylaxis; (ii) those at moderate risk received low-dose (0.625 mg) droperidol or propofol-based intravenous anesthesia without droperidol; and (iii) those in the high-risk group received propofol-based intravenous anesthesia, dexamethasone 4 mg and droperidol 0.625 mg. Rates of PONV were reduced from 50% to 14% ($P < 0.001$). Such risk-guided antiemetic regimens are likely to be a cost-effective strategy. This concept has further support from another continuous quality improvement (QI) program aimed at lowering PONV in the PACU[55]. A multimodal PONV management protocol that standardized the anesthetic technique and antiemetic regimen was used, according to the Apfel PONV risk scoring system[56]. There were three stages to the QI program: (1) a prospective analysis of existing practice; (2) protocol implementation; (3) active feedback to staff and evaluation of guideline compliance. They found that 37/395 (9.4%) and 151/3,864 (3.9%) patients experienced PONV in the PACU before and after protocol implementation, respectively ($P < 0.001$), demonstrating a successful QI program.

A QI program introduced at the University of Texas MD Anderson Cancer Center and covering 23,279 anesthetics[57] found that compliance was not significantly influenced by a brief education program or in low-risk patients (the latter because of ingrained habits of universal antiemetic prophylaxis), but some improvement occurred when anesthesiologists were provided with brief performance data (59% versus 54%, $P < 0.001$) and most strongly when ongoing compliance data were presented (65% versus 59%, $P < 0.001$). Beneficial effects were strongest for those patients who had at least three risk factors for PONV.

Hill et al.[58] found prophylaxis was more cost-effective than placebo in high-risk patients because of the increased costs associated with nausea and vomiting[59]. The additional costs associated with PONV in placebo patients were up to 100 times higher compared with prophylaxis with a generic antiemetic, and the cost of treating vomiting was three times greater than the cost of treating nausea. Other studies have reported similar findings, but prophylaxis is only marginally more effective than treatment. Tramer et al. [60] did a modeling study and found that treatment of established PONV with ondansetron is more cost-effective and safer than prophylaxis with the same drug when effective doses are used. This was in part due to the weak antinausea effect of prophylactic ondansetron. These findings, however, might not be currently applicable since ondansetron became generic.

Paech et al.[61] included a cost–benefit analysis in a comparison of three 5-HT_3 receptor antagonists in 118 patients undergoing major gynecologic surgery. They found no significant differences between groups, and concluded that the choice between these agents should be based on the lowest available acquisition cost for each agent.

Pueyo et al.[62] compared the cost-effectiveness of three combinations of antiemetics in the prevention of PONV in 90 women undergoing major gynecologic surgery. A decision analysis tree was used to divide each group into nine mutually exclusive subgroups, depending on the incidence of PONV, need for rescue therapy, side effects and their treatment. Direct cost and probabilities were calculated for each subgroup, and then a cost-effectiveness analysis was conducted from the hospital point-of-view. They found that the combination of ondansetron–droperidol was cheaper than and at least as effective as ondansetron–dexamethasone, and was more effective than dexamethasone–droperidol with minimal extra cost.

Chang et al.[15] compared the cost-effectiveness of ondansetron and prochlorperazine in 78 patients undergoing hip or knee arthroplasty. They measured the cost-effectiveness ratio for each antiemetic. Prochlorperazine was more effective at reducing PONV in this study population. The mean total costs of PONV management per patient in the prochlorperazine and ondansetron groups were $13.99 and $51.98, respectively. The cost of successfully treating one patient with prochlorperazine and ondansetron was $31.87 and $275.01, respectively. They concluded that prochlorperazine is a more cost-effective antiemetic compared with ondansetron for the prevention of PONV in their study population. However, ondansetron has since become generic and so those findings might not be applicable to current practice.

There are few pediatric studies evaluating cost-effectiveness of PONV management.

An excellent study by Sennaraj et al.[63] compared the cost-effectiveness of prophylactic ondansetron with early ondansetron treatment in the management of PONV in 150 children undergoing strabismus repair using patient-centered outcome measures. Outcome measures included PONV rates, duration of stay in the PACU, parental satisfaction scores and costs (cost to benefit a child and cost per PONV-free child). Ondansetron prophylaxis was effective in reducing early and late PONV, and resulted in a shorter duration of PACU stay and superior parental satisfaction scores. The cost to benefit a child was more than fourfold less and the cost per PONV-free child was 35% less in the PONV prophylaxis group.

Olutoye et al.[64] evaluated the smallest dose of dolasetron for the prophylaxis of POV in 204 children undergoing ambulatory surgery. Costs were calculated from the perspective of the hospital. The incidence of early (0–6 h) and 24-h emesis was more frequent in the dolasetron 45 μg/kg group compared with the dolasetron 350 and 700 μg/kg groups and with the ondansetron group. They concluded that dolasetron 350 μg/kg IV was the smallest dose that provided acceptable equivalent efficacy and patient satisfaction scores to ondansetron 100 μg/kg.

Parra-Sanchez et al.[11] determined the incremental costs of PONV/PDNV in ambulatory patients with a time-and-motion study in 100 ambulatory surgery patients. They evaluated the incidence of PONV, time staff spent with patients, use of PONV-related supplies, recovery duration, PONV rescue treatments and a quality-of-life metric up to the third postoperative morning. They found that 37% of patients experienced PONV during hospitalization; this increased to 42% by the first postoperative morning and to 49% by the third postoperative morning. Patients with PONV spent 1 h longer in PACU compared with patients without PONV ($P = 0.001$) and more nursing time was required ($P = 0.02$). The total cost of postoperative recovery was significantly greater for patients with PONV/PDNV than for those without (US$730 versus $640; ICER $75, $P = 0.006$). The proportion of those who rated their quality of life high on each of four domains was less in those with PONV/PDNV, 49% versus 94%, respectively ($P < 0.001$). The incremental cost was comparable with the cost patients are willing to pay to avoid PONV.

There are many effective, cheap (generic) antiemetic agents that have been shown to be effective in the prophylaxis and treatment of PONV and PDNV. Lower drug acquisition costs support the cost-effectiveness of PONV prophylaxis in at-risk groups. In general, the decision about whether or not to use PONV prophylaxis is determined by the drug efficacy, risk for PONV, and drug acquisition costs, and these will vary from one setting to another.

References

1. Gan T, Ing R, de L Dear G, et al. How much are patients willing to pay to avoid intraoperative awareness? *J Clin Anesth* 2003; 15: 108–12.
2. Gan TJ, Diemunsch P, Habib AS, et al. SAMBA Consensus guidelines for the management of postoperative nausea and vomiting. *Anesth Analg* 2014; 118: 85–113.
3. Bishof RO, Nash DB. Cost-effectiveness and cost containment. A physician's primer. *Prim Care* 1996; 23: 115–26.
4. Coronini-Cronberg S, Appleby J, Thompson J. Application of patient-reported outcome measures (PROMs) data to estimate cost-effectiveness of hernia surgery in England. *J R Soc Med* 2013; 106: 278–87.
5. Frighetto L, Loewen PS, Dolman J, et al. Cost-effectiveness of prophylactic dolasetron or droperidol vs rescue therapy in the prevention of PONV in ambulatory gynecologic surgery. *Can J Anaesth* 1999; 46: 536–43.
6. Gillespie EL, White CM, Kluger J, et al. A hospital perspective on the cost-effectiveness of beta-blockade for prophylaxis of atrial fibrillation after cardiothoracic surgery. *Clin Ther* 2005; 27: 1963–9.
7. Gomes M, Soares MO, Dumville JC, et al. Cost-effectiveness analysis of general anaesthesia versus local anaesthesia for carotid surgery (GALA Trial). *Br J Surg* 2010; 97: 1218–25.
8. Johnstone R, Martinec C. Anesthesia studies should include costs. *Anesthesiology* 1993; 79: 195–7.
9. Lake AP, Hugo S, Coetzee G, et al. Cost-effectiveness analysis of antiemetic therapy for ambulatory surgery. *J Clin Anesth* 1995; 7: 551–3.
10. McCabe C, Claxton K, Culyer AJ. The NICE cost-effectiveness threshold: what it is and what that means. *Pharmacoeconomics* 2008; 26: 733–44.
11. Parra-Sanchez I, Abdallah R, You J, et al. A time–motion economic analysis of postoperative nausea and vomiting in ambulatory surgery. *Can J Anaesth* 2012; 59: 366–75.
12. Rennie L, Porteous T, Ryan M. Preferences for managing symptoms of differing severity: a discrete choice experiment. *Value Health* 2012; 15: 1069–76.
13. Watcha M. The cost-effective management of postoperative nausea and vomiting (editorial). *Anesthesiology* 2000; 92: 931–3.
14. Watcha MF, Smith I. Cost-effectiveness analysis of antiemetic therapy for ambulatory surgery. *J Clin Anesth* 1994; 6: 370–7.
15. Chang P, Okamoto M, Chen J, et al. Cost-effectiveness analysis of ondansetron and prochlorperazine for the prevention of postoperative nausea and vomiting. *J Manag Care Pharm* 2005; 11: 317–21.
16. Kranke P, Eberhart LH. Possibilities and limitations in the pharmacological management of postoperative nausea and vomiting. *Eur J Anaesthesiol* 2011; 28: 758–65.
17. Kapur PA. The big "little problem". *Anesth Analg* 1991; 73(3):243–5.
18. Gagnon JP, Osterhaus JT. Proposed drug–drug cost effectiveness methodology. *Ann Pharmacother* 2006; 40: 524–8.
19. Drummond MF, Jefferson TO. Guidelines for authors and peer reviewers of economic submissions to the BMJ. The BMJ Economic Evaluation Working Party. *BMJ* 1996; 313: 275–83.
20. Siegel JE, Weinstein MC, Russell LB, et al. Recommendations for reporting cost-effectiveness analyses. Panel on Cost-Effectiveness in Health and Medicine. *JAMA* 1996; 276: 1339–41.
21. Weinstein MC, Siegel JE, Gold MR, et al. Recommendations of the Panel on Cost-Effectiveness in Health and Medicine. *JAMA* 1996; 276: 1253–8.

22. Barshes NR, Chambers JD, Cantor SB, et al. A primer on cost-effectiveness analyses for vascular surgeons. *J Vasc Surg* 2012; 55: 1794–800.

23. Elliot RA. The economics of anaesthesia. *Eur J Anaesthesiol* 2001; 18: 205–7.

24. Carroll NV, Miederhoff PA, Cox FM, et al. Costs incurred by outpatient surgical centers in managing postoperative nausea and vomiting. *J Clin Anesth* 1994; 6: 364–9.

25. Moschetti K, Favre D, Pinget C, et al. Comparative cost-effectiveness analyses of cardiovascular magnetic resonance and coronary angiography combined with fractional flow reserve for the diagnosis of coronary artery disease. *J Cardiovasc Magn Reson* 2014; 16: 13.

26. Berenguer F, Bean RJ, Bozec L, et al. Coherent x-ray imaging of collagen fibril distributions within intact tendons. *Biophys J* 2014; 106: 459–66.

27. Diez L. Assessing the willingness of parents to pay for reducing postoperative emesis in children. *Pharmacoeconomics* 1998; 13: 589–95.

28. Weinstein MC. How much are Americans willing to pay for a quality-adjusted life year? *Med Care* 2008; 46: 343–5.

29. Franken MG, van Gils CW, Gaultney JG, et al. Practical feasibility of outcomes research in oncology: lessons learned in assessing drug use and cost-effectiveness in The Netherlands. *Eur J Cancer* 2013; 49: 8–16.

30. Selby JV, Beal AC, Frank L. The Patient-Centered Outcomes Research Institute (PCORI) national priorities for research and initial research agenda. *JAMA* 2012; 307: 1583–4.

31. Black N, Varaganum M, Hutchings A. Relationship between patient reported experience (PREMs) and patient reported outcomes (PROMs) in elective surgery. *BMJ Qual Saf* 2014; 23: 534–542.

32. Myles PS, Hunt JO, Nightingale CE, et al. Development and psychometric testing of a quality of recovery score after general anesthesia and surgery in adults. *Anesth Analg* 1999; 88: 83–90.

33. Basch E. New frontiers in patient-reported outcomes: adverse event reporting, comparative effectiveness, and quality assessment. *Annu Rev Med* 2014; 65: 307–17.

34. McDowell A, Fothergill JA, Khan A, et al. A cyclodextrin formulation to improve use of the anesthetic tribromoethanol (*Avertin*). *J Pharm Bioallied Sci* 2014; 6: 16–21.

35. Madhusudhan S, Hussain A, Sahni JN. Value of anti-VEGF treatment in choroidal neovascularization associated with autosomal recessive bestrophinopathy. *Digit J Ophthalmol* 2013; 19: 59–63.

36. Hajeer AH, Al Balwi MA, Aytul Uyar F, et al. HLA-A, -B, -C, -DRB1 and -DQB1 allele and haplotype frequencies in Saudis using next generation sequencing technique. *Tissue Antigens* 2013; 82: 252–8.

37. Fritzsche M, Thorogate R, Charras G. Quantitative analysis of ezrin turnover dynamics in the actin cortex. *Biophys J* 2014; 106: 343–53.

38. Institute of Medicine. Evaluation of biomarkers and surrogate endpoints in chronic disease, 2010. www.iomedu/Reports/2010/Evaluation-of-Biomarkers-and-Surrogate-Endpointsin-Chronic-Diseaseaspx

39. Fisher DM. Surrogate outcomes: meaningful not! *Anesthesiology* 1999; 90: 355–6.

40. Ricotta C, Celesti-Grapow L, Kuhn I, et al. Geographical constraints are stronger than invasion patterns for European urban floras. *PLoS ONE* 2014; 9: e85661.

41. Myles PS, Wengritzky R. Simplified postoperative nausea and vomiting impact scale for audit and post-discharge review. *Br J Anaesth* 2012; 108: 423–9.

42. Hall DP, Maccormick IJ, Phythian-Adams AT, et al. Network analysis reveals distinct clinical syndromes underlying acute mountain sickness. *PLoS ONE* 2014; 9: e81229.

43. Royse CF, Newman S, Chung F, et al. Development and feasibility of a scale to assess postoperative recovery: the post-operative quality recovery scale. *Anesthesiology* 2010; 113: 892–905.
44. Myles PS, Weitkamp B, Jones K, et al. Validity and reliability of a postoperative quality of recovery score: the QoR-40. *Br J Anaesth* 2000; 84: 11–5.
45. Stark PA, Myles PS, Burke JA. Development and psychometric evaluation of a postoperative quality of recovery score: the QoR-15. *Anesthesiology* 2013; 118: 1332–40.
46. Berg K, Kjellgren K, Unosson M, et al. Postoperative recovery and its association with health-related quality of life among day surgery patients. *BMC Nurs* 2012; 11: 24.
47. Phillips C, Blakey G, 3rd, Jaskolka M. Recovery after orthognathic surgery: short-term health-related quality of life outcomes. *J Oral Maxillofac Surg* 2008; 66: 2110–5.
48. Gornall BF, Myles PS, Smith CL, et al. Measurement of quality of recovery using the QoR-40: a quantitative systematic review. *Br J Anaesth* 2013; 111: 161–9.
49. Murphy GS, Szokol JW, Greenberg SB, et al. Preoperative dexamethasone enhances quality of recovery after laparoscopic cholecystectomy: effect on in-hospital and postdischarge recovery outcomes. *Anesthesiology* 2011; 114: 882–90.
50. Kim SH, Oh YJ, Park BW, et al. Effects of single-dose dexmedetomidine on the quality of recovery after modified radical mastectomy: a randomised controlled trial. *Minerva Anestesiol* 2013; 79: 1248–58.
51. Carlisle JB, Stevenson CA. Drugs for preventing postoperative nausea and vomiting. *Cochrane Database Syst Rev* 2006: CD004125.
52. Kooij FO, Klok T, Hollmann MW, et al. Decision support increases guideline adherence for prescribing postoperative nausea and vomiting prophylaxis. *Anesth Analg* 2008; 106: 893–8.
53. Pergolizzi JV, Pappagallo M, LeQuang J, et al. New health care measures: emphasis on better management of postsurgical pain and postoperative nausea and vomiting. *Hosp Pract (1995)* 2014; 42: 65–74.
54. Pierre S, Corno G, Benais H, et al. A risk score-dependent antiemetic approach effectively reduces postoperative nausea and vomiting – a continuous quality improvement initiative. *Can J Anaesth* 2004; 51: 320–5.
55. Kolanek B, Svartz L, Robin F, et al. Management program decreases postoperative nausea and vomiting in high-risk and in general surgical patients: a quality improvement cycle. *Minerva Anestesiol* 2014; 80: 337–46.
56. Apfel CC, Laara E, Koivuranta M, et al. A simplified risk score for predicting postoperative nausea and vomiting: conclusions from cross-validations between two centers. *Anesthesiology* 1999; 91: 693–700.
57. Frenzel JC, Kee SS, Ensor JE, et al. Ongoing provision of individual clinician performance data improves practice behavior. *Anesth Analg* 2010; 111: 515–9.
58. Hill R, Lubarsky D, Phillips-Bute B, et al. Cost-effectiveness of prophylactic antiemetic therapy with ondansetron, droperidol or placebo. *Anesthesiology* 2000; 92: 958–67.
59. Hill RP, Lubarsky DA, Phillips-Bute B, et al. Cost-effectiveness of prophylactic antiemetic therapy with ondansetron, droperidol, or placebo. *Anesthesiology* 2000; 92: 958–67.
60. Tramer MR, Phillips C, Reynolds DJ, et al. Cost-effectiveness of ondansetron for postoperative nausea and vomiting. *Anaesthesia* 1999; 54: 226–34.
61. Paech MJ, Rucklidge MW, Banks SL, et al. The efficacy and cost-effectiveness of prophylactic 5-hydroxytryptamine3 receptor antagonists: tropisetron, ondansetron and dolasetron. *Anaesth Intensive Care* 2003; 31: 11–7.

62. Pueyo FJ, Lopez-Olaondo L, Sanchez-Ledesma MJ, et al. Cost-effectiveness of three combinations of antiemetics in the prevention of postoperative nausea and vomiting. *Br J Anaesth* 2003; 91: 589–92.

63. Sennaraj B, Shende D, Ilavajady S, Sadhasivam S, Jagan D. Management of post-strabismus nausea and vomiting in children using ondansetron: a value-based comparison of outcomes. *Br J Anaesth* 2002; 89: 473–8.

64. Olutoye O, Jantzen EC, Alexis R, et al. A comparison of the costs and efficacy of ondansetron and dolasetron in the prophylaxis of postoperative vomiting in pediatric patients undergoing ambulatory surgery. *Anesth Analg* 2003; 97: 390–6.

Chapter 15

Postoperative nausea and vomiting research: methodology, assessment and strength of evidence

John Carlisle

The rate and odds of vomiting and their ratios

Nausea and vomiting are usually reported as a rate present or absent at a given time after surgery or as an incidence during a given period after surgery. The severity of both is less often reported. This chapter therefore concentrates on rates of postoperative nausea and vomiting (PONV).

Specific terminology is used when describing the results of randomized controlled trials (RCTs) and meta-analyses. The *vomit rate* is the number in a group who vomit divided by the total number in the group, and the *vomit odds* is the number in a group who vomit divided by the number in the group who do not vomit; these are different. The *rate ratio* (or "relative risk" or "risk ratio") is the rate in one group divided by the rate in another group, and the *odds ratio* is the odds in one group divided by the odds in another group; these are also different. It is important that you remember that rates, odds and their ratios are different.

Table 15.1 shows the same antiemetic drug being given to two different populations. The first population has a vomit rate in the control group of 40 in 100 and the control rate in the second population is 20 in 100. The rates and odds change, the rate ratio stays the same but the odds ratio changes. It is true that we are interested in what makes the control vomit rates different in different populations and we are also interested in the generalizable effect of a drug. It is important that we separate the two to determine the drug effect. We therefore should characterize the effect of a drug as a rate ratio and not as an odds ratio because it is unaffected by the control rate. Similarly, we should not characterize the generalizable drug effect as either an absolute rate reduction or as the "number needed-to-treat." These measures are very important when determining the expected drug effect in a particular population, but they are not, by definition, generalizable. Rates and their ratios are easily understood. Odds are different, so they are more difficult to understand, particularly their ratios; they are odd.

Nausea and vomiting are not the same. "Nausea" is the premonitory urge to vomit and is usually accompanied by unpleasant autonomic symptoms and signs, for instance sweating, pallor, salivation and gastrointestinal (GI) dysmotility. "Vomiting" is the retrograde expulsion of GI contents. Nausea may not be accompanied by vomiting and – more

Postoperative Nausea and Vomiting: A Practical Guide, eds. Tong Joo Gan and Ashraf S. Habib. Published by Cambridge University Press.

Table 15.1 Antiemetic postoperative vomiting rate reduction by 0.25 (RR of 0.75)

	Vomit	No vomit	Total	Rate		Odds	
			Vomiting rate 40/100				
Group							
Drug	30	70	100	30/100	0.30	30/70	0.43
Control	40	60	100	40/100	0.40	40/60	0.67
Ratio							
Rates	30/40	70/60	1/1	30/40		(3/7)/(4/6)	
Proportion	0.75	1.17	1	0.75		0.64	
Drug benefit	10			ARR = (1 − 0.75) × 40/100 = 0.10			
No drug benefit	90			NNT = 1/0.10 = 10			
			Vomiting rate 20/100				
Group							
Drug	15	85	100	15/100	0.15	15/85	0.18
Control	20	80	100	20/100	0.20	20/80	0.25
Ratio							
Rates	15/20	85/80	1/1	15/20		(15/85)/(20/80)	
Proportion	0.75	1.06	1	0.75		0.71	
Drug benefit	5			ARR = (1 − 0.75) x 20/100 = 0.05			
No drug benefit	95			NNT = 1/0.05 = 20			

ARR, absolute rate reduction; NNT, number needed-to-treat.

rarely – vomiting may not be preceded by nausea. Vomiting may relieve the unpleasantness of nausea. Some patients may want to avoid nausea more than vomiting and other patients may want to avoid vomiting more than nausea. An antiemetic may prevent or relieve nausea more than vomiting and vice versa. It is theoretically possible for an antiemetic to prolong nausea by preventing vomiting. PONV is therefore a composite of two outcomes that differ in rate, duration, perceived severity, undesirability and response to treatment. Composite outcomes should generally be avoided because they do not inform clinicians or patients of the separate probabilities of outcomes that are different. The composite outcome of PONV is superficially attractive because it appears to summarize epidemiology and response to treatment, but given the concerns listed above, the composite should always be accompanied by separate reports of the rate of nausea and the rate of vomiting. The composite must be clearly defined each time it is reported. Without definition it is not apparent what various terms mean, including "PONV," "complete response" (no vomiting or use of rescue antiemetic) and "total response" (no nausea or vomiting or use of rescue antiemetic). The composite outcome cannot usually be calculated from the rate of nausea and the rate of vomiting. For instance, a paper may report that the rate of nausea was 20/100 and that the rate of vomiting was 10/100. One might conclude that the rate of PONV was 20/100, but this calculation assumes that all the patients that vomited were nauseated. If vomiting was not preceded by nausea, the composite rate of PONV would be 30/100.

Chance, association and causation

Nausea and vomiting happen all the time to people of all ages, with or without an operation. "PONV" implies an association between having an operation and subsequent nausea and vomiting. Sometimes nausea and vomiting after surgery will be associated with having had an operation and everything else associated with it, but on other occasions PONV will be a chance event.

Research can quantify the probability that chance accounts for the apparent association of different factors with PONV. A factor that applies to everyone does not interest PONV researchers, e.g., being human or having an operation. Factors that vary or *variables* are of interest. Some variables are fixed for an individual but their value can be different between individuals, for instance genetic sex. Some variables are fixed for an individual at a given moment but can change with time and cannot be changed by someone else, e.g., age. Some variables can be changed through intervention. Although physical fitness changes with time, it can be modified through intervention, unlike age. Physical fitness is intrinsic to someone's body but other variables are not. These extrinsic variables are easiest to modify, e.g., one can give someone a drug. Similarly research can quantify variables associated with the severity or duration of PONV as well as its treatment.

So we have variable patients who experience variable rates of nausea and variable rates of vomiting after variable operations under variable conditions. How are we going to quantify the independent association of a factor with PONV? We want the research to quantify whether the variable is associated with an increase or decrease in the rate of PONV and by how much: we want the answers to be true and precise, i.e., accurate. We are going to be particularly interested in variables that are associated with "big" changes in the rates (or severity) of PONV, whilst we will be unconcerned with variables that are associated with "small" effects. In both cases, we still want accurate answers otherwise we cannot reliably conclude whether there is an association or not and we cannot conclude whether an association is important or unimportant.

The power of most RCTs to detect an effect of antiemetic drugs has been very weak, which has profound implications for how the result of a single trial is viewed[1], as shown in Table 15.1. The relative rate of vomiting with the drug was 0.75. The number who benefited with a control vomit rate of 40% was 10/100 participants and 5/100 with a control rate of 20%. Recent studies have reiterated the consequences of power and *P* value on the four potential outcomes of individual trials, as depicted in Flow Diagram 15.1[2–4].

The variables in the left-hand box might be those we are examining for a prediction model, e.g., age or sex, or they might be interventions we are testing for an effect, e.g., metoclopramide or ondansetron. We want our research to return the light gray boxes and not the dark gray boxes. Sample size calculations quantify the "Yes" boxes: light gray is the power, dark gray is the *P* value. A variable can associate with PONV or fail to associate with PONV, consistently or inconsistently. Inconsistent associations might be more common than consistent associations. It is important to appreciate that a *P* value underestimates the chance of a false discovery for inconsistent associations. Consider a variable that associates with PONV half the time: how often would it be wrong to accept an association if the *P* value was 0.05? Remember that the *P* value is the probability that we incorrectly accept an association when there is no association. So it might be considered that the probability of incorrectly accepting an association is 0.05 or 5% or 1 in 20. But what about the probability

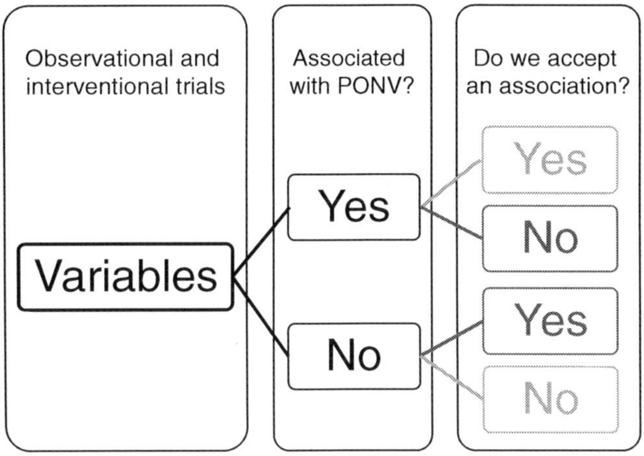

Flow Diagram 15.1 Diagram showing potential outcomes of individual trials for postoperative nausea and vomiting (PONV). The middle column shows whether a variable, such as sex, is associated with PONV, and whether an intervention changes the rate of PONV. The right-hand column depicts the possible results of an experiment, which may correctly or incorrectly identify associations and effects as present or absent. Experiments that correctly identify associations and effects as present (Yes) or absent (No) are colored light gray, whereas false results are colored dark gray.

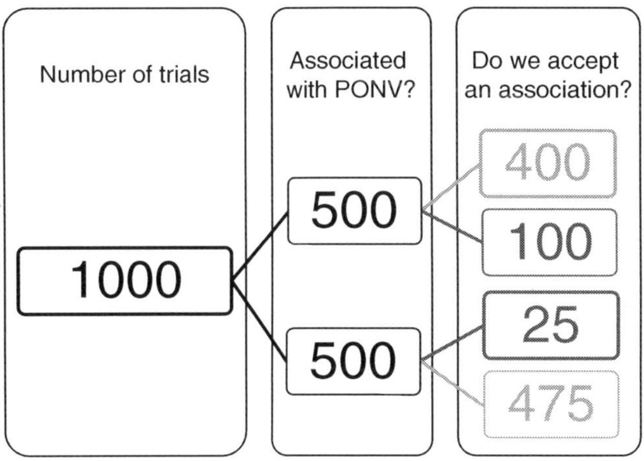

Flow Diagram 15.2 Diagram showing outcomes of trials for postoperative nausea and vomiting (PONV) where the middle column depicts 1000 experiments, in which half have a variable that associates with PONV (or an intervention that affects PONV) and in half there is no association or effect. Sample sizes are calculated using two parameters plus an effect size. One parameter is the power – the probability of correctly accepting an effect – which in this example is equivalent to 400 in the right-hand column divided by the number of experiments where the association exists (500), i.e., 400/500, which is 0.80 or 80%. The other parameter is the statistical threshold for accepting an effect when it does not exist, which in this example is equivalent to the 25 in the right-hand column, divided by the number of experiments in which an effect does not exist (500), i.e., 25/500, which is 0.05. The total number of times that we would declare an effect in this scenario is 400 + 25, which is 425. The proportion of times that this declaration would be wrong is 25/425, or 0.06 or 6%, which is called the "false discovery rate," which means that the P value of 0.05 underestimates the number of times we would incorrectly state that an effect exists.

that we will accept an association when there is an association? Flow Diagram 15.2 depicts 1000 tests each with a power of 80% for which we use a *P* value of 0.05 to accept that a variable is associated with PONV, but the association is true only half of the time.

You can see that the number of times we incorrectly accept an association is 25/425 or 0.059, slightly more than the *P* value of 0.05. This disparity is not particularly worrying. However, the disparity rapidly grows as the association becomes less consistent or as the power weakens. Consider Flow Diagram 15.3 in which a variable associates with PONV 10% of the time, again in trials with a power of 80% and for which we will accept an association at $P = 0.05$.

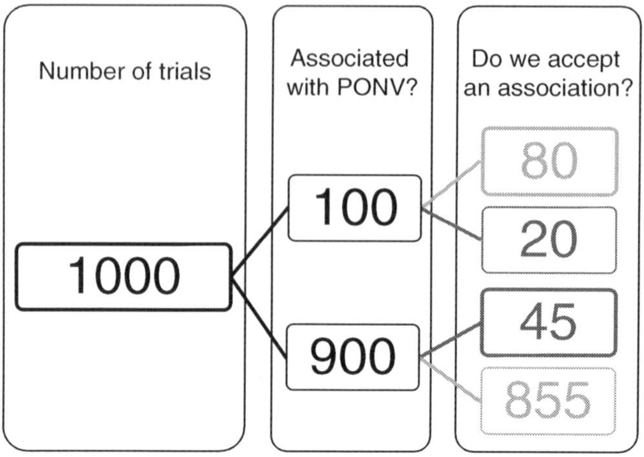

Flow Diagram 15.3 Diagram showing how the principles illustrated in Flow Diagram 15.2 result in worryingly high false discovery rates when an effect is weak, being present in 100/1000 experiments. The total number of times that we would declare an effect in this scenario is 80 + 45, which is 125. The proportion of times that this declaration would be wrong is 45/125, or 0.36 or 36%, which means that the *P* value of 0.05 (45/900) substantially underestimates the number of times we would incorrectly state that an effect exists. PONV, postoperative nausea and vomiting.

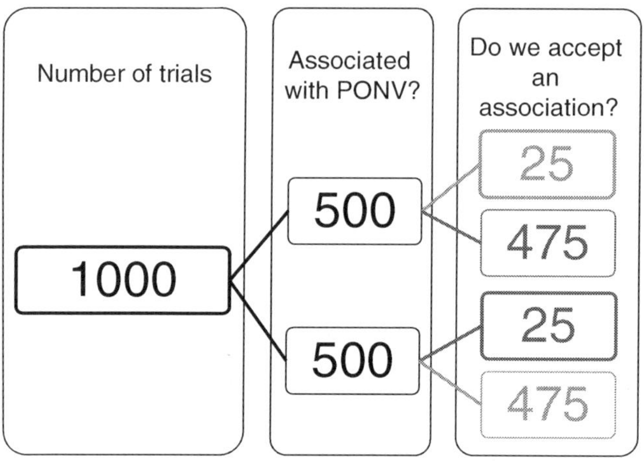

Flow Diagram 15.4 Diagram showing the situation that represents many randomized controlled trials of drugs to prevent nausea and vomiting, in which the relative risk of postoperative nausea and vomiting (PONV) is 0.5 (500/1000) but the power is only 0.05 (25/500), as is the *P* value for statistical significance. The total number of times that we would declare an effect in this scenario is 25 + 25, which is 50. The proportion of times that this declaration would be wrong is 25/50, or 0.50 or 50%, which means that the *P* value of 0.05 (25/500) overestimates 10-fold the proportion of times that there is an effect when we declare there is an effect.

In this case the number of associations that we incorrectly accept is 45/125 or 0.36 or 36%.

Let us take as an example RCTs of metoclopramide. The RR of postoperative vomiting (POV) is reduced by 25% or so by metoclopramide compared with placebo (RR 0.75). The control rate of POV in RCTs of metoclopramide has averaged 40%. About 750 participants would need to be recruited (375 in the control group and 375 in the metoclopramide group) to have a 20% probability (80% power) of falsely rejecting a real association and a 5% probability of incorrectly accepting an absent association (*P* value of 0.05). Unfortunately, researchers have recruited 46 participants on average (23 to each group), a power of about 5%. Let us suppose that metoclopramide has an effect in half of the RCTs (Flow Diagram 15.4).

The rate of wrong acceptance is 25/50, or 0.5 or 50%. A combination of 5% power and a less consistent association with PONV, say 10%, would result in a false detection rate of 45/50 or 90%! It can be noted that the probability of falsely rejecting a true association is also affected by the rate of association and the choices of power and statistical threshold. In

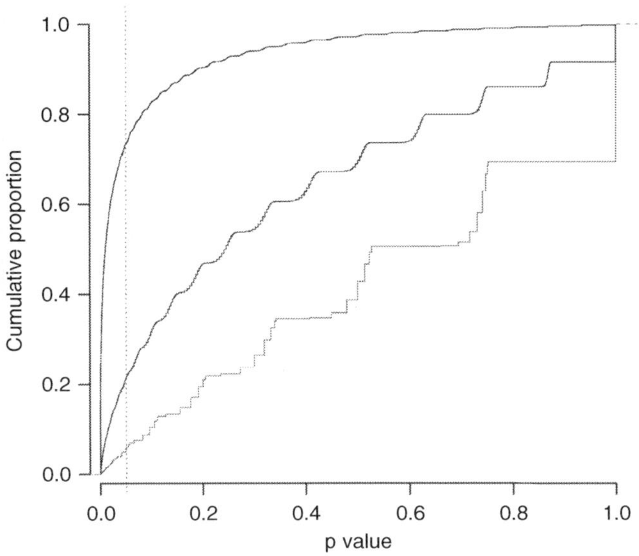

Figure 15.1 A graph showing the proportion of randomized controlled trials (vertical axis) that generate a *P* value less than a given value (horizontal axis). Simulations of experiments of an antiemetic drug were run by this author, which reduced the rate of postoperative nausea and vomiting (PONV) by 0.25, i.e., the relative risk of PONV is 0.75 after the drug, who simulated experiments that recruited 20, 80 or 320 participants to each group, one receiving the antiemetic drug and the other a placebo. The power of these studies to identify an effect were 5%, 21% and 73%, which is the proportion of trials (vertical axis) that generated a *P* value less than 0.05 (horizontal axis).

the first scenario (association 50%, power 80% and *P* value 0.05), the rate of wrong rejection was 100/575, 0.17 or 17%. In the second scenario (association 10%, power 80% and *P* value 0.05), the rate of wrong rejection was 20/875, 0.02 or 2%. In the third scenario (association 50%, power 5% and P value 0.05), the rate of wrong rejection was 475/950, 0.5 or 50%, i.e., in this last scenario, which might be representative of PONV RCTs, half the time we say that there is an association there is not, and half the time we say that there is not an association there is[5].

So trials with low power do not detect true associations but do detect untrue associations. Trials with more power detect more true associations; they generate smaller *P* values that congregate more closely around the true magnitude of the association. Figures 15.1–15.3 illustrate the association of trial power with the accuracy (and precision) of the results. This author has conducted 300,000 simulations of RCTs of metoclopramide in which the average control and intervention PONV rates were 40% and 30%, respectively. Also conducted were 100,000 simulations for trials, which recruited 20, 80 or 320 participants per group, with respective powers of 5%, 21% and 73% (Figure 15.1); the true RR was 30/40 or 0.75. The *P* value sequentially increases with loss of power, and as expected the proportion of simulations that generated *P* values <0.05 were 73.4%, 21.3% and 5.9% at powers of 73%, 21% and 5%.

Half of the RCTs have RRs less than the true value (0.75) and half have values more than 0.75. The 95% confidence interval (CI) for the RR increases around the median of 0.75 as the power decreases: 0.60–0.92, 0.47–1.15 and 0.24–1.80 with powers of 73%, 21% and 5%, respectively (Figure 15.2).

The null hypothesis that is being tested is that differences in rates of PONV between groups are due to chance, i.e. the RR is one. The *P* value is the probability of falsely accepting an effect of metoclopramide, so if the rate of vomiting is the same in the control and metoclopramide groups (RR of 1), we would be very foolish to say that there is a difference, which the *P* value of 1 reflects. The absence of an effect becomes less likely (*P* values become

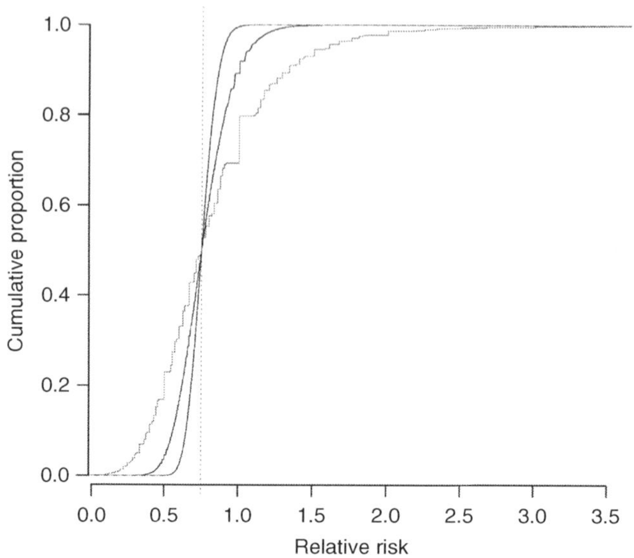

Figure 15.2 The same simulations used to plot Figure 15.1 are used in this graph to illustrate the proportion of randomized controlled trials (vertical axis) that generate a relative risk (RR) less than a given value (horizontal axis). The true effect of the antiemetic is a RR for postoperative nausea and vomiting of 0.75 (dotted vertical line). Experiments that recruit 320 participants to each group generate RRs similar to 0.75, whereas experiments that recruit only 20 participants to each group generate RRs that are often much smaller or larger than 0.75.

smaller) the greater the discrepancy between the observed RR and a RR of 1 (no drug effect). Trials with a power of 5% will generate statistically significant RRs that are smaller than RCTs with powers of 21% or 73%: in simulations, the respective mean (95% CI) RRs for RCTs *P* values <0.05 were 0.49 (0.10–2.33), 0.56 (0.41–0.64) and 0.72 (0.59–0.80). There are relatively few trials that generate RRs in excess of 1, as indicated by the lack of trial density contour lines (Figure 15.3).

What does this all mean for calculating the effect of a drug such as metoclopramide? It is of surprise to note that a more reliable estimate of the effect of an antiemetic drug is obtained if the results of "insignificant" RCTs (*P* >0.05) rather the results of "significant" RCTs (*P* ≤ 0.05) are used, which is a consequence of antiemetic RCTs having powers of 5–30%.

Table 15.2 explains this apparent paradox. We are going to simulate RCTs of an antiemetic in three populations: with mean (95%) rates of vomiting in the control group of 10% (4–16), 20% (12–28) and 40% (30–49). We will generously assume that the antiemetic consistently reduces the vomiting rate to 75% of the control rate, so for every 100 participants given metoclopramide the number that will benefit will be 2.5 (10 subtract 7.5), 5 (10 subtract 15) and 10 (40 subtract 30), respectively. The RCTs recruit 20, 50 or 100 participants to both the control and metoclopramide groups. The RCTs are done perfectly: there is no bias in any methodologic domain (see below). What are our results? It can be seen that the power increases with the rate of vomiting in the control group as well as with the number of participants. As expected, the *P* values decrease as the power increases and the RRs get closer to 0.75. This author used two methods to generate "average" RRs for each trial size in each vomiting rate population: the meta-analysis method is statistically correct, whereas the "mean" value is not, but it might better reflect the average belief of what effect metoclopramide had if the readers were asked, who would have read a sample of RCT results and do not do meta-analyses in their heads. If readers "believed" all results equally, it would be expected for them to believe that the RR of vomiting after metoclopramide was between 0.95 and 0.76, whereas if they only believed statistically significant results, they would think that the RR

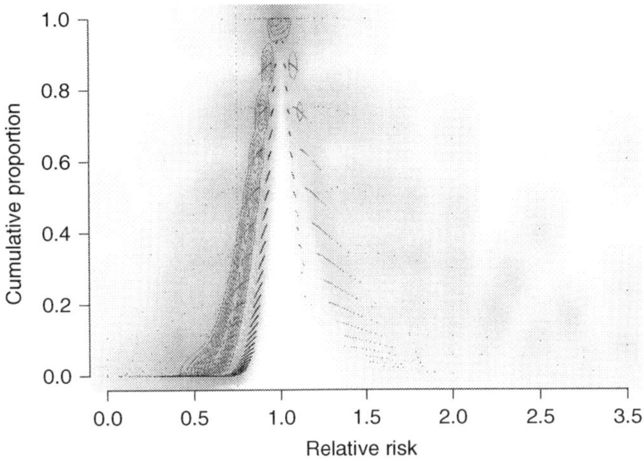

Figure 15.3 Figure combining Figures 15.1 and 15.2, plotting the right-skewed distribution of *P* values versus the relative risk (RR) of each simulated experiment. The *P* values from trials with 20 participants per group, which had a power of 5%, are more widely distributed to the left and right of the other two distributions (black contours). The distribution of *P* values from trials that recruited 80 participants per group (power 21%) forms a narrower band of *P* values between the other two distributions (gray contours). The distribution of *P* values from trials that recruited 320 participants per group (73% power) form a narrow concentrated band of *P* values (white contours), 73% of which are less than 0.05, predominantly around the true RR of 0.75 (vertical dashed line).

was between 0.59 and 0.11, which doubles the number of patients who appeared to benefit. In contrast, the mean RRs of insignificant trials were between 0.97 and 0.82.

In Table 15.2, the same number of participants contributed to results of both RCTs and meta-analyses. Nine different scenarios were simulated from three different control rates (10%, 20% and 40%) and groups that contained 20, 50 or 100 participants. The results of each scenario are presented in three ways – when the RRs are calculated: using all RCTs; using only RCTs with significant results ($P < 0.05$); using only RCTs with "insignificant" results ($P > 0.05$). The points of interest are: meta-analyses more accurately estimate the true RR (0.75) than taking the mean of RCTs that contain the same number of participants; "insignificant" results ($P > 0.05$) are more accurate than "significant" results ($P < 0.05$) when the power of RCTs was 26% or less (the maximum power simulated). Similarly the estimates of the number out of 100 participants who would benefit from the antiemetic are most accurate when all RCTs are analysed but only marginally less so if insignificant RCTs are analysed. Trials with significant results substantially overestimate the benefit derived from the antiemetic.

In summary, trials with unlikely results are unlikely to represent the play of chance, which is better represented by the more numerous trials with likely results. But also, RCTs with unlikely results are unlikely to represent the effect of an intervention as well, which is also better represented by the more numerous RCTs with likely results. So how should we synthesize the significant and insignificant results from unlikely and likely trials? In Table 15.2, it can be seen that the results of meta-analysis are predominantly closer to the true RR of 0.75 than taking a mean of the RRs in all trials; the disparity between the estimated and true benefit of giving metoclopramide to a population of 100 is similarly minimized through meta-analysis. So, we will discuss meta-analysis, but first we will talk about risks of biases.

Biases

A bias is a systematic error as opposed to a chance error. Chance causes the results of trials to vary as the preceding simulations demonstrated. Those simulations also demonstrated that

Table 15.2 Results of simulated RCTs and meta-analyses for an antiemetic drug for which the RR of postoperative vomiting is 0.75

Control rate		**10%**			**20%**			**30%**		
Group size		**20**	**50**	**100**	**20**	**50**	**100**	**20**	**50**	**100**
Power (% *P* values ≤0.05)		**1**	**3**	**6**	**3**	**6**	**12**	**6**	**13**	**26**
Programmed average values										
Does vomit										
Control		2	6	10	4	12	20	6	18	30
Drug		1.5	4.5	7.5	3	9	15	4.5	13.5	22.5
Does not vomit										
Control		18	44	90	16	38	80	14	32	70
Drug		18.5	45.5	92.5	17	41	85	15.5	36.5	77.5
Patients per 100 treated who benefit		2.5	2.5	2.5	5	5	5	10	10	10
Average relative risks of simulated RCTs										
	True value									
RCTs any *P*										
'Mean'	0.75	0.86	0.94	0.84	0.95	0.83	0.78	0.82	0.77	0.76
Meta-analysis	0.75	0.81	0.78	0.77	0.79	0.76	0.76	0.77	0.76	0.75
RCTs *P* ≤ 0.05										
'Mean'	0.75	0.11	0.47	0.43	0.35	0.41	0.45	0.39	0.48	0.59
Meta-analysis	0.75	0.16	0.22	0.33	0.22	0.34	0.44	0.32	0.48	0.59
RCTs *P* > 0.05										
'Mean'	0.75	0.88	0.96	0.86	0.97	0.85	0.83	0.85	0.82	0.82
Meta-analysis	0.75	0.82	0.79	0.80	0.80	0.80	0.81	0.80	0.80	0.82
Overestimate of benefit per 100 (simulated true)										
RCTs any *P*										
'Mean'	0	−1.1	−2.3	−0.9	−4.0	−1.8	−0.7	−2.9	−1.2	−0.5
Meta-analysis	0	−0.6	−0.3	−0.2	−0.7	−0.3	−0.2	−1.0	−0.3	−0.2
RCTs *P* ≤ 0.05										
'Mean'	0	6.4	3.3	3.3	8.0	8.1	6.0	14.3	13.1	6.5
Meta-analysis	0	5.9	6.4	4.2	10.6	9.9	6.2	17.4	13.0	6.3
RCTs *P* > 0.05										
'Mean'	0	−1.3	−2.5	−1.1	−4.4	−2.5	−1.5	−4.1	−3.4	−3.0
Meta-analysis	0	−0.7	−0.5	−0.5	−1.0	−1.0	−1.2	−2.2	−2.4	−2.8

if one relied upon the results from RCTs with small power and small *P* values, one would get a less correct answer than relying upon the results from RCTs with small power and large *P* values. This is ironic, as the emphasis on trials with small *P* values is driven by the desire to get the answer right and is due to the misinterpretation of the *P* value as the likelihood of getting the answer wrong. As an aside, remember that power is synonymous not only with the number of participants, but also higher control rates and intervention effects: an RCT with fewer participants can be more powerful than one with more participants.

The previous simulations did not introduce any bias into the RCTs. What would happen if trial results were intrinsically biased or if their publication was extrinsically biased? The common "domains" of intrinsic bias in RCTs are: selection bias; performance bias; detection bias; attrition bias; and reporting bias[6]. The results of trials are most profoundly biased the earlier the allocation is revealed in the course of the experiment, i.e., in the sequence listed in the preceding sentence. Most of the time we cannot confirm what happened in trials but we can read what the authors report. Trials that clearly report an effective method to prevent people knowing what the next allocation is report weaker effects for interventions, as do trials that maintain allocation blinding during administration of the intervention and control[7,8]. The increase in treatment effect associated with allocation revelation becomes less of a problem with subsequent steps in the course of the experiment, the detection of outcomes and the loss of participants during follow-up. The communication of the harm and benefit of an intervention can also be warped by authors choosing what to report once they know their results, as well as by authors choosing whether or where to submit a paper for publication. The "publication bias" that has stereotyped journal editors as rejecting trials with "statistically insignificant" results is more realistically viewed as an amalgam of behaviors by authors as well as journals.

The results of meta-analyses will be biased if they include biased RCTs. In addition, the authors of meta-analyses can introduce biases in similar methodologic domains as those that affect RCTs, particularly in the prominence given to some results over others and the misinterpretations that authors make.

Meta-analysis

Meta-analysis appears to be the best way to synthesize trials of PONV that predominantly have low power. One large RCT, for instance Wallenborn et al.[9], reduces the utility of a meta-analysis to determine the point estimate of effect, but meta-analysis remains useful in exploring the interaction of antiemetic effect with other variables. There are two related reasons why there is a disparity in Table 15.2 between the primitive mean RR and the point estimate generated by meta-analysis of the same simulated data. The RRs generated by two trials can have very different precisions, a characteristic that is not taken into account by taking their mean: the best estimate of the real effect would be weighted towards the more precise RR. The RR is not a linear scale, in that the error around a RR is only symmetrical as a logarithm, so meta-analysis takes this scaling into account. The pooled estimate of effect generated by a meta-analysis and the error around that estimate depend upon the analysis method and the distribution of variables in the analysed RCTs: the distribution of participant numbers amongst the RCTs, the distribution of power amongst RCTs, the distribution of control rate values in the RCTs and the distribution of effects in the RCTs[10].

This author generated Figure 15.4 from simulated meta-analyses based upon the approximate total number of participants in RCTs of granisetron (left plot, 2,800) and of metoclopramide (right plot, 16,000). In order to show the effects of total participant number and their distribution between RCTs, 0.75 (vertical black dotted line) was used as the rate ratio in all simulations. The graph shows the cumulative distribution pooled RRs (95% CI) from 1,000 meta-analyses with participants distributed in a few large RCTs (black lines) or in

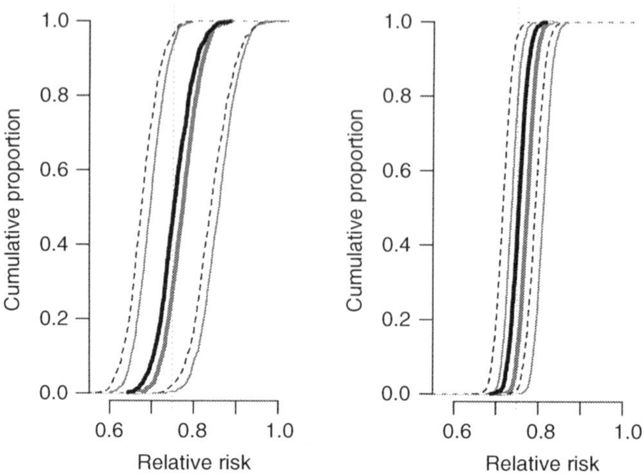

Figure 15.4 Simulations of meta-analyses of randomized controlled trials. There are fewer participants in the meta-analyses in the left-hand plot (2,800) and more in the meta-analyses in the right-hand plot (16,000). The true relative risk (RR) of postoperative nausea and vomiting with the antiemetic in both plots is 0.75 (horizontal axis). There are three pairs of lines: the center pair are the cumulative RRs; the pairs either side are the 95% confidence interval, the 2.5 percentile (left) and 97.5 percentile (right). The left of each pair of cumulative lines is generated by simulations of meta-analyses containing a few large studies; the right of each pair is from meta-analyses of many smaller studies. As Figures 15.1–15.3 have shown, larger studies more accurately measure the true RR of 0.75, with accuracy being better with more participants in the simulated meta-analyses (right plot).

many small RCTs (grey lines). More total participants generate more precise estimates of the RR (right plot). Distribution of the same number of participants into more but smaller RCTs (grey lines) slightly reduces accuracy, but this effect is less than the improvement in precision that results from having more participants.

These simulations show that a consistent antiemetic effect is compatible with a range of estimated effects, even when large numbers of patients and RCTs are analyzed. There is no single "truth." So the result of a single meta-analysis is consistent with a range of "true" antiemetic effects that is estimated by the 95% CI of the median simulation (0.5 on the vertical "cumulative proportion" axis). However, when there is a single meta-analysis one does not know how close to the median value the result is, an example of "meta-uncertainty." There are many meta-analytical statistics but only two standard models to weight the results of different RCTs: random-effects and fixed-effect. The random-effects model assumes that the antiemetic can have many effects and the fixed-effect model assumes that the antiemetic always has the same effect, with differences in results between RCTs being due to sampling variation and known interactions with covariables. The principle of the random-effects model is more attractive as it does not depend upon a special unique effect and it does not assume that one knows all the different variables that can interact with the antiemetic effect. Unfortunately, trials with lower power are given more weight by the random-effects model. As discussed previously, RCTs with low power are inaccurate. An accurate pooled estimate depends upon "statistically insignificant" low-powered RCTs because "statistically significant" low-powered RCTs will give inaccurate results. An imbalance in the proportions of significant and insignificant RCTs will skew the results.

A meta-analysis is an observational study of trial results. The results of a meta-analysis are sensitive to the assumptions one makes in the analysis of trial data that are usually only available as summary measures of populations, rather than the much more powerful analyses that can be conducted on the data from individual participants in multiple trials. It is therefore reasonable to analyze the same results in multiple ways to assess the consistency of the results in the face of different analytical methods. Importantly the prominence given to a result generated by one method at the expense of a result generated by a different method should not be determined by the result, otherwise researchers will just pick the result that they "like." This is one reason why protocols for any trial, whether an RCT or a meta-analysis, should be published before the trial starts. There are a number of online facilities for registering trials, whilst the Cochrane library and a number of journals publish protocols. One can also check the data of trials to determine whether the correct analyses have been performed. Authors of RCTs rarely make their raw data public, although this is changing. Conversely, the "raw" data used in systematic reviews are already in the public domain. This author spends much of his time checking the retrieval and analyses of data in systematic reviews that are submitted to the journal for which he edits, which is also what he did as an editor for the Cochrane collaboration. As an author of a Cochrane systematic review, this author has retrieved and analysed nearly 1,000 RCTs, which led to an interest in the work of Fujii et al. and his subsequent work on fraud[11].

Fraud

We have seen that chance and bias overestimate treatment effects. Invented data could have any effect, but one might reasonably suppose that fabricated data would also contribute to overestimating an effect. We do not know how much published research has been fabricated. We do know that 0.004% of biomedical papers have been retracted, over half of which for fraud.

The most profligate biomedical fraudster is Dr. Yoshitaka Fujii, who authored 193 RCTs. Investigations by his various employers failed to confirm the validity of 183 RCTs[12,13]. Dr. Fujii et al. authored most of the RCTs that investigated granisetron for PONV, for instance 40/63 RCTs that reported postoperative vomiting. Granisetron's effect in these fraudulent papers was 1.3–2.5 more than the effect in RCTs published by authors other than Fujii et al. Dr. Fujii also overestimated the effect of ramosetron in fraudulent RCTs[14].

We know that others have fabricated biomedical research, anesthesiologists amongst them. There is evidence that there remain unretracted fabricated papers, and there are likely to be many more. Given Dr. Fujii's fraudulent overestimate of effect, combined with similar findings for Drs Boldt, Poldermans and Reuben[15–17], this author concludes that fraud contributes to the overestimation of effect that already results from chance and biases.

Summary

Most individual antiemetic RCTs have little power. For most single antiemetic RCTs, it would be incorrect half the time if a P value <0.05 was used to indicate an antiemetic effect and a P value >0.05 to indicate its absence. If only RCTs with P values <0.05 are used to calculate an antiemetic effect, it could be believed that the antiemetic prevents nearly twice as much PONV as it really does. If, unusually, only RCTs with P values >0.05 are used to calculate an antiemetic effect, this would be closer to the truth, and it could be believed that the antiemetic prevents 80% of the PONV that it does.

The meta-analytic result least likely to be misinterpreted is the rate ratio (risk ratio or RR). If the odds ratio from a meta-analysis is thought to be the antiemetic effect, it could be believed that both the relative and absolute effects increase with the control PONV rate, and the relative antiemetic effect would be overestimated by 5–40%, the exact amount depending upon the control rate and antiemetic intervention. However, the rate ratio also probably overestimates the antiemetic effect due to the intrinsic and extrinsic biases that affect published RCTs, as well as because of fraudulent data. Overestimation of effect may be further compounded by the weights given to small RCTs in the random-effects model. The antiemetic effects of newer drugs will be generally less precise and will be overestimated, a problem contributed to by commercial sponsorship, publication bias and early truncation of trials.

Over 1,000 RCTs have tested drugs to prevent PONV in over 150,000 participants, so the total number of RCTs that have tested prophylactic interventions and interventions to treat PONV probably exceeds 2,000 with over 300,000 participants. PONV is amongst the most extensively studied medical events. Anesthesiologists and other researchers should default to the belief that PONV does not require more primary research, at least not until we have examined better the research that has already been done and, perhaps, not ever. Further research might slightly increase the precision of how uncertain we are about the effects of interventions. We would spend our time more effectively instituting reliable methods of delivering the antiemetic prophylaxis and treatment that people want.

References

1. Carlisle J, Stevenson CA. Drugs for preventing postoperative nausea and vomiting. *Cochrane Database Syst Rev* 2006; (3): CD004125.
2. Colquhuon D. An investigation of the false discovery rate and the misinterpretation of P values. *R Soc Open Sci* 2014; 1: 140216.
3. Ioannidis JPA. Why most published research findings are false. *PLoS Med* 2005; 2: e124.
4. Ioannidis JPA. How to make more published true. *PLoS Med* 2014; 11: e1001747.
5. Kault D. False negatives in evidence based medicine. *J Med Stat Inform* 2014; 2: 5.
6. Higgins JPT, Altman DG, Sterne JAC. Assessing risk of bias in included studies. In: Higgins JPT, Green S, eds. *Cochrane Handbook for Systematic Reviews of Interventions, version 5.0.2*. The Cochrane Collaboration, 2009. www.cochrane-handbook.org (accessed November 2, 2014).
7. Schulz KF, Chalmers I, Hayes RJ, et al. Dimensions of methodological quality associated with estimates of treatment effects in controlled trials. *JAMA* 1995; 273: 408–12.
8. Dechartres A, Altman DG, Trinquart L, et al. Association between analytic strategies and estimates of treatment outcomes in meta-analyses. *JAMA* 2014; 312: 623–30.
9. Wallenborn J, Gelbrich G, Bulst D, et al. Prevention of postoperative nausea and vomiting by metoclopramide combined with dexamethasone: randomised double blind multicentre trial. *BMJ* 2006; 333: 324.
10. Trikalinos TA, Trow P, Schmid CH. Simulation-based comparison of methods for meta-analysis of proportions and rates. *AHRQ Publication* 2013; 13: EHC084–EF. www.effectivehealthcare.ahrq.gov/reports/final.cfm (accessed November 2, 2014).
11. Carlisle JB. The analysis of 168 randomised controlled trials to test data integrity. *Anaesthesia* 2012; 67: 521–37.
12. Sumikawa K on behalf of the Japanese Society of Anaesthesiologists. The results of investigation into Dr. Yoshitaka Fujii's papers. http://www.anesth.or.jp/english/pdf/news20120629.pdf (accessed November 2, 2014).
13. Klein AA, ed. Special Collection: Research Misconduct. External announcements: Fujii case.

Anaesthesia http://onlinelibrary.wiley.com/journal/10.1111/(ISSN)1365-2044/homepage/-_research_misconduct.htm (accessed November 2, 2014).

14. Carlisle JB. A meta-analysis of prevention of postoperative nausea and vomiting: randomised controlled trials by Fujii et al. compared with other authors. *Anaesthesia* 2012; 67: 1076–90.
15. Wilkes MM Navickis RJ. The Boldt affair: a quandary for meta-analysts. *Anesthesiol News* 2013; 39: 4.
16. Shafer SL. Anesthesia & Analgesia – Notice of retractions, February 20, 2009. http://www.aaeditor.org/HWP/Retraction.Notice.pdf (accessed November 2, 2014).
17. RetractionWatch.com. Critics of Poldermans' work baffled by NEJM stance on DECREASE papers. http://retractionwatch.com/2014/09/29/critics-of-poldermans-work-baffled-by-nejm-stance-on-decrease-papers/#more-22958 (accessed November 2, 2014).

Chapter 16

Implementing postoperative nausea and vomiting management guidelines

Peter Kranke

Why it is important to prevent postoperative nausea and vomiting

More than 230 million major surgical procedures are performed worldwide each year[1]. Postoperative nausea and vomiting (PONV) is among the most frequently observed adverse events associated with anesthesia. Moreover, it is distressing to patients and impairs the quality of recovery as judged by the patients and anesthesiologists alike. Despite pharmacologic prophylaxis, the rate of PONV remains about 20–30%, and is often even higher[2]. Unresolved PONV may result in prolonged facility stay (e.g., in the postanesthesia care unit (PACU)) and unanticipated hospital admission or even readmission in adults and children, which has the potential to significantly increase overall healthcare costs[3,4]. Further, PONV significantly affects patient's well-being and is among the important determinants of patient satisfaction with perioperative care[5]. The goal of PONV prophylaxis is therefore to decrease the risk of PONV with its associated patient-related distress and to reduce healthcare costs.

PONV prevention, however, invariably involves costs. Since these interventions exert a beneficial effect only if there is a certain event rate for PONV ("no pain, no gain"), the restriction of preventive measures to patient populations with increased risk makes intuitive sense from an economic point of view, and also to only expose patients to risks (e.g., adverse reactions to drug exposure) if there is justification to do so due to an associated gain in patient satisfaction or quality of recovery, or the avoidance of more severe morbidity.

Consequently, in the 2003 Society for Ambulatory Anesthesia (SAMBA) PONV guidelines[6], there was more or less general agreement with the advice in Guideline 6 to "*use prophylaxis* in patients at high risk for PONV and *consider prophylaxis* in patients at moderate risk for PONV." This principle that prophylaxis is likely to be useful only for patients at moderate-to-high risk for PONV was based on two main assumptions.

(1) The ability to correctly predict who will develop PONV.
(2) If a treatment effect in a population is low or below a defined threshold, the administration of an antiemetic may not be justified.

Postoperative Nausea and Vomiting: A Practical Guide, eds. Tong Joo Gan and Ashraf S. Habib. Published by Cambridge University Press.

Traditionally applied efficacy hurdles for prophylactic interventions

Historically, the use of prophylactic antiemetics is generally considered futile if the number needed-to-treat (NNT) of such an intervention exceeded the value of "5." In this context, an NNT indicates the number of patients who needed to receive a particular antiemetic intervention to prevent one emetic event that would have occurred had the patient not received the intervention[7].

Considering the variable control event rate (CER) observed in different institutional settings, transferring the concept of the NNT as a parameter to classify the efficacy of prophylactic antiemetics may be misleading. The NNT depends on two figures: the CER in a given patient population in which the antiemetic prevention is applied, and the efficacy of an intervention or combined (multiple) interventions. In any real-world scenario, further determinants skew this simple calculation and contribute to the gap between efficacy of a defined strategy in randomized trials and the effectiveness observed in routine clinical practice. Among others, these determinants are:

- the ability to correctly identify the risk of patients to suffer from PONV
- the guideline adherence, and thus the proportion of patients who actually receive prophylactic antiemetics according to a suggested algorithm
- further variables, such as discrepancies in response rate between study populations and real-world patient populations.

The average event rate of PONV varies widely as reported in observational studies, randomized controlled trials (RCTs) and systematic reviews. In one very large multifactorial trial of six prophylactic antiemetic interventions, 26 of 44 (59%) patients receiving no active interventions had PONV[8,9]. Although in shorter procedures, e.g., ambulatory patients receive less emetogenic anesthesia with little exposure to opioids, the overall prevalence may only be 5% or 10%[10]. Thus, in a comprehensive Cochrane review of drugs for the prevention of PONV, the CER (placebo or no treatment) varied widely from almost nil to close to 100%[11].

Moreover, the reported PONV prevalence is highly dependent on the duration of observation[12]. For example, the prevalence in a recent observational study was 15% (86/560) in the PACU, but was 31% (172/560) during the first 24 postoperative hours[13]. Additionally, PONV appears to be underreported in routine clinical care. In the same observational report, only about 40% (36/86) of those with PONV immediately after surgery were recorded as such by the responsible nursing staff[13]. This does not necessarily represent substandard care, but highlights the fact that many other issues could have distracted the attention of the responsible staff so that complaints of potentially minor importance, such as a patient feeling mildly nauseated, fall into oblivion.

Another aspect that adds complexity to these estimates is the fact that the severity of PONV is not a binary outcome and there may be a greater burden to some patients than others. Recent reports suggest that approximately one-third to one-half of those with PONV are severely affected, with negative impact on quality of life and convalescence as well as delayed discharge after ambulatory surgery[14].

Risk-based approaches to prevent PONV

Recommendations for the administration of antiemetic interventions traditionally support the application of a "valid assessment of the patient's risk for postoperative vomiting (POV) or PONV"[15]. Further, according to various guidelines, when developing a management strategy for each individual patient, the choice should be based on patient preference, cost-efficiency, level of PONV risk and patient's pre-existing condition (e.g., avoid QT prolonging antiemetics in patients with prolonged QT syndrome and transdermal scopolamine in closed-angle glaucoma patients). Such recommendations are based on the premise that antiemetics and other interventions effectively reduce the baseline risk for PONV in "high-risk patients," i.e., patients who actually need antiemetic prevention. This would save costs and prevent pharmacologic exposure, and eventually the occurrence of adverse effects, among patients who will not vomit anyway. Assuming that each antiemetic intervention is associated with a defined relative risk reduction (RRR) that has been determined by clinical trials and meta-analyses, this RRR translates into an absolute risk reduction (ARR) that depends mainly on the CER in a given patient population. If the CER is high (e.g., 60%), then an antiemetic with an RRR of 30% reduces the incidence in that population to 42%. Consequently, the ARR would be 18%. This means that approximately six patients (1/0.18) need to be treated with antiemetics for one to stay completely free from PONV. If, using the same antiemetic with similar efficacy, in a cohort of patients with a CER in the range of 10%, the ARR would equal 3%, and approximately 33 (33 = 1/0.03) patients need to be treated for one to benefit from the administration of antiemetics in that population. With such a high NNT of "33" it seems at first sight hard to justify the exposure of many patients who do not need the prophylactic antiemetic anyway for the sake of one patient who stays completely free from PONV[16].

The problem, however, with such a reasoning is that there remain many imponderables. The most influencing factors rendering these assumptions in a clinical scenario as valid or not are the ability to correctly classify the PONV risk, the acquisition costs of antiemetics, the potential of antiemetics to cause adverse effects as well as the clinical applicability and compliance with guidelines depending on their structure (e.g., general multimodal prevention versus various risk-adapted approaches or a combination of these approaches).

A major determinant in such an approach is the validity of prognostic factors.

Prognostic factors to guide antiemetic prophylaxis

A risk factor for PONV is any factor that is associated in one or more studies with either a higher or lower risk. Since the beginning of anesthesia provision, many risk factors have been associated with PONV. Even though there is strong evidence for some risk factors, none of those risk factors taken in isolation is clinically sufficient for a risk assessment. Several factors, such as female gender and history of PONV and/or motion sickness, were published as early as 1960 using simple cross-classification methods[17,18]. Starting in the 1990s, following the development of widely available statistical software for automatic variable selection, studies have been performed using stepwise logistic regression analysis to prospectively identify risk factors for PONV in various cohorts of patients. Koivuranta et al.[19] and Apfel et al.[20] identified some important risk factors that form the basis for scoring systems: female gender, history of PONV/motion sickness, non-smoking status, the use of postoperative opioids and the duration of surgery or anesthesia[21]. However, many other risk factors have been identified and summarized by Apfel et al.[22], and these can be divided into patient risk factors, anesthetic technique and surgical procedure. Patient risk factors, for instance, include female gender, non-smoking status, previous history of PONV/motion sickness, and genetic predisposition (e.g., metabolizer status with respect to opioid metabolism or degradation of antiemetics). Anesthetic factors include the use of inhalation agents, nitrous oxide and intraoperative and postoperative opioid use. Surgical factors include longer duration of surgery and different operative procedures.

Eberhart et al. identified slightly different risk factors in children than in adults, which included duration of surgery >30 min, age >3 year, strabismus surgery and a history of POV in the patient or in a parent or sibling[23].

Relying on a single prognostic factor usually leads to undertreatment in a large cohort of patients without that specific factor. For instance, restricting antiemetics to female patients (the prognostic factor associated with the highest risk in many investigated populations[24]) would lead to undertreatment in male patients. Therefore, the combination of multiple prognostic factors summarized in prognostic models gained some popularity[25,26].

Prognostic models to stratify antiemetic prevention

A prognostic model for PONV is a numeric representation estimating the likelihood of this event given a set of prognostic factors. A probability prediction rule assigns a probability to a patient for the occurrence of a specified event. The raw materials for developing a probability prediction rule on PONV are covariates recorded prior to and sometimes during surgery and anesthesia, or are supposed to occur in the postoperative period (e.g., postoperative opioid consumption). Essentially, the same commonly used method (stepwise logistic regression) to identify risk factors can estimate a statistical model relating a linear combination of the covariates to the binary outcome. Multiple prognostic models have been published and are in use[27]. The extent of internal and external validation of the discrimination and calibration properties, however, varies considerably. These questions are currently investigated in an ongoing Cochrane project on prognostic factors and prediction models for PONV[28].

Stratified medicine by a risk-based PONV prevention

Stratified management is the tailoring of therapeutic decisions to specific groups of patients based on their relative risk of an event[29]. The baseline risk of PONV in an individual having a specified surgical and anesthetic may be assessed using a validated risk score that is based on the (weighted) sum of independent predictors. In turn, prognostic models have been used to adopt guidelines for preventative therapy[30]. There are conflicting results on the use of PONV risk scores to significantly reduce the institutional rates of PONV[31].

Following an enthusiastic uptake of totally risk-adapted approaches to prevent PONV with zero prevention in supposed low-risk patients[25], there has been an intense debate and discussion about whether these approaches actually work in a busy and varied clinical environment[32–34].

Shortcomings and pitfalls of strictly risk-based PONV-prevention algorithms

Although the general principle that prophylactic antiemetic prevention confers benefit in patients with increased baseline risk, as recommended by the current SAMBA consensus guidelines, is valid, there are some concerns raised in adopting a strictly risk-based approach.

In the revised 2014 SAMBA guidelines[35], Guideline 7 states that clinicians should "ensure PONV prevention and treatment is implemented in the clinical setting." Taking into account that study settings (ideal world) and clinical routine (real-life setting) often differ to a large extent, sometimes more pragmatic approaches are needed in busy clinical environments.

The most recent guidelines stated that "measures must be put in place to determine whether suggested algorithms for the management of PONV are actually implemented as standard operating procedure in clinical settings and that these practices lead to improvement of PONV management."

Of note: it should be kept in mind that these new recommendations do not intend to discredit the value of prognostic models for various purposes. Clinical risk models have made substantial contributions to eliminate presumed risk factors so that more reasonable risk assessment is now feasible for patients and especially patient cohorts[19,21,23].

It is important to note, however, that no risk model can accurately predict the likelihood of an individual having PONV (which can essentially only be "yes" or "no") rather, they allow us to estimate the risk for PONV among patient groups[36].

As already outlined, the overall performance and validity of stratified approaches mainly rest upon:

- the ability to correctly classify the PONV risk
- the potential of antiemetics to cause adverse effects
- the acquisition costs of antiemetics
- the clinical applicability and compliance with strictly stratified algorithms.

Ability to correctly classify the PONV risk

Problems and ambiguities may arise, for instance, in the prospective determination of what constitutes "postoperative opioid therapy." Should 2 mg of morphine equivalent given in the PACU be considered as a risk factor? Should feeling sick during a bumpy helicopter flight be considered as motion sickness, or not until the patient confirms that even sitting on the co-driver's seat evokes feeling of nausea or even vomiting? Assessing "smoking status" seems simple at first sight. But should smoking one cigarette once a week be considered the same as one pack per day? And how about a past history of smoking? Should this fact be considered a valid argument to down-score the individual risk assessment? Whilst the dichotomous assessment of the "PONV history" per se is straightforward, the interpretation remains a matter of debate. If we consider a patient who developed PONV after one of a previous four anesthetics, it is more than questionable whether this fact is truly a risk factor or whether we should rather consider the fact that three out of four anesthetics passed uneventfully so could be viewed as a sign for being less susceptible towards an emetogenic stimulus. Further, patients can rarely report whether this outcome has been achieved without or with (multiple) antiemetic prophylaxis that further complicates easy judgment. These shortcomings should not discredit the reliability of a risk score based approach. In fact, observational trials have shown that:

- the allocation of patients to risk groups has been successful, and the predicted risk corresponded to an observed incidence of PONV in the patient cohorts[37], and
- a risk-adapted PONV protocol may effectively reduce the institutional PONV incidence[25].

The acquisition costs of antiemetics

The costs of most antiemetics have decreased dramatically during recent years as generic versions have become available. Further, the respective acquisition costs vary to a large extent from country to country and among different institutions. Acquisition costs also depend on the amount of ordered quantities, which means that a more liberal prophylaxis may result in lower costs per patient. Published analyses suggest that "PONV prophylaxis is cost-effective with the older, less expensive drugs when patients have a 10% or more risk of emesis"[38]. Lower drug acquisition costs may even support PONV prophylaxis in patient groups at a lower risk for PONV. Newer antiemetics are associated with greater costs, but older drugs should not per se constitute a relevant obstacle to a liberal administration of antiemetics. However, the argument to use well-proven drugs with moderate costs and to save more costly interventions for treatment (if available as an IV formulation) remains valid.

Potential for antiemetics to cause adverse effects

The safety of antiemetics is well established considering the huge amount of clinical data available and their summary in valid meta-analyses[11]. Limited adverse effects have been associated with antiemetics if minimum effective doses are used. It is, however, of utmost importance that awareness exists for real contraindications for the use of the available substances (e.g., dopamine D_2-antagonists and Parkinsonism, and corticosteroids in patients at risk for tumor lysis syndrome), and to have a look at potential contraindications in patients with prolonged QT interval and consider alternative preventive measures. But these precautions need to be in place irrespective of a restrictive or rather liberal antiemetic prevention.

Clinical applicability and compliance with guidelines

It is accepted knowledge that a risk-adapted PONV protocol may effectively reduce the institutional PONV incidence[25]. When transferring such results to routine care of patients, it has to be considered that the results of such a protocol were obtained in a clinical study that had good compliance with the proposed algorithms, which is in contrast to most clinical settings with less strict adherence to suggested pathways[39,40].

Clinical effectiveness of PONV protocols

As observed with other settings and pharmacologic preventive measures, effectiveness may be different from efficacy evaluations. The latter may be partly due to poor compliance with existing protocols. This is especially true in the area of PONV prevention and treatment, where irrespective of tremendous amounts of research findings in RCTs, observational studies have shown that existing clinical guidelines for PONV prevention (even if present in the intranet or in the format of a booklet) are poorly implemented. This phenomenon was demonstrated for adults[41] and pediatric patients[42]. Therefore, some studies suggest the introduction of electronic reminders to improve compliance with standard operating procedures[43,44].

The argument that poor education is the root cause for the reluctance to administer appropriate antiemetic prophylaxis seems to be invalid, since a study has shown that the problem may even persist after intense educational activities[40]. In this study, even after training and continuous provider feedback, only 47% of the patients at moderate risk (two risk factors present) and 37% of the patients at high risk (three risk factors present) actually received the scheduled prophylactic treatment using a very simple algorithm, which suggested administering one antiemetic per risk factor. In contrast, almost all patients received single antiemetic prophylaxis, which was the de facto standard at the site where the study took place. The message here is that "keep it simple" does not seem enough; a sufficient PONV prevention needs to be self-evident and fully accepted in the clinical routine.

Is "early treatment" a better alternative to manage PONV?

Arguing that treating PONV only after symptoms occur is as effective and as appropriate for patients as prevention – which may be true for a clinical trial scenario[45] – disregards the findings of a recent trial showing that PONV symptoms, and nausea in particular, are frequently missed in a busy clinical scenario[13]. This observational study shows that only 42% and 29% of PONV episodes were actually detected by the nursing staff in the PACU and on the ward, respectively. It should be noted that indeed there are some arguments in favor of an aggressive (maybe multimodal) treatment. However, such a concept would clearly demand a very alert environment in which patients are:

- adequately informed and encouraged to report any signs of nausea, and
- prompt treatment is ensured.

These two arguments prohibit an approach based on aggressive treatment rather than multimodal prevention in children, where symptom assessment, especially with respect to the feeling of nausea, is restricted. Further, such an approach is incompatible with busy environments where nursing staff and physicians are busy and a close monitoring of PONV symptoms and an appropriate response (instant and effective treatment) cannot be ensured.

In summary, the clinical applicability of fully risk-adapted approaches with zero prevention in presumably low-risk cohorts may be impaired and appear questionable due to the following factors.

- Even well-established risk scores are imprecise when it comes to the prediction of individuals at-risk to suffer from PONV. This may be in part explained by the ambiguity regarding the prognostic ability of some of the risk factors.
- The potential of antiemetics to cause adverse effects is low for most of the standard antiemetics given in an appropriate (low) dose and provided contraindications are considered.
- The acquisition costs of antiemetics have declined in recent years so that the acquisition cost, and thus the argument to withhold antiemetics due to this factor, plays a less important role.
- Unfortunately, even in clinical trials, the compliance with strictly stratified algorithms is surprisingly low, constituting an argument for a more liberal use of prophylactic (multimodal) antiemetics.

Although the actual use of antiemetics may not be considerably different between a risk-adapted PONV-prevention algorithm with zero prevention in low-risk patients (Table 16.1) and a PONV-prevention algorithm with multimodal prevention in all patients, including low-risk patients plus additional interventions for high-risk patients (Table 16.2), the latter may be better suited in a busy clinical setting and is more likely to ensure that research results actually translate into clinical benefit for patients. The given example algorithms may help to set up an institutional PONV policy, by replacing the wildcards ("A," "B," "C," etc.) with specific antiemetics from different classes.

Table 16.1 Risk-adapted PONV-prevention algorithm with no prevention in low-risk patients[35]

	Estimated risk for PONV (e.g., as determined by a risk score)		
	Low	**Medium**	**High**
Interventions for prophylaxis	No prevention ("wait-and-see")	Drug A + Drug B or TIVA	Drug A + Drug B + TIVA On a case-by-case decision: further interventions
Interventions for treatment	1. Drug B 2. Drug C (in case of ineffectiveness of treatment in stage 1) (i.e., Drug B)	1. Drug C 2. Drug D (in case of ineffectiveness of treatment in stage 1) (i.e., Drug C)	1. Drug C 2. Drug D (in case of ineffectiveness of treatment in stage 1) (i.e., Drug C)

Example interventions: Drug A = dexamethasone 4 mg in adults/0.15 mg/kg of body weight in children; Drug B = ondansetron 4 mg in adults/0.1 mg/kg of body weight in children; Drug C = droperidol 1 mg in adults/10 to 15 ng/kg of body weight in children; Drug D = dimenhydrinate 1 mg/kg of body weight in adults/0.5 to 1.0 mg/kg of body weight in children. The given drug examples are used to illustrate how the algorithm may be implemented but may not represent the most favorable approach. The latter may be context-sensitive (children, adults or other issues). In the event of treatment failure, a timely assessment and alternative antiemetics should be used. A multimodal treatment approach may be appropriate to increase the likelihood of success. TIVA = total intravenous anesthesia, that is, propofol induction and maintenance, no nitrous oxide.

Of note: when replacing "wildcards" with actual drug names, it is important to judge whether the specific option makes sense from a pharmacokinetic point of view. For instance, it would not be a suitable option to use dexamethasone as Drug B in the algorithms being scheduled for single rescue treatment (slow onset of action).

Table 16.2 Combination PONV-prevention algorithm in all patients including low-risk patients *plus* additional interventions for high-risk patients[35]

	Estimated risk for PONV, for example, as determined by a risk score		
	Low	**Medium**	**High**
Interventions for prophylaxis	Drug A + (Drug B or TIVA)	Drug A + (Drug B or TIVA)	Drug A + Drug B + TIVA On a case-by-case decision: further interventions
Interventions for treatment	1. Drug C 2. Drug D (in case of ineffectiveness of treatment in stage 1) (i.e., Drug C)	1. Drug C 2. Drug D (in case of ineffectiveness of treatment in stage 1) (i.e., Drug C)	1. Drug C 2. Drug D (in case of ineffectiveness of treatment in stage 1) (i.e., Drug C)

Example interventions: Drug A = dexamethasone 4 mg in adults/0.15 mg/kg of body weight in children; Drug B = ondansetron 4 mg in adults/0.1 mg/kg of body weight in children; Drug C = droperidol 1 mg in adults/10 to 15 μg/kg of body weight in children; Drug D = dimenhydrinate 1 mg/kg of body weight in adults/0.5 to 1.0 mg/kg of body weight in children.

The given drug examples are used to illustrate how the algorithm may be implemented but may not represent the most favorable approach. The latter may be context-sensitive (children, adults or other issues). In the event of treatment failure, a timely assessment and alternative antiemetics should be used. A multimodal treatment approach may be appropriate to increase the likelihood of success. TIVA = total intravenous anesthesia, that is, propofol induction and maintenance, no nitrous oxide.

Of note: when replacing "wildcards" with actual drug names, it is important to judge whether the specific option makes sense from a pharmacokinetic point of view. For instance, it would not be a suitable option to use dexamethasone as Drug B in the algorithms being scheduled for single rescue treatment (slow onset of action).

Liberal general multimodal prevention algorithms

The factors mentioned under the previous subheadings as shortcomings for strictly risk-based prevention protocols, including a "wait-and-see approach" for patients at low risk, gave rise to a more liberal recommendation in an updated PONV consensus recommendation[35].

The new SAMBA PONV consensus Guideline 8 advises clinicians to "use general multimodal prevention to facilitate implementation of PONV policies." With this new section, the shortcomings of strictly risk-based protocols, and particularly the undertreatment in low-risk patients receiving no prevention and the appropriate prevention in high-risk patients, were tackled. The recommendation of the expert panel states that "in view of the poor guideline compliance with risk-adapted approaches and no general preventive measures, multimodal prevention strategy (adjusted with additional measures in high-risk patients) may be an option to facilitate clinical implementation." Many observational data gathered to assess whether standard operating procedures work in busy clinical environments support this shift in paradigm. This is particularly true for high-risk patients in which the latter procedure may overcome the hurdle to provide multimodal prevention, since e.g., two antiemetics are given anyway, which lowers the threshold for the overall administration of three or four preventive measures. In a setting where two antiemetics are given on a routine basis, a third intervention (e.g., a total intravenous anesthesia) should be added if there are hints for an increased risk. This approach will result in a significant benefit.

Some evidence highlighting the inherent trend towards undertreatment has already been reported. In a recent study, despite intense educational strategies that resulted in lower incidence of PONV, it was surprising to note that no significant difference in the rate of administration of antiemetic prophylaxis was observed between the overall "before" and "after" patient populations (31.4% versus 36.8%)[46]. The only difference was in the rate of administration of antiemetic prophylaxis in the high-risk group (with an Apfel simplified score of >2), which reached statistical significance (36.4–52.8%). Such observational data underscore the observed extremely low compliance with institutional PONV policies. In another report, it was stated that only 37% of medium- and high-risk patients received the specified prophylaxis, leading to suboptimal PONV prevention in moderate- and high-risk patients[47]. Interestingly, the report was intended to highlight that PONV prediction actually works! In this context, we should bear in mind that as long as the change in practice does not translate into a significant increase in patient benefit, such implementation should not be recommended.

Not surprisingly, fast-track or enhanced recovery protocols often incorporate multimodal preventive PONV strategies[48,49]. General multimodal strategies may well be a starting point to facilitate clinical implementation of better PONV protection of patients[50]. Such approaches may prove more effective than strictly risk-based approaches that rely on no prevention in low-risk patients.

It is reassuring and encouraging to note that the current SAMBA guidelines explicitly state the goal for antiemetic multimodal prevention to become an integral part of anesthesia[35,51]. At the end of the day, anesthesia care providers should view PONV prevention as self-evident as preventing and treating pain.

Challenges for everyday practice

PONV has been extensively studied and there is excellent evidence to guide clinical practice. Perhaps the biggest problem is that many anesthesia providers fail to translate this knowledge into changes in practice, and thus patient benefit[33,52].

We need to accept that some of the adverse events occurring during the course of anesthesia are difficult to cope with or cannot be controlled in a sufficient manner. However, we should accept and be happy that some of the oldest problems associated with anesthesia, i.e., PONV, where there is excellent evidence based on myriads of clinical trials, can be managed quite effectively, provided we apply the attitude of "zero tolerance" and do not accept that PONV is a surrogate outcome that does not bother our patients.

The PONV-free hospital should be a realistic goal as long as we devote effort into the clinical implementation of PONV protocols. The rule of thumb and paradigm for creating and implementing PONV protocols should be "the simpler, the better," with a more liberal use of preventive measures than a too restrictive one.

References

1. Weiser TG, Regenbogen SE, Thompson KD, et al. An estimation of the global volume of surgery: a modelling strategy based on available data. *Lancet* 2008; 372: 139–44.
2. Habib AS, Gan TJ. Postoperative nausea and vomiting: then & now. *Anesth Analg* 2012; 115: 493–5.
3. Blacoe DA, Cunning E, Bell G. Paediatric day-case surgery: an audit of unplanned hospital admission Royal Hospital for Sick Children, Glasgow. *Anaesthesia* 2008; 63: 610–5.
4. Gold BS, Kitz DS, Lecky JH, et al. Unanticipated admission to the hospital following ambulatory surgery. *JAMA* 1989; 262: 3008–10.
5. Eberhart LH, Mauch M, Morin AM, et al. Impact of a multimodal anti-emetic prophylaxis on patient satisfaction in high-risk patients for postoperative nausea and vomiting. *Anaesthesia* 2002; 57: 1022–7.
6. Gan TJ, Meyer T, Apfel CC, et al. Consensus guidelines for managing postoperative nausea and vomiting. *Anesth Analg* 2003; 97: 62–71.
7. Tramer M, Moore A, McQuay H. Meta-analytic comparison of prophylactic antiemetic efficacy for postoperative nausea and vomiting: propofol anaesthesia vs omitting nitrous oxide vs total i.v. anaesthesia with propofol. *Br J Anaesth* 1997; 78: 256–9.
8. Apfel CC, Korttila K, Abdalla M, et al. An international multicenter protocol to assess the single and combined benefits of antiemetic interventions in a controlled clinical trial of a 2×2×2×2×2×2 factorial design (IMPACT). *Control Clin Trials* 2003; 24: 736–51.
9. Apfel CC, Korttila K, Abdalla M, et al. A factorial trial of six interventions for the prevention of postoperative nausea and vomiting. *N Engl J Med* 2004; 350: 2441–51.
10. Cillo JE, Jr. Analysis of propofol and low-dose ketamine admixtures for adult outpatient dentoalveolar surgery: a prospective, randomized, positive-controlled clinical trial. *J Oral Maxillofac Surg* 2012; 70: 537–46.
11. Carlisle JB, Stevenson CA. Drugs for preventing postoperative nausea and vomiting. *Cochrane Database Syst Rev* 2006: CD004125.

12. Eberhart LHJ, Frank S, Lange H, et al. Systematic review on the recurrence of postoperative nausea and vomiting after a first episode in the recovery room – implications for the treatment of PONV and related clinical trials. *BMC Anesthesiol* 2006; 6: 14.

13. Franck M, Radtke FM, Apfel CC, et al. Documentation of post-operative nausea and vomiting in routine clinical practice. *J Int Med Res* 2010; 38: 1034–41.

14. Apfel CC, Philip BK, Cakmakkaya OS, et al. Who is at risk for postdischarge nausea and vomiting after ambulatory surgery? *Anesthesiology* 2012; 117: 475–86.

15. Gan TJ, Meyer TA, Apfel CC et al. Society for Ambulatory Anesthesia guidelines for the management of postoperative nausea and vomiting. *Anesth Analg* 2007; 105: 1615–28.

16. Kranke P, Eberhart LH, Gan TJ, et al. Algorithms for the prevention of postoperative nausea and vomiting: an efficacy and efficiency simulation. *Eur J Anaesthesiol* 2007; 24: 856–67.

17. Burtles R, Peckett BW. Postoperative vomiting; some factors affecting its incidence. *Br J Anaesth* 1957; 29: 114–23.

18. Bellville JW, Bross ID, Howland WS. Postoperative nausea and vomiting. IV. Factors related to postoperative nausea and vomiting. *Anesthesiology* 1960; 21: 186–93.

19. Koivuranta M, Laara E, Snare L, et al. A survey of postoperative nausea and vomiting. *Anaesthesia* 1997; 52: 443–49.

20. Apfel CC, Greim CA, Haubitz I, et al. The discriminating power of a risk score for postoperative vomiting in adults undergoing various types of surgery. *Acta Anaesthesiol Scand* 1998; 42: 502–9.

21. Apfel CC, Laara E, Koivuranta M, et al. A simplified risk score for predicting postoperative nausea and vomiting: conclusions from cross-validations between two centers. *Anesthesiology* 1999; 91: 693–700.

22. Apfel CC, Heidrich FM, Jukar-Rao S, et al. Evidence-based analysis of risk factors for postoperative nausea and vomiting. *Br J Anaesth* 2012; 109: 742–53.

23. Eberhart LHJ, Geldner G, Kranke P, et al. The development and validation of a risk score to predict the probability of postoperative vomiting in pediatric patients. *Anesth Analg* 2004; 99: 1630–7.

24. Apfel CC, Kranke P, Greim CA, et al. What can be expected from risk scores for predicting postoperative nausea and vomiting? *Br J Anaesth* 2001; 86: 822–7.

25. Pierre S, Corno G, Benais H, et al. A risk score-dependent antiemetic approach effectively reduces postoperative nausea and vomiting – a continuous quality improvement initiative. *Can J Anaesth* 2004; 51: 320–5.

26. Biedler A, Wermelt J, Kunitz O, et al. A risk adapted approach reduces the overall institutional incidence of postoperative nausea and vomiting. *Can J Anaesth* 2004; 51: 13–9.

27. Apfel CC, Kranke P, Eberhart LH, et al. Comparison of predictive models for postoperative nausea and vomiting. *Br J Anaesth* 2002; 88: 234–240.

28. Pace NL, Carlisle J, Eberhart LHJ, et al. Prediction models for the risk of postoperative nausea and vomiting. Cochrane Library, September 2014.

29. Hingorani AD, Windt DA, Riley RD, et al. Prognosis research strategy (PROGRESS) 4: stratified medicine research. *BMJ (Clin Res Ed)* 2013; 346: e5793.

30. Rusch D, Eberhart L, Biedler A, et al. Prospective application of a simplified risk score to prevent postoperative nausea and vomiting. *Can J Anaesth* 2005; 52: 478–4.

31. Kappen TH, Moons KG, van Wolfswinkel L, et al. Impact of risk

assessments on prophylactic antiemetic prescription and the incidence of postoperative nausea and vomiting: a cluster-randomized trial. *Anesthesiology* 2014; 120: 343–54.

32. Eberhart LHJ, Morin AM. Risk scores for predicting postoperative nausea and vomiting are clinically useful tools and should be used in every patient: con – 'life is really simple, but we insist on making it complicated'. *Eur J Anaesthesiol* 2011; 28: 155–9.

33. Kranke P. Effective management of postoperative nausea and vomiting: let us practise what we preach! *Eur J Anaesthesiol* 2011; 28: 152–4.

34. Pierre S. Risk scores for predicting postoperative nausea and vomiting are clinically useful tools and should be used in every patient: pro – 'don't throw the baby out with the bathwater'. *Eur J Anaesthesiol* 2011; 28: 160–3.

35. Gan TJ, Diemunsch P, Habib AS, et al. Consensus guidelines for the management of postoperative nausea and vomiting. *Anesth Analg* 2014; 118: 85–113.

36. van den Bosch JE, Kalkman CJ, Vergouwe Y, et al. Assessing the applicability of scoring systems for predicting postoperative nausea and vomiting. *Anaesthesia* 2005; 60: 323–31.

37. Pierre S, Benais H, Pouymayou J. Apfel's simplified score may favourably predict the risk of postoperative nausea and vomiting. *Can J Anaesth* 2002; 49: 237–42.

38. Watcha MF, Smith I. Cost-effectiveness analysis of antiemetic therapy for ambulatory surgery. *J Clin Anesth* 1994; 6: 370–7.

39. Franck M, Radtke FM, Baumeyer A, et al. [Adherence to treatment guidelines for postoperative nausea and vomiting. How well does knowledge transfer result in improved clinical care?]. *Der Anaesthesist* 2010; 59: 524–8.

40. Frenzel JC, Kee SS, Ensor JE, et al. Ongoing provision of individual clinician performance data improves practice behavior. *Anesth Analg* 2010; 111: 515–9.

41. Franck M, Radtke FM, Baumeyer A, et al. Adherence to treatment guidelines for postoperative nausea and vomiting. How well does knowledge transfer result in improved clinical care? *Der Anaesthesist* 2010; 59: 524–8.

42. Klotz C, Philippi-Hohne C. Prophylaxis of postoperative nausea and vomiting in pediatric anesthesia: recommendations and implementation in clinical routine. *Der Anaesthesist* 2010; 59: 477–8.

43. Kooij FO, Klok T, Hollmann MW, et al. Automated reminders increase adherence to guidelines for administration of prophylaxis for postoperative nausea and vomiting. *Eur J Anaesthesiol* 2010; 27: 187–91.

44. Kooij FO, Klok T, Hollmann MW, et al. Decision support increases guideline adherence for prescribing postoperative nausea and vomiting prophylaxis. *Anesth Analg* 2008; 106: 893–8.

45. Scuderi PE, James RL, Harris L, et al. Antiemetic prophylaxis does not improve outcomes after outpatient surgery when compared to symptomatic treatment. *Anesthesiology* 1999; 90: 360–71.

46. Sigaut S, Merckx P, Peuch C, et al. Does an educational strategy based on systematic preoperative assessment of simplified Apfel's score decrease postoperative nausea and vomiting? *Ann Fr Anesthes Reanim* 2010; 29: 765–9.

47. Kumar A, Brampton W, Watson S, et al. Postoperative nausea and vomiting: simple risk scoring does work. *Eur J Anaesthesiol* 2012; 29: 57–9; author reply 59–60.

48. Jensen K, Kehlet H, Lund CM. Post-operative recovery profile after laparoscopic cholecystectomy: a prospective, observational study of a

multimodal anaesthetic regime. *Acta Anaesthesiol Scand* 2007; 51: 464–71.

49. Bergland A, Gislason H, Raeder J. Fast-track surgery for bariatric laparoscopic gastric bypass with focus on anaesthesia and peri-operative care. Experience with 500 cases. *Acta Anaesthesiol Scand* 2008; 52: 1394–9.

50. Scuderi PE. PRO: Anatomical classification of surgical procedures improves our understanding of the mechanisms of postoperative nausea and vomiting. *Anesth Analg* 2010; 110: 410–1.

51. Kranke P, Eberhart LHJ. Possibilities and limitations in the pharmacological management of postoperative nausea and vomiting. *Eur J Anaesthesiol* 2011; 28: 758–65.

52. Curran JA, Grimshaw JM, Hayden JA, et al. Knowledge translation research: the science of moving research into policy and practice. *J Contin Educ Health Prof* 2011; 31: 174–80.

Index

Made in United States
Orlando, FL
21 October 2026

89529439R00111